Pediatric Obesity: Causes, Prevention, and Treatment

Editors

ELIANA M. PERRIN
GITANJALI SRIVASTAVA

PEDIATRIC CLINICS
OF NORTH AMERICA

www.pediatric.theclinics.com

Consulting Editor
TINA L. CHENG

October 2024 • Volume 71 • Number 5

ELSEVIER

1600 John F. Kennedy Boulevard • Suite 1800 • Philadelphia, Pennsylvania, 19103-2899

http://www.theclinics.com

THE PEDIATRIC CLINICS OF NORTH AMERICA Volume 71, Number 5
October 2024 ISSN 0031-3955, ISBN-13: 978-0-443-29630-7

Editor: Kerry Holland
Developmental Editor: Anirban Mukherjee

The Pediatric Clinics of North America (ISSN 0031-3955) is published bimonthly by Elsevier Inc., 360 Park Avenue South, New York, NY 10010-1710. Months of issue are February, April, June, August, October, and December. Periodicals postage paid at New York, NY and additional mailing offices. Subscription prices are $290.00 per year (US individuals), $368.00 per year (Canadian individuals), $440.00 per year (international individuals), $100.00 per year (US students and residents), $100.00 per year (Canadian students and residents), and $165.00 per year (international residents and students). For institutional access pricing please contact Customer Service via the contact information below. To receive students/resident rare, orders must be accompanied by name of affiliated institution, date of term, and the signature of program/residency coordinator on institution letterhead. Orders will be billed at individual rate until proof of status is received. Foreign air speed delivery is included in all *Clinics* subscription prices. All prices are subject to change without notice. Orders, claims, and journal inquiries: Please visit our Support Hub page https://service.elsevier.com for assistance.

Reprints. For copies of 100 or more, of articles in this publication, please contact the Commercial Reprints Department, Elsevier Inc., 360 Park Avenue South, New York, NY 10010-1710. Tel.: 212-633-3874; Fax: 212-633-3820; E-mail: reprints@elsevier.com.

The Pediatric Clinics of North America is also published in Spanish by McGraw-Hill Inter-americana Editores S.A., Mexico City, Mexico; in Portuguese by Riechmann and Affonso Editores, Rua Comandante Coelho 1085, CEP 21250, Rio de Janeiro, Brazil; and in Greek by Althayia SA, Athens, Greece.

The Pediatric Clinics of North America is covered in *MEDLINE/PubMed (Index Medicus), Excerpta Medica, Current Contents, Current Contents/Clinical Medicine, Science Citation Index, ASCA, ISI/BIOMED*, and *BIOSIS*.

JOURNAL TITLE: *Pediatric Clinics of North America*
ISSUE: 71.5

PROGRAM OBJECTIVE

The goal of the *Pediatric Clinics of North America* is to keep practicing physicians and residents up to date with current clinical practice in pediatrics by providing timely articles reviewing the state-of-the-art in patient care.

TARGET AUDIENCE

All practicing pediatricians, physicians, and healthcare professionals who provide patient care to pediatric patients.

LEARNING OBJECTIVES

Upon completion of this activity, participants will be able to:
1. Review how the Built Environment can influence community health.
2. Discuss strategies for promoting healthier food environments.
3. Recognize pediatric obesity as a disease with multifactorial origins.

ACCREDITATION

The Elsevier Office of Continuing Medical Education (EOCME) is accredited by the Accreditation Council for Continuing Medical Education (ACCME) to provide continuing medical education for physicians.

The EOCME designates this journal-based activity for a maximum of 15 *AMA PRA Category 1 Credit*(s)™. Physicians should claim only the credit commensurate with the extent of their participation in the activity.

All other healthcare professionals requesting continuing education credit for this journal-based activity will be issued a certificate of participation.

DISCLOSURE OF RELEVANT FINANCIAL RELATIONSHIPS

The EOCME evaluates the relevancy of financial relationships with its instructors, faculty, planners, and other individuals who are in a position to control the content of CME activities. The EOCME will review all identified disclosures and mitigate financial relationships with ineligible companies, as applicable. An ineligible company is any entity whose primary business is producing, marketing, selling, re-selling, or distributing healthcare products used by or on patients. For specific examples of ineligible companies visit accme.org/standards. EOCME is committed to providing its learners with CME activities that promote improvements or quality in healthcare and not a specific proprietary business or a commercial interest.

The authors and editors listed below have identified no financial relationships or relationships to products or devices they have with ineligible companies related to the content of this CME activity:
Amy Beck, MD, MPH; Julie Benard, MD; Amy Braddock, MD, MsPH; Rochelle L. Cason-Wilkerson, MD, MPH; Rebecca Chasnovitz, MD; Eileen Chaves, PhD, MSc; Stephen Cook, MD, MPH; Angel DiPangrazio, RD, LD; Wesley P. Dutton, MD; Ihuoma Eneli, MD, MS; Kori B. Flower, MD, MS, MPH; Maida P. Galvez, MD, MPH, FAAP; Michelle C. Gorecki, MD, MPH; Sarah E. Hampl, MD; Joan C. Han, MD; Jessica Hart, MD; Faith Anne N. Heeren, BA; Pamela Hu, MD; Awab Ali Ibrahim, MD; Amrik Singh Khalsa, MD, MSc, FAAP, FACP; Clint E. Kinney, PhD; Jennifer O. Lambert, MD, MHS; Nicole Larson, PhD, MPH, RD; Melissa N. Laska, PhD, RD; Jacqueline Maya, MD; Katharine McCarthy, PhD, MPH; Alison Mears, AIA LEED AP; Carmen Monthe-Dreze, MD; Colin J. Orr, MD, MPH; Nina Paddu, DO; Matthew Paponetti, PT, DPT; Keeley J. Pratt, PhD; Kenneth Resnicow, PhD; Stephanie Samuels, MD; Chethan Sarabu, MD, FAMIA, FAAP; Mona Sharifi, MD, MPH; Nakiya N. Showell, MD, MHS, MPH; Juwairriyyah Siddiqui, MD; Fatima Cody Stanford, MD, MPH, MPA, MBA; Griffin Stout, MD; Brooke Sweeney, MD, FAAP, FACP, DABOM; Juliet Villegas, MA; Brooke E. Wagner, PhD; Stephanie W. Waldrop, MD, MPH; Ashley E. Weedn, MD, MPH; Heather Wright Williams, MD; Megan Winkler, PhD, RN; Jennifer A. Woo Baidal, MD, MPH; Charles Wood, MD, MPH, FAAP; Susan J. Woolford, MD, MPH, FAAP, DipABLM

The authors and editors listed below have identified financial relationships or relationships to products or devices they have with ineligible companies related to the content of this CME activity:
Joan C. Han, MD: Researcher: Rhythm Pharmaceuticals Fatima Cody Stanford, MD, MPH, MPA, MBA: Consultant: Calibrate, GoodRx, Pfizer, Lilly, Boehringer Ingelheim, Gelesis, Vida Health, Lifeforce, Ilant Health, MelliCell, Novo Nordisk Brooke Sweeney, MD, FAAP, FACP, DABOM: Researcher: Rhythm Pharmaceuticals

The Clinics staff listed below have identified no financial relationships or relationships to products or devices they have with ineligible companies related to the content of this CME activity:
Kerry Holland; Shyamala Kavikumaran; Michelle Littlejohn; Patrick J. Manley; Anirban Mukherjee

UNAPPROVED/OFF-LABEL USE DISCLOSURE
The EOCME requires CME faculty to disclose to the participants:
1. When products or procedures being discussed are off-label, unlabelled, experimental, and/or investigational (not US Food and Drug Administration [FDA] approved); and
2. Any limitations on the information presented, such as data that are preliminary or that represent ongoing research, interim analyses, and/or unsupported opinions. Faculty may discuss information about pharmaceutical agents that is outside of FDA-approved labelling. This information is intended solely for CME and is not intended to promote off-label use of these medications. If you have any questions, contact the medical affairs department of the manufacturer for the most recent prescribing information.

TO ENROLL
To enroll in the *Pediatric Clinics of North America* Continuing Medical Education program, call customer service at 1-800-654-2452 or sign up online at http://www.pediatric.theclinics.com/cme/home. The CME program is available to subscribers for an additional annual fee of USD 313.00.

METHOD OF PARTICIPATION
In order to claim credit, participants must complete the following:
1. Complete enrolment as indicated above.
2. Read the activity.
3. Complete the CME Test and Evaluation. Participants must achieve a score of 70% on the test. All CME Tests and Evaluations must be completed online.

CME INQUIRIES/SPECIAL NEEDS
For all CME inquiries or special needs, please contact elsevierCME@elsevier.com.

Contributors

CONSULTING EDITOR

TINA L. CHENG, MD, MPH
BK Rachford Professor and Chair of Pediatrics, University of Cincinnati, Director, Cincinnati Children's Research Foundation, Chief Medical Officer, Cincinnati Children's Hospital Medical Center, Cincinnati, Ohio

EDITORS

ELIANA M. PERRIN, MD, MPH
Bloomberg Distinguished Professor, Division of General Pediatrics, Department of Pediatrics, School of Medicine, School of Nursing, Johns Hopkins University, Baltimore, Maryland

GITANJALI SRIVASTAVA, MD
Professor of Medicine, Pediatrics, and Surgery, Division of Diabetes, Endocrinology, and Metabolism, Vanderbilt University School of Medicine, Nashville, Tennessee

AUTHORS

AMY BECK, MD, MPH
Associate Professor of Pediatrics, Department of Pediatrics, School of Medicine and Co-director of San Francisco General Hospital's Healthy Lifestyles Clinic, University of California San Francisco, San Francisco, California

JULIE BENARD, MD
Pediatrician, Obesity Medicine Specialist, Cape Physician Associates, Saint Francis Healthcare System, Cape Girardeau, Missouri

AMY BRADDOCK, MD, MSPH
Associate Professor, Department of Family and Community Medicine, University of Missouri, Columbia, Missouri

ROCHELLE L. CASON-WILKERSON, MD, MPH
Assistant Professor, Department of Pediatrics, Section of Nutrition, University of Colorado Anschutz Medical Campus, Aurora, Colorado

REBECCA CHASNOVITZ, MD
Associate Professor, Pediatric Division of General Pediatrics and Adolescent Medicine, University of North Carolina School of Medicine, North Carolina

EILEEN CHAVES, PhD, MSc
Pediatric Psychologist, Division of Neuropsychology and Pediatric Psychology, Center for Healthy Weight and Nutrition, Nationwide Children's Hospital, The Ohio State University, College of Medicine, Columbus, Ohio

STEPHEN COOK, MD, MPH
Director for Center for Healthy Weight and Nutrition, Nationwide Children's Hospital, Columbus, Ohio; formerly Associate Professor, Department of Pediatrics, Internal Medicine and Center for Community Health, Golisano Children's Hospital, University of Rochester School of Medicine, Rochester, New York

ANGEL DIPANGRAZIO, RD, LD
Registered Dietitian, Center for Healthy Weight and Nutrition, Nationwide Children's Hospital, Columbus, Ohio

WESLEY P. DUTTON, MD
Instructor, Department of Medicine, Harvard Medical School; Assistant, Department of Medicine and Pediatrics, Massachusetts General Hospital; Director, Weight Center at Massachusetts General Hospital, Boston, Massachusetts

IHUOMA ENELI, MD, MS
Professor, Department of Pediatrics, Head, Section of Nutrition, University of Colorado Anschutz Medical Campus, Aurora, Colorado

KORI B. FLOWER, MD, MS, MPH
Professor and Division Chief, General Pediatrics and Adolescent Medicine, Department of Pediatrics, University of North Carolina at Chapel Hill, Chapel Hill, North Carolina

MAIDA P. GALVEZ, MD, MPH, FAAP
Professor, Department of Environmental Medicine and Climate Science, and Department of Pediatrics, Icahn School of Medicine at Mount Sinai, New York

MICHELLE C. GORECKI, MD, MPH
Academic General Pediatrics Research Fellow, Department of General and Community Pediatrics, Cincinnati Children's Hospital Medical Center, Cincinnati, Ohio

SARAH E. HAMPL, MD
Professor of Pediatrics at Department of Pediatrics, Children's Mercy Kansas City, Center for Children's Healthy Lifestyles & Nutrition, Kansas City, Missouri

JOAN C. HAN, MD
Chief, Division of Pediatric Endocrinology and Diabetes, Professor, Department of Pediatrics, Mount Sinai Hospital, Diabetes, Obesity, and Metabolism Institute, Mindich Child Health and Development Institute, Icahn School of Medicine at Mount Sinai, New York

JESSICA HART, MD
Assistant Professor, Division of General Pediatrics and Adolescent Medicine, University of North Carolina at Chapel Hill, Chapel Hill, North Carolina

FAITH ANNE N. HEEREN, BA
Doctoral Candidate, Department of Health Outcomes and Biomedical Informatics, University of Florida College of Medicine, Gainesville, Florida

PAMELA HU, MD
Assistant Professor of Pediatrics (Endocrinology and Diabetes), Section of Endocrinology, Diabetes and Metabolism, Yale University School of Medicine, New Haven, Connecticut

AWAB ALI IBRAHIM, MD
Instructor, Division of Pediatric Gastroenterology and Nutrition, Department of Pediatrics, Massachusetts General Hospital, Boston, Massachusetts

AMRIK SINGH KHALSA, MD, MSc, FAAP, FACP
Assistant Professor, Division of Primary Care Pediatrics, Center for Child Health Equity and Outcomes Research, The Abigail Wexner Research Institute, Nationwide Children's Hospital, The Ohio State University College of Medicine, Columbus, Ohio

CLINT E. KINNEY, PhD
Postdoctoral Fellow, Division of Pediatric Endocrinology and Diabetes, Department of Pediatrics, Mount Sinai Hospital, Diabetes, Obesity, and Metabolism Institute, Mindich Child Health and Development Institute, Icahn School of Medicine at Mount Sinai, New York

JENNIFER O. LAMBERT, MD, MHS
Academic General Pediatrics Fellow, Department of Pediatrics, Johns Hopkins University School of Medicine, Baltimore, Maryland

NICOLE LARSON, PhD, MPH, RD
Senior Research Associate, Division of Epidemiology and Community Health, School of Public Health, University of Minnesota, Minneapolis, Minnesota

MELISSA N. LASKA, PhD, RD
McKnight Distinguished University Professor, Division of Epidemiology and Community Health, School of Public Health, University of Minnesota, Minneapolis, Minnesota

JACQUELINE MAYA, MD
Instructor, Department of Pediatrics, Division of Pediatric Endocrinology, Massachusetts General Hospital Weight Center, Massachusetts General Hospital, Boston, Massachusetts

KATHARINE MCCARTHY, PhD, MPH
Assistant Professor, Department of Population Health Science and Policy, and Department of Gynecology and Reproductive Science, Blavatnik Family Women's Health Research Institute, Icahn School of Medicine at Mount Sinai, New York

ALISON MEARS, AIA LEED AP
Associate Professor of Architecture and Director, Healthy Materials Lab, Parsons School of Design, New York

CARMEN MONTHE-DREZE, MD
Attending Neonatologist, Newborn Intensive Care Unit (NICU), Brigham and Women's Hospital; Instructor, Department of Pediatrics, Harvard Medical School, Boston, Massachusetts

COLIN J. ORR, MD, MPH
Assistant Professor, Department of Pediatrics, Vanderbilt University Medical Center, Nashville, TN; formerly Assistant Professor, Department of Pediatrics, University of North Carolina at Chapel Hill School of Medicine, Chapel Hill, North Carolina

NINA PADDU, DO
Obesity Medicine Fellow, Vanderbilt University Medical Center, Nashville, Tennessee

MATTHEW PAPONETTI, PT, DPT
Board-Certified Clinical Specialist in Orthopedic Physical Therapy, Center for Healthy Weight and Nutrition, Sports and Orthopedic Therapies, Nationwide Children's Hospital, Columbus, Ohio

KEELEY J. PRATT, PhD
Associate Professor, Department of Human Sciences, College of Education and Human Ecology, Departments of Surgery and Pediatrics, College of Medicine, The Ohio State University, Columbus, Ohio

KENNETH RESNICOW, PhD
Professor, Department of Health Behavior and Health Education, School of Public Health, University of Michigan, Ann Arbor, Michigan

STEPHANIE SAMUELS, MD
Assistant Professor of Pediatrics (Endocrinology and Diabetes), Yale University School of Medicine, New Haven, Connecticut

CHETHAN SARABU, MD, FAMIA, FAAP
Director of Clinical Innovation, Health Tech Hub, Cornell Tech, New York; Clinical Assistant Professor of Pediatrics, Stanford Medicine Children's Health, Stanford, California

MONA SHARIFI, MD, MPH
Associate Professor of Pediatrics (General Pediatrics) and of Biomedical Informatics and Data Science; Associate Professor of Biostatistics (Health Informatics), Yale University School of Medicine, New Haven, Connecticut

NAKIYA N. SHOWELL, MD, MHS, MPH
Assistant Professor of Pediatrics and Medical Director of Harriet Lane Clinic, Johns Hopkins University School of Medicine, Baltimore, Maryland

JUWAIRRIYYAH SIDDIQUI, MD
Pediatric Endocrinology Fellow, Division of Pediatric Endocrinology and Diabetes, Department of Pediatrics, Mount Sinai Hospital, Diabetes, Obesity, and Metabolism Institute, Mindich Child Health and Development Institute, Icahn School of Medicine at Mount Sinai, New York, New York

FATIMA CODY STANFORD, MD, MPH, MPA, MBA
Associate Professor of Medicine and Pediatrics, Division of Endocrinology-Neuroendocrine, Department of Medicine, Massachusetts General Hospital, Massachusetts General Hospital Weight Center; Department of Pediatrics, Division of Endocrinology, Nutrition Obesity Research Center at Harvard (NORCH), Boston, Massachusetts

GRIFFIN STOUT, MD
Psychiatrist, Division of Child and Adolescent Psychiatry, College of Medicine, The Ohio State University; Medical Director of Eating Disorders, Nationwide Children's Hospital, Columbus, Ohio

BROOKE SWEENEY, MD, FAAP, FACP, DABOM
Professor, Department of Internal Medicine/Pediatrics, University of Missouri Kansas City; Medical Director - Weight Management Services, Department of Pediatrics, Center for Children's Healthy Lifestyles & Nutrition, Children's Mercy Kansas City, Missouri

JULIET VILLEGAS, MA
Associate Professor, Department of Pediatrics, Susan B. Meister Child Health Evaluation and Research Center, University of Michigan, Ann Arbor, Michigan

BROOKE E. WAGNER, PhD
Postdoctoral Associate, Department of Population Health Sciences, Duke Center for Childhood Obesity Research, Duke University School of Medicine, Durham, North Carolina

STEPHANIE W. WALDROP, MD, MPH
Instructor, Fellow of Pediatrics, Section on Nutrition, Department of Pediatrics, Anschutz Medical Campus, Nutrition Obesity Research Center (NORC), University of Colorado, Aurora, Colorado

ASHLEY E. WEEDN, MD, MPH
Assistant Professor, Department of Pediatrics, University of Oklahoma Health Sciences Center, Oklahoma City, Oklahoma

HEATHER WRIGHT WILLIAMS, MD
Assistant Professor, Department of General Pediatrics and Adolescent Medicine, University of North Carolina at Chapel Hill, Chapel Hill, North Carolina

MEGAN R. WINKLER, PhD, RN
Assistant Professor, Department of Behavioral, Social and Health Education Sciences, Rollins School of Public Health, Emory University, Atlanta, Georgia

JENNIFER A. WOO BAIDAL, MD, MPH
Associate Professor, Department of Pediatrics, Stanford University, Palo Alto, California

CHARLES WOOD, MD, MPH, FAAP
Assistant Professor, Department of Pediatrics, Division of General Pediatrics and Adolescent Health, Duke Center for Childhood Obesity Research, Duke University School of Medicine, Durham, North Carolina

SUSAN J. WOOLFORD, MD, MPH, FAAP, DipABLM
Associate Professor, Department of Pediatrics, Susan B. Meister Child Health Evaluation and Research Center, University of Michigan, Ann Arbor, Michigan

Contents

> The authors highlight well-known and hypothesized pathophysiologic
> mechanistic links underlying obesity and the various pediatric disorders
> across multiple organ systems with which it is associated. Obesity is attrib-
> uted to an imbalance in energy intake versus expenditure; there is growing
> knowledge regarding its multifactorial origins, dysfunctional physiologic
> processes, and adverse health consequences. Individuals with obesity ex-
> hibit variations in metabolic rate, genetic predisposition, and hormonal
> regulation, influencing diverse responses in regulating energy balance.
> Understanding the complex mechanistic relationships surrounding the
> pathophysiology of obesity assists in its consideration as a disease proc-
> ess, allowing pediatric health practitioners to manage its sequelae more
> effectively.

> Despite a long history of advances in measuring body size and composi-
> tion, body mass index (BMI) has remained the most commonly used clin-
> ical measure. We explore the advantages and disadvantages of using BMI
> and other measures to estimate adipose tissue, recognizing that no meas-
> ure of body size or adiposity has fulfilled the goal of differentiating health
> from disease. BMI and waist circumference remain widely-used clinical
> screening measures for appropriate risk stratification as it relates to
> obesity.

> Obesity is a major public health problem that frequently begins in early
> childhood and persists into later life. While obesity's multifactorial causes
> and solutions largely lie outside of the individual and family levels, pediatric
> clinicians can support families with infants in preventing obesity and pro-
> moting long-term health and well-being. They can do so by focusing on
> counseling during well visits on exclusive breastfeeding, limiting bottle
> size, delaying solid food introduction, avoiding juice and sugar-sweetened

beverages, limiting screen time, and promoting physical activity and healthy sleep.

The etiology of pediatric obesity is complex and multifactorial. This article encourages pediatric clinicians to consider patient's socioenvironmental context and structural discrimination as drivers of pediatric obesity. Viewing pediatric obesity through an equity lens can inform clinical practice, advocacy, and policy to promote equity.

Weight stigma is pervasive during childhood and adolescent years. Well-established physical and psychosocial health consequences of weight stigma, like disordered eating behaviors, low self-esteem, and higher depressive symptoms, make it especially harmful during a critical period of development for youth. Lasting negative health impacts of these experiences highlight the importance of addressing weight stigma early on. The pediatric health care setting, both physical and social components, can be one of many sources of weight-stigmatizing experiences for youth. This observation has prompted calls for action in the health care setting to reduce weight biases and stigmatizing behavior among pediatric providers.

Counseling on physical activity (PA) to promote a child's overall growth, development, and wellness is a routine part of a well child visit. Given less than a quarter of children in the United States ages 6 to 17 years get 60 minutes of PA daily, there is increased focus on the built environment, that is, neighborhood level supports and barriers to PA and risk for obesity. Broad-based consideration of the built environment's contribution to childhood obesity can inform public health prevention strategies at the individual, family, community, and societal levels that promote children's health, especially in high-risk communities.

This article explores how food and beverage environments influence child health and obesity risk and addresses institutional settings, retail environments, food assistance programs, and food and beverage industry marketing. It emphasizes social determinants of health, evidence-based interventions, and policy recommendations to promote healthier food options and reduce inequities. Pediatric health care providers play a critical role in addressing the need for systemic changes to eliminate inequities in food environments and the systems that support these inequities.

Obesity is a complex and chronic disease that can affect the entire body. The review of systems and physical examination are important components of the evaluation. Laboratory assessment is directed toward known cardiometabolic comorbidities. Regular follow-up visits with repeated review of systems, physical examination, and laboratory testing can facilitate early detection and management of comorbidities of this chronic disease.

Children and youth with overweight and obesity are at an increased risk for the development of an eating disorder. Previous research has shown that disordered eating behaviors are prevalent in this population. Screening for disordered eating behaviors in children and youth with overweight and obesity is necessary to determine the course of the treatment. In children and youth with obesity and comorbid disordered eating behaviors, treatment should be multidisciplinary and include psychological, medical, nutrition, and physical activity care.

Understanding the genetic causes of obesity permits anticipatory guidance and targeted treatments. Children with hyperphagia and severe early-onset obesity should receive genetic testing for rare monogenic and syndromic disorders caused by pathogenic variants involving a single gene or single chromosomal region. Gene panels covering the leptin pathway, the key regulator of energy balance, are becoming more widely available and at lower cost. Polygenic obesity is much more common and involves multiple genes throughout the genome, although the overlap in genes for rare and common disorders suggests a spectrum of severity and the potential of shared precision medicine approaches for treatment.

In 2023, the American Academy of Pediatrics (AAP) published its first clinical practice guideline (CPG) for the treatment of obesity. The CPG is organized by key action statements (KAS) and consensus recommendations that address screening, diagnosis and evaluatin of children and adolescents with obesity, assessment of comorbidities and evidence-based treatment options. The evidence base for each KAS and recommendation is detailed alongside care recommendations. Alongsde the publication of the CPG, the AAP published many resources for pediatric clinicians to support implementation of these recommendations to daily practice.

Motivational interviewing (MI), which is recommended for prevention and treatment of pediatric obesity, is a patient-centered counseling style used to modify behaviors. When using MI, pediatric providers generally avoid direct attempts to convince or persuade. Instead, they help patients or parents think about and verbalize their reasons for and against change and how their behavior aligns with their values and goals. MI relies on specific techniques, including reflective listening, to strategically balance the need to "comfort the afflicted" and "afflict the comfortable"; to balance the expression of empathy with the need to build discrepancy for change, thereby encouraging "change talk".

Pediatric clinicians should offer guidance on age-appropriate nutrition, physical activity, sleep and screen time for families of children and adolescents with obesity. They should build rapport with families, ask permission before discussing obesity-related health concerns, use preferred terminology, and recommend whole family change. Using principles of shared decision-making, pediatric clinicians and families should set individualized goals for lifestyle changes, prioritizing reducing sugar-sweetened beverage intake, increasing physical activity, and reducing screen time. Families of children and adolescents with obesity should be connected to the highest level of support accessible to and desired by the family, including intensive health behavior and lifestyle treatment programs.

The recent advent of highly effective anti-obesity medications (AOM) provides pediatric clinicians a powerful tool to augment the treatment of obesity and improve outcomes. The 2023 American Academy of Pediatrics guidelines state clinicians "should offer adolescents 12 years and older with obesity weight loss pharmacotherapy, according to medication indications, risks, and benefits, as an adjunct to health behavior and lifestyle treatment". This article will provide an update on the integration of AOM into practice, emphasizing clinical pearls and practical tips.

Obesity is a chronic, complex, and multifactorial disease. Currently, approximately 6% have severe obesity with higher rates seen among racial/ethnic minority subgroups and in rural communities. Severe obesity is associated with cardiometabolic, psychologic, and musculoskeletal comorbidities. Metabolic and bariatric surgery is an effective treatment option for adolescents endorsed by major pediatric organizations. The most common procedure is the vertical sleeve gastrectomy. Pre-operative evaluation includes an in-depth medical, nutrition, physical activity and psychosocial assessment, with a care plan developed by a multidicplinary team with the adolescent and caregiver. The post-operative plan should include monitoring for surgical complications, weight regain, micronutrient deficiencies, psychologic challenges, and transition to adult care.

PEDIATRIC CLINICS OF
NORTH AMERICA

THE CLINICS ARE AVAILABLE ONLINE!
Access your subscription at:
www.theclinics.com

PEDIATRIC CLINICS OF
NORTH AMERICA

Foreword

A New Era in Obesity Medicine: What About the Kids?

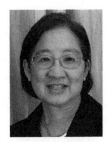

Tina L. Cheng, MD, MPH
Consulting Editor

It is an exciting and important time in addressing the global obesity epidemic. First, the COVID-19 pandemic exacerbated the obesity epidemic. The World Obesity Atlas 2024[1] warned that by 2035 more than one in two adults will be living with overweight and obesity. For young people aged 5 to 19 years, 22% experienced a high body mass index (BMI) (430 million) in 2020, and this is expected to increase to over 39% (770 million) by 2035 with disparities in prevalence across ethnic and racial groups. The pandemic accelerated the obesity epidemic, especially among children, and may prove hard to reverse. The Centers for Disease Control and Prevention reported that among a cohort of 432,302 children and youth aged 2 to 19 years, the rate of BMI increase approximately doubled during the pandemic compared with before the pandemic. The largest increases were seen in children who were overweight prior to the pandemic and younger school-aged children.[2] While preventing and treating obesity requires financial investment, the cost of failing to prevent and treat obesity is far higher. It has been estimated that high BMI will reduce the global economy by over US$4 trillion in 2035, nearly 3% of the global gross domestic product.[3]

Second, the American Academy of Pediatrics[4] updated its clinical practice guidelines on the evaluation and treatment of obesity in 2023, documenting the physical, metabolic, and psychological consequences in childhood and the growing research showing that early childhood is a critical and relatively narrow window predicting sustained obesity into adulthood.[5–7] These guidelines recognize the multifactorial and complex nature of obesity and address management with a policy statement on prevention in the works.

Finally, the Food and Drug Administration has approved new drugs for chronic weight management, with skyrocketing demand. *Science* magazine[8] named glucagon-like peptide-1 receptor agonists as their 2023 Breakthrough of the Year, noting "they are

https://doi.org/10.1016/j.pcl.2024.07.007
0031-3955/24/© 2024 Published by Elsevier Inc.
pediatric.theclinics.com

reshaping medicine, popular culture, and even global stock markets in ways both electrifying and discomfiting." More drugs are on the horizon.[9] This new era of obesity treatment is likely to influence how we think about weight in our society, starting in childhood.

This *Pediatric Clinics of North America* issue comes at a time of needed focus and great change. It focuses on what we know today about pediatric obesity, its measurement, contexts, prevention, and treatment, so we can harness a healthier future for our children.

DISCLOSURES

The author has no conflicts of interest to disclose.

Tina L. Cheng, MD, MPH
Cincinnati Children's Hospital Medical Center
University of Cincinnati
Cincinnati Children's Research Foundation
3333 Burnet Avenue MLC 3016
Cincinnati, OH 45229-3026, USA

E-mail address:
Tina.cheng@cchmc.org

REFERENCES

1. World Obesity Federation. World Obesity Atlas 2024. London: World Obesity Federation; 2024. Available at: https://data.worldobesity.org/publications/?cat=22. [Accessed 10 July 2024].
2. Lange SJ, Kompaniyets L, Freedman DS, et al. Longitudinal trends in body mass index before and during the COVID-19 pandemic among persons aged 2-19 years—United States, 2018-2020. MMWR Morb Mortal Wkly Rep 2021;70(37): 1278–83.
3. World Obesity Federation. World Obesity Atlas 2024. London: World Obesity Federation; 2024. Available at: https://data.worldobesity.org/publications/?cat=22, [Accessed 10 July 2024].
4. Hampl SE, Hassink SG, Skinner AC, et al. Clinical practice guideline for the evaluation and treatment of children and adolescents with obesity. Pediatrics 2023; 151(2):e2022060640.
5. Geserick M, Vogel M, Gausche R, et al. Acceleration of BMI in early childhood and risk of sustained obesity. N Engl J Med 2018;379:1303–12.
6. Ward ZJ, Long MW, Resch SC, et al. Simulation of growth trajectories of childhood obesity into adulthood. N Engl J Med 2017;377(22):2145–53. PMID: 29171811; PMCID: PMC9036858.
7. Simmonds M, Llewellyn A, Owen CG, et al. Predicting adult obesity from childhood obesity: a systematic review and meta-analysis. Obes Rev 2016;17(2):95–107. Epub 2015 Dec 23. PMID: 26696565.
8. Couzin-Frankel J. Obesity meets its match. Science 2023;382(6676):1226–7. Epub 2023 Dec 14. PMID: 38096291.
9. Stanford FC. A new era in obesity management. Nat Rev Gastroenterol Hepatol 2024;21:80–1.

Preface

Pediatric Obesity: Causes, Prevention, and Treatment

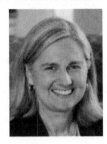 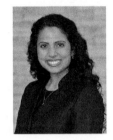

Eliana M. Perrin, MD, MPH   Gitanjali Srivastava, MD

Editors

As Guest Editors and faculty professors with expertise in pediatric care, we are honored to introduce this comprehensive issue of *Pediatric Clinics of North America*. In this issue, we examine pediatric obesity's multifaceted origins and impact on young lives and future health. Our goal is to provide a thorough exploration of the epidemiologic, biological, clinical, and societal aspects of childhood obesity, which affects millions of children and adolescents and the adults they will become. In so doing, we will equip readers with essential knowledge to improve prevention and treatment of childhood obesity through their understanding.

Childhood obesity prevalence has dramatically increased, leading to significant consequences. These consequences include biological, metabolic, cardiovascular, behavioral, and psychosocial conditions during childhood, as well as an increased risk of developing other chronic diseases later in life. The burden of childhood obesity extends beyond physical health, affecting mental well-being and overall quality of life. In addition, childhood obesity often persists into adulthood, making it crucial to address prevention and early treatment. By prioritizing effective prevention and early and appropriate treatment as well as continuing to promote policies that promote health and equity in communities, we can mitigate the disease burden associated with childhood obesity and improve long-term health of our patients and their communities.

We have organized the articles such that readers learn about an overview of obesity and how it's measured, primary prevention, environmental and social context that's important to remember, individual behavioral and medical assessment, followed by treatment strategies. We start off with an article by Waldrop and colleagues that reviews obesity as a multisystem disease with multifactorial origins and calls for an interdisciplinary approach in prevention and management. We then dive into assessment of

Pediatr Clin N Am 71 (2024) xxi–xxiii
https://doi.org/10.1016/j.pcl.2024.07.008
0031-3955/24/© 2024 Published by Elsevier Inc.

pediatric.theclinics.com

obesity with an article by Wood and Khalsa on BMI and other ways of screening for obesity. Early on in our issue, Flower and colleagues present the importance of prevention and key strategies. An article by Orr and colleagues then reviews the importance of an equity lens in evaluating both the causes and the management of obesity. Wagner and Cook then remind us of the remarkable stigma about obesity and what providers can do to avoid stigma with their care. Two articles—one by Galvez and colleagues on the built environment (reviewing urban planning, neighborhood design, and access to recreational spaces) and one by Laska and colleagues on the food and beverage environment (reviewing the importance of marketing and food policies)—speak to the barriers that families face to growing up healthy and lend context to the origins of our obesity epidemic.

Before we launch into treatment approaches, Weedn and colleagues share best practices for the physical examination of a young person with obesity, and then we share some special assessments related to disordered eating by Chaves and colleagues and genetics by Siddiqui and colleagues.

The last set of articles in this issue concentrates on treatment and management best practices. Hu and colleagues share an overview of treatment and the American Academy of Pediatrics' 2023 Clinical Practice Guidelines. Woolford and colleagues discuss the practical tools of motivational interviewing. Lambert and colleagues discuss lifestyle approaches, including physical activity, dietary practices, and other behavioral changes. Dutton and colleagues overview pharmacology options (and their benefits and risks). And we close our issue by reviewing metabolic surgery for adolescents with severe obesity by Eneli and colleagues.

Throughout this issue, we discuss how some populations are disproportionately affected by obesity as a result of historical and structural disadvantage, and we advocate for equitable access to resources and interventions.

As we embark on this journey through the pages of *Pediatric Clinics of North America*, we invite readers to engage critically, learn, and collaborate. Together, we can make a meaningful impact on the health and well-being of our youngest generation and empower the next generation to lead healthier lives.

DISCLOSURES

E.M. Perrin has no disclosures. G. Srivastava discloses advisory fees with Novo Nordisk, Rhythm, and Eli Lilly. G. Srivastava receives research grant support from Eli Lilly. G. Srivastava is on Speakers Bureau for Novo Nordisk and Rhythm.

Eliana M. Perrin, MD, MPH
Division of General Pediatrics
Department of Pediatrics, School of Medicine
School of Nursing, Johns Hopkins University
200 North Wolfe Street
Rubenstein Building #2075
Baltimore, MD 21287, USA

Gitanjali Srivastava, MD
Division of Diabetes, Endocrinology & Metabolism
Department of Medicine; Department of Pediatrics
Vanderbilt University School of Medicine
Vanderbilt Weight Loss Clinic
719 Thompson Lane Suite 22200
Nashville, TN 37204, USA

E-mail addresses:
eperrin@jhmi.edu (E.M. Perrin)
gitanjali.srivastava@vumc.org (G. Srivastava)

Overview of Pediatric Obesity as a Disease

Stephanie W. Waldrop, MD, MPH[a],*, Awab Ali Ibrahim, MD[b],
Jacqueline Maya, MD[c], Carmen Monthe-Dreze, MD[d],
Fatima Cody Stanford, MD, MPH, MPA, MBA[e,f]

KEYWORDS

• Pediatric obesity • Pathophysiology • Metabolic dysfunction • Inflammation

KEY POINTS

- Obesity is a multisystem disease with multifactorial origins and results in dysfunctional and detrimental physiologic processes that generate adverse effects on multiple aspects of health.
- Because pediatric obesity is complex, it warrants an interdisciplinary treatment approach.
- Viewing obesity as a disease emphasizes the need for medical attention, research, and comprehensive prevention and management strategies to address its multifaceted nature.

INTRODUCTION

The conceptualization of pediatric obesity as a disease represents a critical paradigm shift in understanding and addressing the multifaceted challenges with which it is

Funded by: NIHHYB. *Grant number(s):* NIDDK U24 DK132733; NIDDK, United States, UE5 DK 137285; P30 DK040561. Funding sources of support: Funding for this research was provided by the National Institute of Diabetes, Digestive and Kidney Disease of the National Institutes of Health (National Institutes of Health NIDDK U24 DK132733, UE5 DK137285, and P30 DK040561 [F.C. Stanford] and NIH, United States/NIDDK 2T32DK007658-32S1 [S.W. Waldrop]). J. Maya was supported by a T32 Training Grant for Endocrinology (3T32DK007028-47S1). The funding bodies had no role in the conceptualization, interpretation, or writing of the article.
 a Section on Nutrition, Department of Pediatrics, Anschutz Medical Campus, Nutrition Obesity Research Center (NORC), University of Colorado, Aurora, CO, USA; b Department of Pediatrics, Division of Pediatric Gastroenterology and Nutrition, Massachusetts General Hospital, 55 Fruit Street, Boston, MA 02114, USA; c Department of Pediatrics, Division of Pediatric Endocrinology, MGH Weight Center, Massachusetts General Hospital, 55 Fruit Street, Boston, MA 02115, USA; d Division of Newborn Medicine, Department of Pediatrics, Brigham and Women's Hospital, 75 Francis Street, Boston, MA 02115, USA; e Division of Endocrinology–Neuroendocrine, Department of Medicine, Massachusetts General Hospital, MGH Weight Center, 50 Staniford Street, Suite 430, Boston, MA 02115, USA; f Department of Pediatrics, Division of Endocrinology, Nutrition Obesity Research Center at Harvard (NORCH), Boston, MA, USA
* Corresponding author. 12700 East 19th Avenue, Mail Stop C-225, Research Complex II, Aurora, CO 80045.
E-mail address: stephanie.waldrop@cuanschutz.edu
Twitter: @askdrfatima (F.C.S.)

associated. This new perspective transcends the conventional view of obesity as a lifestyle choice under individual control. Instead, obesity is considered a complex medical condition involving interactions among genetic, environmental, and behavioral factors, resulting in an altered physiologic state with significant health implications. This evolution in the understanding of obesity, particularly among children and adolescents, will help patients, their families, and health care professionals in addressing its complexities with tailored interventions and treatments.[1] In addition, such an understanding establishes common ground rooted in pathophysiology and potentially improves discussion and collaboration with those possessing diverse perspectives (eg, Health at Every Size movement). In this narrative review, the authors have endeavored to showcase some of the well-known and hypothesized pathophysiologic mechanistic links that underlie obesity and the various disorders across multiple organ systems with which it is associated to provide a more comprehensive perspective of obesity as an "adiposity-based chronic disease" or ABCD.[2]

PATHOPHYSIOLOGY OF OBESITY

Hypothalamic regulation of energy balance occurs through control of appetite and satiety via interactions with the metabolic, endocrine, and nervous systems and is influenced by environmental factors.[3,4] Obesity is a chronic neurobehavioral disorder characterized by dysregulation of this complex interaction and is complicated by an individual predisposition to increase energy intake when placed in an obesogenic environment.[5,6] These definitions go beyond body mass index (BMI) and its potential flaws in assessing metabolic risk across racial and ethnic groups and individuals with greater lean body mass,[6,7] while placing greater focus on the pathophysiologic mechanisms driving and perpetuating obesity. In later discussion, the authors focus on describing the pathophysiology of pediatric obesity as it affects different organ systems.

PHYSIOLOGIC EFFECTS BY ORGAN SYSTEM
The Cardiovascular System

The clustering of cardiovascular risk factors (CVRFs), such as hypertension (HTN), dyslipidemia, vascular changes, subclinical inflammation, and insulin resistance, is highly prevalent in youth with obesity.[8] These CVRFs correlate significantly with early atherosclerosis and left ventricular remodeling, which persist into adulthood.[8] In addition, obesity during adolescence along with multiple other CVRFs is associated with a 14.6-fold increased risk of developing cardiovascular disease (CVD) before the age of 50 years.[9]

The prevalence of childhood HTN is significantly higher among children with obesity, with estimates as high as 25% among children and youth with obesity compared with 10% in children with normal weight.[9,10] Furthermore, those with obesity from childhood to adulthood have a ~3.8-fold greater risk for adult HTN.[9] Combined dyslipidemia (CD) is now the most predominant abnormal lipid pattern in childhood. It is characterized by moderate to severe elevation in triglyceride levels (age <10 years: >100 mg/dL; age 10–18 years: >130 mg/dL) and/or non–high-density lipoprotein (HDL) -cholesterol (>145 mg/dL), plus reduced HDL-cholesterol at less than 40 mg/dL.[11] CD prevalence increases with increasing BMI and is observed in 43% of youth with obesity.[11] Moreover, the risk of developing lipid disorders is 2.8 times higher in children with obesity than in children with normal body weight.[12] Childhood obesity also plays a significant role in the development of metabolic syndrome (MetS), characterized by increased abdominal obesity, dyslipidemia, HTN, and dysglycemia. Studies have shown that childhood MetS at the age of ~5 years is a significant predictor of adulthood MetS.[13] Finally, compared with normal-weight youth, obesity is associated with left ventricular hypertrophy (14% vs 3.6%), left ventricular diastolic dysfunction (5% vs 2%), and carotid intimal media thickness (cIMT), all of which can persist into adulthood and contribute to increased risk of CVD and mortality.[9,13,14] The underlying pathophysiology of HTN, CD, MetS, and structural heart damage with coronary heart disease in children with obesity is complex and interrelated, involving multiple mechanisms, as shown in **Fig. 1**.

The Endocrine System

Obesity is a known risk factor for developing glucose intolerance leading to prediabetes and Type 2 Diabetes Mellitus (T2DM). A prospective cohort study of more than 6000 people found that those with persistently higher BMI from childhood to adulthood had a 5 times greater risk of developing T2DM.[15] Even in children with type 1 diabetes, studies suggest that body size plays a causal role in developing the disease.[16] Initially, patients develop impaired glucose tolerance with increased peripheral and hepatic insulin resistance and compensatory hyperinsulinemia. Higher insulin resistance is associated with more severe obesity.[17] Adolescents have greater insulin resistance and insulin hypersecretion, which are associated with worse clinical outcomes and faster progression of disease compared with adults, leading to insufficient compensation and hyperglycemia.[18,19] The relationship of various adipokines, transcription factors, enzymes, and hormones relating obesity to insulin resistance and cardiometabolic disease is shown in **Fig. 1**.

Another endocrine condition closely related to insulin resistance and obesity is polycystic ovarian syndrome (PCOS). The prevalence of PCOS in individuals of reproductive age ranges from 5% to 10%, depending on the criteria used for diagnosis. The diagnosis in adolescence is challenging, given the overlap between age-appropriate

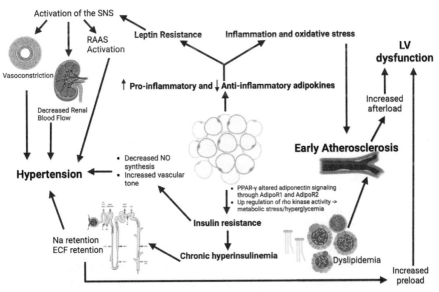

Fig. 1. Pathophysiologic mechanisms linking obesity to CVD. ECF, extracellular fluid; LV, left ventricular; Na, sodium; NO, nitric oxide; RAAS, renin-angiotensin aldosterone system; SNS, sympathetic nervous system.

findings and those considered normative for certain ethnic populations. PCOS in adolescence is defined as irregular menses that persist 2 years after menarche in the presence of clinical and/or biochemical hyperandrogenism. Comorbidities in PCOS include increased insulin resistance at lower BMIs, T2DM, CD, HTN, MetS, and metabolic-associated steatotic liver disease (MASLD), among others. Although obesity is not always present in individuals with PCOS, the risk of PCOS is higher in adolescents with obesity (OR, 7.86; 95% CI, 3.09–19.96) compared with those with overweight (OR, 5.32; 95% CI, 2.99–9.45).[20] With obesity, chronic hyperglycemia and increased triglyceride and fatty acid deposition in adipose cells lead to hyperinsulinism, insulin resistance, and decreased adiponectin.[21] The consequence is ovarian stroma stimulation and hypertrophy and increased theca cell production of androgens, which manifest as typical signs and symptoms (ie, acanthosis nigricans, hirsutism, acne, irregular periods, and infertility).[21]

Aside from its specific associations with T2DM and PCOS, obesity has effects on the hypothalamic-pituitary-gonadal and -growth axes. For example, leptin, produced by adipose tissue and found to be higher in individuals with obesity, is also elevated in children with central precocious puberty.[22] Some suggest that obesity may interfere with the timing of activation of the hypothalamic-pituitary-gonadal axis[23] by exacerbating the insulin resistance and hyperinsulinism that characterizes normal puberty.[24] Several hormones and peptides are involved in this process. The intricate positive feedback relationship proposed between energy control and reproduction is illustrated in **Fig. 2**.[23,25,26] Furthermore, high free-fatty-acid levels and hyperinsulinemia in obesity inhibit growth hormone (GH) secretion, leading to low GH levels.[27,28] Children with obesity undergoing growth stimulation testing demonstrate blunted GH secretion responses,[29] and compared with their normal weight

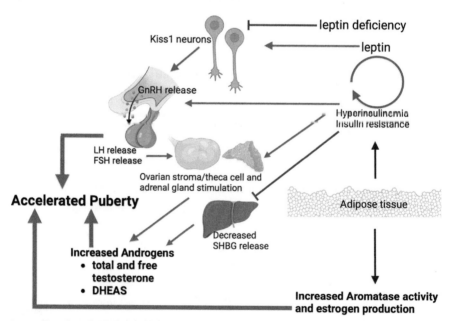

Fig. 2. Postulated relationships between energy balance and accelerated puberty. DHEAS, dehydroepiandosterone sulfate; FSH, follicle-stimulating hormone; GnRH, gonadotropin-releasing hormone; Kiss, kisspeptin; LH, luteinizing hormone; SHBG, sex hormone binding globulin.

counterparts, have greater height velocity in childhood but less pronounced growth during puberty.[30]

Behavior and Mental Health

Obesity has been characterized as a determinant of poor psychological outcomes.[31] More recent analyses, however, have revealed the mediating role that weight bias internalization (ie, negative stereotypes and attitudes associated with excess weight) by some with obesity plays in contributing to the development of adverse psychological symptoms, independent of weight status, and acting through internalized stress, hypothalamic-pituitary-adrenal axis activation, and maladaptive eating behaviors.[32–34] According to some, the relationships between weight stigma and subsequent weight bias internalization, psychological distress, disordered eating, and weight gain/weight status may be more of a cyclical and reinforcing process.[34] Some of the most common comorbid mental health disorders associated with obesity among pediatric patients include depression, anxiety, attention-deficit/hyperactivity disorder (ADHD), and eating disorders (eg, Loss of Control–Eating Disorder).[31,35]

The estimated prevalence of depression or depressive symptoms among children and adolescents with obesity is higher compared with those with normal weight across childhood and adolescence in various geographically diverse populations. Children and adolescents with obesity, but not overweight, had significantly higher odds (OR, 1.85; CI, 1.41–2.42) of major depressive disorder when compared with healthy controls.[36] However, among girls with obesity, there was 1.4 higher odds of depression compared with girls with normal weight.[37] These results echo literature on weight bias internalization, self-esteem, and stigma, which indicate a greater adverse influence on girls with obesity. Furthermore, several studies have shown that dissatisfaction with body image appears to mediate the relationship between BMI and depression in girls.[38–40] Finally, depression in self-identified black and white adolescents in the United States has been significantly associated with elevated BMI as well as increased adiposity, with early stressful life events, visceral adiposity, and adiponectin concentrations predicting the severity of depression experienced.[41]

Pediatric patients with obesity have also been shown to have an increased risk of developing anxiety compared with normal or lower-weight peers.[42] However, associations overall appear to be less strong and less consistent compared with depression.[35,43] One systematic review and meta-analysis evaluating more than 3000 individuals looked at several psychological outcomes, and in those for which the outcome was anxiety, a significant relationship with obesity was identified, but only when using the most specific assessment scale (ie, the Spielberger State–Anxiety Inventory).[44] Their results indicated a 30% greater likelihood of anxiety for both girls and boys with obesity. The full meta-analysis, however, found no association between obesity and risk of anxiety,[44] findings similar to other studies revealing obesity and overweight either to not be associated with anxiety[35] or to be only modestly so.[45]

The association between ADHD and obesity is well described throughout the literature. In 2016, Cortese[46,47] and others noted the prevalence of obesity in children with ADHD to be ~40% higher compared with those without ADHD, and evidence from meta-analyses indicates a significant association between the 2 disorders despite confounding factors. Some evidence suggests a shared genetic background for both[47,48] with familial coaggregation of ADHD and obesity described.[49] The presence of ADHD and a genetic profile indicative of increased dopamine receptor activation within the reward system has been associated with elevated BMI and reward-based eating patterns.[48] **Fig. 3** illustrates the shared neurobiological pathways that suggest a link between energy and attentional dysregulation.

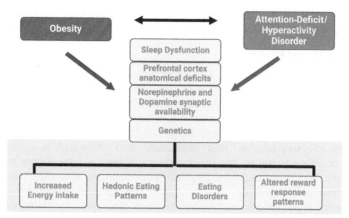

Fig. 3. Shared neurobiological pathways and outcomes linking energy balance and attentional dysregulation.

The Immune System

Innate and adaptive immunity is impaired in the chronic, inflammatory state of obesity.[50] Changes in the innate immune system include increased neutrophils with decreased bactericidal capacity, increased mast cells, decreased eosinophils in adipose tissue, decreased natural killer cells, and increased proinflammatory factors.[50,51] Furthermore, there is decreased number and altered function of CD8 and CD4 T and B cells.[50,51] Increased leptin and other proinflammatory cytokines (eg, interleukin-1 [IL-1], IL-6, IL-12, IL-17, tumor necrosis factor-alpha [TNF-α], migration inhibitory factor) and decreased anti-inflammatory molecules, such as adiponectin, over sustained periods contribute to low-grade systemic inflammation.[51–53] Peroxisome proliferator–activated receptor transcription factors (eg, PPAR-α and PPAR-β/δ), which are less expressed in obesity, have an inverse relationship with levels of proinflammatory markers (TNF-α and IL-8, respectively).[54]

Obesity has been associated with different cancer types as well as autoimmune diseases[50] and inflammation.[55] In childhood and adolescence, patients with acute lymphoblastic leukemia and obesity have worse outcomes, including higher likelihood of hyperlipidemia, abdominal complications requiring surgery, intracranial or other severe bleeding episodes, and liver and kidney failure.[56] Excess weight in childhood increases the risk of type 1 diabetes,[16] and other autoimmune disorders, including multiple sclerosis, Crohn disease, rheumatoid arthritis, systemic lupus erythematosus, inflammatory bowel disease, Hashimoto thyroiditis, and psoriasis.[57]

The Skin

Systemic diseases can often have dermatologic manifestations, and obesity is no exception (**Box 1**). Obesity predisposes to skin disorders owing to physiologic alterations in skin barrier integrity, collagen structure, sebaceous and sweat gland production, and abnormalities of lymphatic and circulatory function.[58] In addition, the systemic inflammatory, hormonal, and metabolic dysfunction accompanying obesity can influence dermatologic signs and symptoms. The chronic low-grade proinflammatory environment associated with obesity has been linked with more severe atopic dermatitis and psoriasis in children with obesity[59,60] as well as the more severe forms of acne (ie, inflammatory pustular, nodular)[61] seen in adolescence. **Fig. 4** showcases

---

Box 1
Common skin disorders associated with pediatric obesity

1. Disorders of skin barrier integrity
   Acquired plantar hyperkeratosis
   Noninfectious intertrigo
   Striae distensae
   Xerosis cutis

2. Hormonally induced skin disorders
   Acanthosis nigricans
   Acrochordons
   Keratosis pilaris
   Inflammatory acne vulgaris

3. Infectious skin disorders
   Fungal infections
     Seborrhea (eg, *Pityrosporum* sp)
     Tinea corporis, tinea cruris, tinea pedis (eg, *Tinea* sp)
     Onychomycosis (eg, Dermatophytes)
     Intertrigo (eg, *Candida* sp)
   Bacterial infections
     Intertrigo (eg, staphylococcal, streptococcal)
     Erythrasma (eg, corynebacterial)
     Folliculitis (eg, staphylococcal, streptococcal)
     Cellulitis (eg, staphylococcal, streptococcal)

4. Inflammatory skin disorders
   Psoriasis
   Hidradenitis suppurativa
   Atopic dermatitis

Hasse L, Jamiolkowski D, Reschke F, Kapitzke K, Weiskorn J, Kordonouri O, Biester T, Ott H. Pediatric obesity and skin disease: cutaneous findings and associated quality-of-life impairments in 103 children and adolescents with obesity. Endocr Connect. 2023 Aug 2;12(9):e230235. https://doi.org/10.1530/EC-23-0235. PMID: 37410088; PMCID: PMC10448574; and Sunkwad, A. and M. Sunanda. Cutaneous manifestations in overweight and obese children and adolescent. Intrnl J of Cont Pediatrics. 2021 Oct 8(10). doi: https://doi.org/10.18203/2349-3291.ijcp20213726.

---

dermatologic manifestations of obesity and their proposed pathophysiologic mechanisms.

The Renal System

The renal impairment associated with obesity begins early in childhood before the signs and symptoms of diabetes, HTN, or associated comorbidities are clinically evident.[62] Studies show children with obesity have larger kidneys and increased renal blood flow. This chronic state of hyperfiltration later induces glomerulomegaly, cellular remodeling, fibrotic scarring, and a progressive decline in glomerular filtration rate. However, the pathophysiology of renal injury in children with obesity continues to be under investigation given mixed findings. Some investigators report positive correlations between measures of obesity and glomerular filtration rate (GFR), reflecting a hyperfiltration state, whereas others have found lower or no differences in GFR levels in children with BMI in the overweight/obesity category.[62] Furthermore, pediatric obesity is associated with a significantly increased risk for all-cause end-stage renal disease later in life.[62] Several observational cohort studies demonstrate significant positive associations between higher BMI in early life and greater renal disease risk in later life (hazard risk range: 1.39 to 6.89).[63]

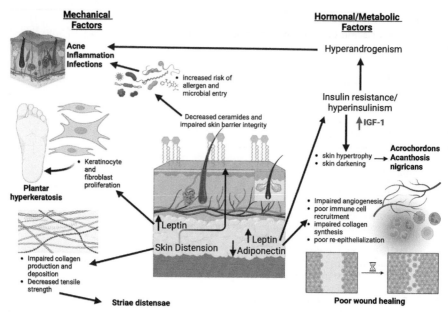

Fig. 4. Dermatologic manifestations of obesity.

The Musculoskeletal System

Obesity significantly impacts bone physiology through its association with MetS and inflammation,[64] negatively affecting growing bone by adversely influencing osteoblast and osteoclast function through modulation of leptin concentrations.[65] Leptin has an inhibitory effect on cortical bone size and fosters accelerated bone resorption and diminished bone formation potentially contributing to osteopenia and osteoporosis.[66] Moreover, vitamin D sequestered in adipose tissue reduces its circulating availability for bone remodeling, which is concerning because the prevalence of vitamin D deficiency increases with excess weight[67] and nutritionally inadequate diets.[65] Consequently, children with obesity face an elevated risk of fractures, particularly in weight-bearing areas, attributable to increased skeletal mechanical stress and potential alterations in bone geometry and density.[68] Moreover, pediatric obesity may contribute to delayed fracture healing owing to compromised blood flow, altered cytokine production, and concurrent conditions, such as type 2 diabetes.[64] The response of bone tissue to trauma is also affected, with biomechanical forces and the proinflammatory environment associated with obesity influencing the efficiency of reparative processes.[66,69] **Table 1** highlights some specific musculoskeletal disorders associated with pediatric obesity.

The Gastrointestinal System

Pediatric obesity is closely linked to an increased risk of numerous gastrointestinal (GI) disorders. These conditions can lead to a range of GI symptoms, including abdominal pain, discomfort, and altered bowel habits. Furthermore, insulin resistance and MetS are both independently associated with GI complications.[70,71] The most common GI disorders associated with pediatric obesity are discussed later.

Gastroesophageal reflux disease (GERD) is characterized by chronic and recurrent symptoms of regurgitation or "acid burn." Longitudinal studies have identified obesity

Table 1
Musculoskeletal disorders associated with obesity in children

Disorder	Cause/Pathophysiology	Relationship to Obesity
Blount disease[88]	Characterized by abnormal growth of the medial aspect of the proximal tibia, leading to varus deformity of the lower limbs	• The increased load on the developing skeleton, especially during weight-bearing activities, contributes to abnormal growth plate development and subsequent alterations in the alignment of the lower extremities • Inflammatory and metabolic changes of obesity exacerbate the pathophysiologic mechanisms involved in Blount disease
Slipped Capital Femoral Epiphysis (SCFE)[89]	Characterized by displacement of the femoral epiphysis relative to the femoral neck through the growth plate	• Excess body weight contributes to increased mechanical stress on the proximal femoral growth plate, potentially influencing the onset and progression of SCFE • Genetic, hormonal, and mechanical factors (eg, ancestry, variations in bone geometry) also contribute
Osteoarthritis[65]	Characterized by breakdown of bone cartilage leading to increased friction and wear within the affected joint. This results in increased pain and reduced mobility	• With obesity, added weight places extra stress on the joints, especially in weight-bearing areas. This exacerbates the wear and tear associated with this condition
Osteoporosis[68]	Characterized by weakened and porous bones, typically associated with aging, is now increasingly recognized as a concern in the context of pediatric obesity	• Pediatric obesity has been linked to alterations in bone metabolism, which influences bone mineral density, increased mechanical loading on bone • Bone development and integrity are adversely affected, potentially predisposing individuals to fractures later in life
Low back pain and lordosis[66]	The altered distribution of body fat, particularly in the abdominal region, can affect the natural curvature of the spine, leading to changes consistent with lordosis and contributing to risk of spondylolisthesis spondylolysis and risk of low back pain	• Excessive body weight places an increased mechanical load on the spine, influencing the biomechanics of the lumbar region and placing stress on the intervertebral discs and facet joints

as a significant risk factor for GERD, with increased abdominal pressure relaxing the lower esophageal sphincter and facilitating gastric content reflux.[72] Waist-hip ratio and particularly visceral fat emerge as stronger predictors for pathologic acid exposure.[73] Weight loss has proven effective in alleviating GERD symptoms, emphasizing the intricate interplay between obesity and GERD pathophysiology.[72]

Functional Gastrointestinal Disorders (FGIDs) represent a complex interplay of physiologic and neurobiological factors contributing to altered GI function.[74] Obesity is associated with an increased prevalence of FGIDs, such as functional constipation, irritable bowel syndrome, and functional abdominal pain.[75] The pathophysiologic mechanisms underlying these associations are multifaceted, involving altered gut motility, visceral hypersensitivity, and dysregulation of the brain-gut axis and the gut microbiome. Adipose tissue, particularly visceral adipose, acts as an endocrine organ, secreting adipokines and proinflammatory mediators that influence gut function and hyperalgesia.[76] In addition, obesity-related changes in gut microbiota composition, immune system activation, and hormonal fluctuations further contribute to the manifestation of FGIDs.[74]

MASLD replaces the previously used term, nonalcoholic fatty liver disease or NAFLD, and signifies a shift in understanding the intricate relationship between metabolic dysregulation and liver pathologic condition.[77] MASLD encompasses a range of hepatic manifestations, from simple steatosis to steatohepatitis, fibrosis, cirrhosis, and hepatocellular carcinoma. The pathogenesis of MASLD involves the interplay of obesity, insulin resistance, and dyslipidemia.[78] The accumulation of triglycerides within hepatocytes, primarily derived from increased free-fatty-acid influx and de novo lipogenesis, initiates hepatocellular injury and inflammation. In addition, adipose tissue dysfunction and the release of adipokines contribute to hepatic inflammation and fibrosis progression.[78] Genetic predisposition and gut microbiota alterations further influence disease susceptibility and progression.[77]

Pediatric obesity also contributes to the development of cholelithiasis and choledocholithiasis through several mechanisms, including altered bile composition, impaired gallbladder motility, and disturbances in cholesterol metabolism. The risk is further compounded by the prevalence of MetS and insulin resistance in children with obesity.[79] The heightened incidence of acute pancreatitis associated with obesity can be attributed to an elevated risk of gallstones, hypertriglyceridemia, diabetes, medications, and bariatric surgery for weight loss interventions.[80] In addition, obesity exacerbates the severity of acute pancreatitis by permitting uncontrolled lipolysis of visceral fat, which is abundant in unsaturated triglycerides. These metabolic alterations are crucial in the onset of necrosis associated with the condition.[70]

Pulmonary, Otolaryngology, and Sleep

Obesity in children and adolescents has been reported to be associated with deleterious changes in lung function, even in the absence of diagnosed respiratory disease, although the complete role of obesity on lung function in children and adolescents has not yet been fully elucidated. Some studies suggest consistent trends toward a lower ratio of functional expiratory velocity over 1 minute to functional velocity capacity (FEV_1/FVC), as well as lower functional residual capacity, expiratory reserve volume, and residual volume.[81–83] These changes are postulated to be mediated by both subclinical inflammation and mechanical factors, such as airway dysanapsis, leading to an obstructive defect.[81,82] In dysanapsis, more commonly seen in children with excess weight, the lung parenchyma grow out of proportion to the airways such that normal or increased values of FEV1 and FVC are seen, although the FEV1/FVC ratio is lowered.[84,85] Relatedly, children with obesity also show a decline in their forced expiratory

Table 2
Pediatric respiratory and otorhinolaryngologic disorders associated with obesity

Disorder	Epidemiology	Cause/Pathophysiology/Contributing Factors Related to Obesity	Clinical Considerations
Asthma	• Obesity increases the relative risk for asthma by 29% • A quarter of asthma cases in children are due to obesity • Higher BMI contributes to more severe asthma phenotype • Obesity is an independent risk factor in asthma development • Visceral or central obesity may better predict pediatric asthma incidence and poor lung function than overall BMI[85]	*Altered anatomy:* Decreased chest wall compliance due to excess fat mass • Dysanapsis increases proportionally with BMI resulting in worsening severity of asthma symptoms and reduced response to treatment[84] • Decreased functional residual capacity • Decreased tidal volumes • Alveolar hypoventilation • Increased airway resistance and hyperresponsiveness[85] *Systemic inflammation and altered immune response:* Asthma in patients with obesity is associated with a T1-helper-cell lymphocytic response instead of the typical T2-helper-cell response more often seen in lean counterparts[59] *Altered metabolism:* Low adiponectin levels are seen in pediatric patients with obesity and asthma[86] *High oxidative stress:* Impairs lung function and contributes to corticosteroid resistance[84]	In the context of obesity, asthma is consistent with a phenotype that is • Less responsive to classical anti-inflammatory treatments • Portends a more severe course with increased use of oral steroids, emergency department visits, and hospitalizations • Reduced response to traditional therapies, such as beta-agonist bronchodilators as well as inhaled corticosteroid[84] Weight loss is considered a significant intervention for improving asthma disease severity and prevalence[84]

(continued on next page)

Table 2
(continued)

Disorder	Epidemiology	Cause/Pathophysiology/Contributing Factors Related to Obesity	Clinical Considerations
Acute Otitis Media and Otitis Media with Effusion	Higher prevalence of OME in children with obesity Increased frequency of acute otitis media in American school-aged children with obesity compared with their lean counterparts[87]	Contributing pathophysiologic factors include: • Chronic systemic inflammation caused by increased production of inflammatory cytokines and adipokines (ie, IL-6, TNF-alpha, IL-1beta, and leptin) • Mechanical dysfunction predisposing to eustachian tube obstruction, negative middle ear pressures and fluid accumulation, laryngopharyngeal reflux, and GERD[87]	Higher concentrations of inflammatory mediators found in middle ear fluid of children with obesity[87]
Obstructive Sleep Apnea Syndrome	Higher incidence of adenoidal and tonsillar hypertrophy in children with obesity compared with those with normal weight[87] Sixty percent of pediatric patients with obesity have OSA, whereas the prevalence of OSA in children without obesity ranges from 1% to 5%[83,87]	Shared factors in the association between OSAS and obesity include: • Increased respiratory work at night due to extrathoracic and intrabdominal excess adiposity, oxidative stress, systemic inflammation, and alterations in the intestinal microbiota[84] • Increased lymphoid tissue size secondary to endocrine-mediated somatic growth predisposing to larger tonsils, fat pads, the soft palate, and tongue[87] • Obesity's synergistic effects on neuroanatomy (eg, upper airway UAJ loading) and UA neuromotor function (eg, altered UA neuromotor reflexes impairing responses to hypercapnia).[87]	OSA risk can persist after adenotonsillectomy and approximately 4 times higher in those with obesity compared with those with normal weight[87] In association with adenotonsillectomy, pediatric patients with obesity compared with their normal weight counterparts have higher risk of: • Bleeding • Airway obstruction • Intraoperative hypoxemia repeated laryngoscopy attempts • Difficult bag mask ventilation[87] • Acute or chronic respiratory insufficiency in the perioperative period • Longer hospitalizations stays[84]

flow rate (25%–75%), a measure of clinically relevant reversible airflow compromise within the smaller airways and a correlate of bronchodilator responsiveness.[82,84]

Mechanical mechanisms suggested to explain the association between obesity and respiratory symptoms include obesity-induced lung compression and reduced lung compliance, diaphragmatic heightening owing to abdominal adiposity, and decreased chest wall compliance, all of which lead to low lung volumes, low expiratory flow rates, and impaired gas exchange.[84] Inflammatory mechanisms that contribute include increased adipocyte mass, which promotes altered secretion of proinflammatory and anti-inflammatory cytokines and mediators, such as leptin (increased) and adiponectin (decreased), which influence M1 proinflammatory and M2 anti-inflammatory macrophage polarization, respectively.[59,84,86] The importance of adipokines, such as leptin and adiponectin, in lung function stems in part from the presence of their receptors within lung tissue.[86] In murine models of chronic asthma, for example, low adiponectin has been shown to increase allergic inflammation and affect pulmonary vascular remodeling. In contrast, exogenous adiponectin appears to alleviate oxidative stress and airway inflammation.[86]

Obesity's effects are also noted in the risk of otorhinolaryngologic disease, including obstructive sleep apnea syndrome. Factors linking the conditions include increased inflammation, mechanical obstruction, and T-helper-cell immune response modifications.[87] **Table 2** details the pathophysiologic effects of excess adiposity on the major respiratory and otorhinolaryngologic disorders commonly affecting pediatric patients with obesity.

SUMMARY

From a semantic perspective, a "disease," as defined by the *Oxford Medical Dictionary*, is "a disorder with specific cause (which may or may not be known) and recognizable signs and symptoms; or any bodily abnormality or failure to function properly, except that resulting directly from physical injury that may open the way for disease." Consistent with this definition and as discussed in this review, childhood obesity has multiple established specific causes, recognizable signs and symptoms, and associated abnormal bodily functions. There are pathophysiologic mechanisms driven by the metabolic and hormonal dysfunction and chronic inflammation accompanying the state of obesity, which in turn result in increased prevalence and risk of numerous secondary diseases across multiple organ systems. "Adiposity-based chronic disease," defined by Steele and Finucane,[2] is an apt description to classify this disease based on its origin, time course, and sequelae. Like many chronic diseases, obesity is multifactorial, with genetic, biological, behavioral, sociocultural, economic, and environmental factors contributing, but that does not diminish the significance of the dysfunctional and detrimental physiologic processes the state generates or the overwhelming adverse effects it engenders on multiple aspects of health, especially among youth.

CLINICS CARE POINTS

- Pediatric patients with obesity face an increased risk of sequelae of disorders that affect almost all organ systems.

- Although cardiovascular disease risk factors are individually associated with obesity, the clustering of these risk factors in adolescence is an important clinical predictor of cardiovascular events in adulthood. Because clustering of risk factors begins in early life, primordial prevention should be embedded in routine pediatric care, beginning in the first 2 years of life, especially in those with family history of obesity, insulin resistance, dyslipidemia, and premature cardiovascular disease.

- Obesity can adversely affect the gastrointestinal tract, increasing the risk of conditions like gastroesophageal reflux disease, nonalcoholic fatty liver disease, and disorders of the gut-brain axis.

- Obesity can impact the normal development of bones and joints, potentially causing long-term issues, such as early-onset osteoarthritis and structural abnormalities, that may persist into adulthood.

- Asthma is often of increasing severity in those with obesity because of altered mechanical and inflammatory/immune system factors (eg, T1-helper-cell/M1 macrophage predominant inflammation) that place these children and adolescents at increased risk of exacerbations, hospitalizations, and poor control with traditional therapies (eg, inhaled corticosteroids, inhaled bronchodilators) that primarily focus on addressing the T2-helper-cell/M2 macrophage inflammatory response.

- The potential common ground between mental health disorders (eg, depression and attention-deficit/hyperactivity disorder) and obesity may have implications for effective treatments as well as understanding the lack of success with intensive lifestyle/behavior change for some patients with both conditions.

DISCLOSURE

F.C. Stanford has served as a consultant to Calibrate, GoodRx, Pfizer, Eli Lilly, Boehringer Ingelheim, Gelesis, Vida Health, Life Force, Ilant Health, Melli Cell, Novo Nordisk.

Other sources of support: University of Colorado School of Medicine–Anschutz Medical Campus and the University of Colorado Nutrition Obesity Research Center, The Nutrition Obesity Research Center at the University of Colorado, Harvard University School of Medicine, Harvard University (NORCH), and the NORCH Diversity Scholars Program.

Authors' contributions: S.W. Waldrop, A.A. Ibrahim, J. Maya, and C. Monthe-Dreze contributed equally to writing and editing this work. F.C. Stanford provided editorial and supervisory expertise.

REFERENCES

1. Farpour-Lambert NJ, Baker JL, Hassapidou M, et al. Childhood Obesity Is a Chronic Disease Demanding Specific Health Care–a Position Statement from the Childhood Obesity Task Force (COTF) of the European Association for the Study of Obesity (EASO). Obes Facts 2015;8(5):342–9.
2. Steele M, Finucane FM. Philosophically, is obesity really a disease? Obes Rev 2023;24(8):e13590. https://doi.org/10.1111/obr.13590.
3. Hall KD, Farooqi IS, Friedman JM, et al. The energy balance model of obesity: beyond calories in, calories out. Am J Clin Nutr 2022;115(5):1243–54.
4. Cypess AM. Reassessing Human Adipose Tissue. N Engl J Med 2022;386(8):768–79.
5. Bays HE, Burridge K, Tondt J, et al. Obesity Algorithm eBook. Obesity Medical Association 2021. Available at: https://obesitymedicine.org/obesity-algorithm/. [Accessed 26 December 2023].
6. Hampl SE, Hassink SG, Skinner AC, et al. Clinical Practice Guideline for the Evaluation and Treatment of Children and Adolescents With Obesity. Pediatrics 2023; 151(2). https://doi.org/10.1542/peds.2022-060640.

7. Weber DR, Moore RH, Leonard MB, et al. Fat and lean BMI reference curves in children and adolescents and their utility in identifying excess adiposity compared with BMI and percentage body fat. Am J Clin Nutr 2013;98(1):49–56.

8. Caprio S, Santoro N, Weiss R. Childhood obesity and the associated rise in cardiometabolic complications. Nat Metab 2020;2(3):223–32.

9. McPhee PG, Singh S, Morrison KM. Childhood Obesity and Cardiovascular Disease Risk: Working Toward Solutions. Can J Cardiol 2020;36(9):1352–61.

10. Sabri M, Gheissari A, Mansourian M, et al. Essential hypertension in children, a growing worldwide problem. J Res Med Sci 2019;24:109.

11. Kavey RW. Combined Dyslipidemia in Children and Adolescents: a Proposed New Management Approach. Curr Atheroscler Rep 2023;25(5):237–45.

12. Nielsen TRH, Lausten-Thomsen U, Fonvig CE, et al. Dyslipidemia and reference values for fasting plasma lipid concentrations in Danish/North-European White children and adolescents. BMC Pediatr 2017;17(1):116.

13. Delvecchio M, Pastore C, Valente F, et al. Cardiovascular Implications in Idiopathic and Syndromic Obesity in Childhood: An Update. Front Endocrinol (Lausanne) 2020;11:330.

14. Burden S, Weedon B, Whaymand L, et al. The effect of overweight/obesity on diastolic function in children and adolescents: A meta-analysis. Clin Obes 2021; 11(5):e12476. https://doi.org/10.1111/cob.12476.

15. Juonala M, Magnussen CG, Berenson GS, et al. Childhood adiposity, adult adiposity, and cardiovascular risk factors. N Engl J Med 2011;365(20):1876–85.

16. Richardson TG, Crouch DJM, Power GM, et al. Childhood body size directly increases type 1 diabetes risk based on a lifecourse Mendelian randomization approach. Nat Commun 2022;13(1):2337.

17. Tagi VM, Chiarelli F. Obesity and insulin resistance in children. Curr Opin Pediatr 2020;32(4):582–8.

18. Arslanian SA, El Ghormli L, Kim JY, et al. OGTT Glucose Response Curves, Insulin Sensitivity, and β-Cell Function in RISE: Comparison Between Youth and Adults at Randomization and in Response to Interventions to Preserve β-Cell Function. Diabetes Care 2021;44(3):817–25.

19. Bacha F, Gungor N, Lee S, et al. Progressive deterioration of β-cell function in obese youth with type 2 diabetes. Pediatr Diabetes 2013;14(2):106–11.

20. Dobbie LJ, Pittam B, Zhao SS, et al. Childhood, adolescent, and adulthood adiposity are associated with risk of PCOS: a Mendelian randomization study with meta-analysis. Hum Reprod 2023;38(6):1168–82.

21. Siddiqui S, Mateen S, Ahmad R, et al. A brief insight into the etiology, genetics, and immunology of polycystic ovarian syndrome (PCOS). J Assist Reprod Genet 2022;39(11):2439–73.

22. Zurita-Cruz JN, Villasís-Keever MA, Manuel-Apolinar L, et al. Altered cardiometabolic profile in girls with central precocious puberty and adipokines: A propensity score matching analysis. Cytokine 2021;148:155660. https://doi.org/10.1016/j. cyto.2021.155660.

23. Shi L, Jiang Z, Zhang L. Childhood obesity and central precocious puberty. Front Endocrinol (Lausanne) 2022;13:1056871. https://doi.org/10.3389/fendo.2022. 1056871.

24. Ouyang L, Yang F. Combined diagnostic value of insulin-like growth factor-1, insulin-like growth factor binding protein-3, and baseline luteinizing hormone levels for central precocious puberty in girls. J Pediatr Endocrinol Metab 2022;35(7): 874–9.

25. Burcelin R, Thorens B, Glauser M, et al. Gonadotropin-releasing hormone secretion from hypothalamic neurons: stimulation by insulin and potentiation by leptin. Endocrinology 2003;144(10):4484–91.

26. Reinehr T, Roth CL. Is there a causal relationship between obesity and puberty? Lancet Child Adolesc Health 2019;3(1):44–54.

27. Bang P. Pediatric implications of normal insulin-GH-IGF-Axis physiology. In: Feingold KR, Anawalt B, Blackman MR, et al, editors. Endotext. South Dartmouth, MA: MDText.com, Inc; 2000. Copyright © 2000-2024, MDText.com, Inc.

28. Hjelholt A, Høgild M, Bak AM, et al. Growth Hormone and Obesity. Endocrinol Metab Clin North Am 2020;49(2):239–50.

29. Abawi O, Augustijn D, Hoeks SE, et al. Impact of body mass index on growth hormone stimulation tests in children and adolescents: a systematic review and meta-analysis. Crit Rev Clin Lab Sci 2021;58(8):576–95.

30. Putri RR, Danielsson P, Marcus C, et al. Height and Growth Velocity in Children and Adolescents Undergoing Obesity Treatment: A Prospective Cohort Study. J Clin Endocrinol Metab 2023;109(1):e314–20.

31. Small L, Aplasca A. Child Obesity and Mental Health: A Complex Interaction. Child Adolesc Psychiatr Clin N Am 2016;25(2):269–82.

32. Alimoradi Z, Golboni F, Griffiths MD, et al. Weight-related stigma and psychological distress: A systematic review and meta-analysis. Clin Nutr 2020;39(7):2001–13.

33. Gmeiner MS, Warschburger P. Simply too much: the extent to which weight bias internalization results in a higher risk of eating disorders and psychosocial problems. Eat Weight Disord 2022;27(1):317–24.

34. Barnhart WR, Cui S, Cui T, et al. Relationships between weight bias internalization and biopsychosocial health outcomes: A prospective study in Chinese adolescents. Int J Eat Disord 2023;56(5):1021–33.

35. Kokka I, Mourikis I, Bacopoulou F. Psychiatric Disorders and Obesity in Childhood and Adolescence-A Systematic Review of Cross-Sectional Studies. Children (Basel) 2023;10(2). https://doi.org/10.3390/children10020285.

36. Rao WW, Zong QQ, Zhang JW, et al. Obesity increases the risk of depression in children and adolescents: Results from a systematic review and meta-analysis. J Affect Disord 2020;267:78–85.

37. Sutaria S, Devakumar D, Yasuda SS, et al. Is obesity associated with depression in children? Systematic review and meta-analysis. Arch Dis Child 2019;104(1):64–74.

38. Lewis-Smith H, Bray I, Salmon D, et al. Prospective Pathways to Depressive Symptoms and Disordered Eating in Adolescence: A 7-Year Longitudinal Cohort Study. J Youth Adolesc 2020;49(10):2060–74.

39. Czepielewski LS. Childhood BMI, adolescent depression, and body dissatisfaction. Lancet Psychiatr 2024;11(1):3–4.

40. Blundell E, De Stavola BL, Kellock MD, et al. Longitudinal pathways between childhood BMI, body dissatisfaction, and adolescent depression: an observational study using the UK Millennium Cohort Study. Lancet Psychiatr 2024;11(1):47–55.

41. McLachlan C, Shelton R, Li L. Obesity, inflammation, and depression in adolescents. Front Psychiatry 2023;14:1221709. https://doi.org/10.3389/fpsyt.2023.1221709.

42. Rankin J, Matthews L, Cobley S, et al. Psychological consequences of childhood obesity: psychiatric comorbidity and prevention. Adolesc Health Med Ther 2016;7:125–46.

43. Sheinbein DH, Stein RI, Hayes JF, et al. Factors associated with depression and anxiety symptoms among children seeking treatment for obesity: A social-ecological approach. Pediatr Obes 2019;14(8):e12518. https://doi.org/10.1111/ijpo.12518.

44. Moradi M, Mozaffari H, Askari M, et al. Association between overweight/obesity with depression, anxiety, low self-esteem, and body dissatisfaction in children and adolescents: a systematic review and meta-analysis of observational studies. Crit Rev Food Sci Nutr 2022;62(2):555–70.

45. O'Hara VM, Curran JL, Browne NT. The Co-occurrence of Pediatric Obesity and ADHD: an Understanding of Shared Pathophysiology and Implications for Collaborative Management. Curr Obes Rep 2020;9(4):451–61.

46. Landau Z, Pinhas-Hamiel O. Attention Deficit/Hyperactivity, the Metabolic Syndrome, and Type 2 Diabetes. Curr Diab Rep 2019;19(8):46.

47. Cortese S. The Association between ADHD and Obesity: Intriguing, Progressively More Investigated, but Still Puzzling. Brain Sci 2019;9(10). https://doi.org/10.3390/brainsci9100256.

48. Martins-Silva T, Vaz JDS, Genro JP, et al. Obesity and ADHD: Exploring the role of body composition, BMI polygenic risk score, and reward system genes. J Psychiatr Res 2021;136:529–36.

49. Chen Q, Hartman CA, Kuja-Halkola R, et al. Attention-deficit/hyperactivity disorder and clinically diagnosed obesity in adolescence and young adulthood: a register-based study in Sweden. Psychol Med 2019;49(11):1841–9.

50. Muscogiuri G, Pugliese G, Laudisio D, et al. The impact of obesity on immune response to infection: Plausible mechanisms and outcomes. Obes Rev 2021;22(6):e13216. https://doi.org/10.1111/obr.13216.

51. Fang X, Henao-Mejia J, Henrickson SE. Obesity and immune status in children. Curr Opin Pediatr 2020;32(6):805–15.

52. Wrann CD, Laue T, Hübner L, et al. Short-term and long-term leptin exposure differentially affect human natural killer cell immune functions. Am J Physiol Endocrinol Metab 2012;302(1):E108–16.

53. Zhao Y, Lin L, Li J, et al. CD4(+) T cells in obesity and obesity-associated diseases. Cell Immunol 2018;332:1–6.

54. Vargas-Sánchez K, Vargas L, Urrutia Y, et al. PPARα and PPARβ/δ are negatively correlated with proinflammatory markers in leukocytes of an obese pediatric population. J Inflamm (Lond) 2020;17(1):35.

55. Skinner AC, Steiner MJ, Henderson FW, et al. Multiple markers of inflammation and weight status: cross-sectional analyses throughout childhood. Pediatrics 2010;125(4):e801–9.

56. Egnell C, Heyman M, Jónsson ÓG, et al. Obesity as a predictor of treatment-related toxicity in children with acute lymphoblastic leukaemia. Br J Haematol 2022;196(5):1239–47.

57. Versini M, Jeandel PY, Rosenthal E, et al. Obesity in autoimmune diseases: not a passive bystander. Autoimmun Rev 2014;13(9):981–1000.

58. Hirt PA, Castillo DE, Yosipovitch G, et al. Skin changes in the obese patient. J Am Acad Dermatol 2019;81(5):1037–57.

59. Stefani C, Pecoraro L, Flodmark CE, et al. Allergic Diseases and Childhood Obesity: A Detrimental Link? Biomedicines 2023;11(7). https://doi.org/10.3390/biomedicines11072061.

60. Steele CE, Morrell D, Evans M. Metabolic syndrome and inflammatory skin conditions. Curr Opin Pediatr 2019;31(4):515–22.

61. Darlenski R, Mihaylova V, Handjieva-Darlenska T. The Link Between Obesity and the Skin. Front Nutr 2022;9:855573. https://doi.org/10.3389/fnut.2022.855573.

62. Correia-Costa L, Azevedo A, Caldas Afonso A. Childhood Obesity and Impact on the Kidney. Nephron 2019;143(1):8–11.

63. Pourghazi F, Mohammadi S, Eslami M, et al. Association Between Childhood Obesity and Later Life Kidney Disorders: A Systematic Review. J Ren Nutr 2023;33(4):520–8.

64. O'Malley GC, Shultz SP, Thivel D, et al. Neuromusculoskeletal Health in Pediatric Obesity: Incorporating Evidence into Clinical Examination. Curr Obes Rep 2021; 10(4):467–77.

65. Nowicki P, Kemppainen J, Maskill L, et al. The Role of Obesity in Pediatric Orthopedics. J Am Acad Orthop Surg Glob Res Rev 2019;3(5):e036. https://doi.org/10.5435/JAAOSGlobal-D-19-00036.

66. Korkmaz HA, Özkan B. Impact of Obesity on Bone Metabolism in Children. J Pediatr Endocrinol Metab 2022;35(5):557–65.

67. Turer CB, Lin H, Flores G. Prevalence of vitamin D deficiency among overweight and obese US children. Pediatrics 2013;131(1):e152–61.

68. Tisano B, Anigian K, Kantorek N, et al. The Insidious Effects of Childhood Obesity on Orthopedic Injuries and Deformities. Orthop Clin North Am 2022;53(4):461–72.

69. Fintini D, Cianfarani S, Cofini M, et al. The Bones of Children With Obesity. Front Endocrinol (Lausanne) 2020;11:200.

70. Emerenziani S, Guarino MPL, Trillo Asensio LM, et al. Role of Overweight and Obesity in Gastrointestinal Disease. Nutrients 2019;12(1). https://doi.org/10.3390/nu12010111.

71. Phatak UP, Pashankar DS. Obesity and gastrointestinal disorders in children. J Pediatr Gastroenterol Nutr 2015;60(4):441–5.

72. Yadlapati R, Pandolfino JE, Alexeeva O, et al. The Reflux Improvement and Monitoring (TRIM) Program Is Associated With Symptom Improvement and Weight Reduction for Patients With Obesity and Gastroesophageal Reflux Disease. Am J Gastroenterol 2018;113(1):23–30.

73. Stein DJ, El-Serag HB, Kuczynski J, et al. The association of body mass index with Barrett's oesophagus. Aliment Pharmacol Ther 2005;22(10):1005–10.

74. Tambucci R, Quitadamo P, Ambrosi M, et al. Association Between Obesity/Overweight and Functional Gastrointestinal Disorders in Children. J Pediatr Gastroenterol Nutr 2019;68(4):517–20.

75. Galai T, Moran-Lev H, Cohen S, et al. Higher prevalence of obesity among children with functional abdominal pain disorders. BMC Pediatr 2020;20(1):193.

76. Taylor SA, Himes R, Hastings E, et al. Gastrointestinal Conditions in the Obese Patient. Adolesc Med State Art Rev. Spring 2016;27(1):93–108.

77. Czepiel KS, Stanford FC. The Many Names of Fatty Liver Disease: Strengths and Limitations of Metabolic (Dysfunction)-Associated Fatty Liver Disease. Child Obes 2023;19(1):1–2.

78. Nassir F. NAFLD: Mechanisms, Treatments, and Biomarkers. Biomolecules 2022; 12(6). https://doi.org/10.3390/biom12060824.

79. Rothstein DH, Harmon CM. Gallbladder disease in children. Semin Pediatr Surg 2016;25(4):225–31.

80. Thavamani A, Umapathi KK, Roy A, et al. The increasing prevalence and adverse impact of morbid obesity in paediatric acute pancreatitis. Pediatr Obes 2020; 15(8):e12643. https://doi.org/10.1111/ijpo.12643.

81. Ferreira MS, Marson FAL, Wolf VLW, et al. Lung function in obese children and adolescents without respiratory disease: a systematic review. BMC Pulm Med 2020;20(1):281.
82. Forno E, Han YY, Mullen J, et al. Overweight, Obesity, and Lung Function in Children and Adults-A Meta-analysis. J Allergy Clin Immunol Pract Mar-Apr 2018; 6(2):570–81.e10.
83. Xanthopoulos M, Tapia IE. Obesity and common respiratory diseases in children. Paediatr Respir Rev 2017;23:68–71.
84. di Palmo E, Filice E, Cavallo A, et al. Childhood Obesity and Respiratory Diseases: Which Link? Children (Basel) 2021;8(3). https://doi.org/10.3390/children8030177.
85. Hay C, Henrickson SE. The impact of obesity on immune function in pediatric asthma. Curr Opin Allergy Clin Immunol 2021;21(2):202–15.
86. Vezir E, Civelek E, Dibek Misirlioglu E, et al. Effects of Obesity on Airway and Systemic Inflammation in Asthmatic Children. Int Arch Allergy Immunol 2021;182(8): 679–89.
87. Krajewska Wojciechowska J, Krajewski W, Zatoński T. The Association Between ENT Diseases and Obesity in Pediatric Population: A Systemic Review of Current Knowledge. Ear Nose Throat J 2019;98(5):E32–43.
88. Janoyer M. Blount disease. Orthop Traumatol Surg Res 2019 Feb;105(1S):S111–21. Epub 2018 Feb 23. PMID: 29481866. (29481866).
89. Perry DC, Metcalfe D, Lane S, et al. Childhood Obesity and Slipped Capital Femoral Epiphysis. Pediatrics 2018 Nov;142(5):e20181067. https://doi.org/10.1542/peds.2018-1067. Epub 2018 Oct 22. PMID: 30348751. (30348751).

Overview of BMI and Other Ways of Measuring and Screening for Obesity in Pediatric Patients

Charles Wood, MD, MPH[a],*, Amrik Singh Khalsa, MD, MSc[b]

KEYWORDS

- Body mass index • Screening • Adiposity • Measurement • Hydrodensitometry
- Air displacement plethysmography • MRI • Dual-energy x-ray absorptiometry

KEY POINTS

- Body mass index (BMI) has been as measure of adiposity for more than a century.
- While there are several other measures of adiposity, they have varying clinical usefulness and correlation to adipose tissue volume.
- No measure of adiposity assesses adipose tissue pathophysiology, thought to be a precursor to obesity-related comorbidities.
- BMI is strongly correlated to obesity-related co-morbidities.
- BMI is also a strong measure of adiposity in children less than 2 years.

HISTORY OF BODY MASS INDEX AND OTHER MEASURES OF ADIPOSITY

Although obesity has been observed in humankind for millennia, the attempt to quantify body size, specifically, weight independent of height, appears to have been initiated by Belgian scientist, Adophe Quetelet in the early 1830s.[1,2] Quetelet's goal was to better describe the periods of development; starting his quest with periods of pediatric growth, he cited the need to estimate a child's age with verifiable physical elements that could "substitute precise characters and exact data for conjectural estimates, which are always vague and often faulty."[3] So, Quetelet's investigation began

a Department of Pediatrics, Division of General Pediatrics and Adolescent Health, Duke Center for Childhood Obesity Research, Duke University School of Medicine, 3116 N. Duke Street, Durham, NC 27704, USA; b Division of Primary Care Pediatrics, Center for Child Health Equity and Outcomes Research, The Abigail Wexner Research Institute, Nationwide Children's Hospital, The Ohio State University College of Medicine, 700 Children's Drive, Columbus, OH 43205, USA
* Corresponding author. 3116 North Duke Street, Durham, NC 27704.
E-mail address: charles.wood@duke.edu

Pediatr Clin N Am 71 (2024) 781–796
https://doi.org/10.1016/j.pcl.2024.07.002
0031-3955/24/© 2024 Elsevier Inc. All rights reserved, including those for text and data mining, AI training, and similar technologies.

by analyzing weight and height data from various sources beginning at birth. Body mass index (BMI) is still occasionally referred to as "Quetelet's index," by his observation of "weight of developed persons, of different heights, is nearly as the square of the stature."[3] However, it is important to recognize that, in childhood, Quetelet found dynamic changes in how children grow until the age of 25. His observations suggested that there is not one suitable ratio that describes body size during the dynamic periods of growth, with weight and height increasing both proportionally and disproportionally, throughout childhood, even concluding that "during development, the squares of weight at different ages are as the fifth powers of height."[3] Recent investigations of different ratios of weight to height during pubertal changes suggest a simple number across child and adolescent development cannot capture body fat in an accurate manner.[4]

How could such a simplistic measure of body size become the most commonly used proxy for adiposity? Independent of its ease of use, Quetelet's 19th Century discovery of BMI has been repeatedly tested against other indices for its validity as a proxy of adiposity. Ancel Keys's study of over 7000 men across 5 countries, correlating skinfold thickness to body size indices showed BMI (a term he first coined in the article) was better than weight or height ratio or weight or height[3] (also known as ponderal index or tri-ponderal index).[5] Since then, BMI has been used most commonly to capture population variation among adults and track trends over time.[6,7] The individual connections between BMI and health are complex, and guidance has focused on BMI's rightful place as a screening tool and a priority for tracking population trends. Although BMI may be the best simple, non-invasive measure of adiposity, it has significant limitations in individual phenotypes or specific pathophysiology of obesity. As focus on the pathophysiology of obesity has intensified, many other measures of adiposity have emerged. The next section focuses on alternative measures to BMI and returns to discuss BMI's advantages and disadvantages as it persists as the proxy of choice for adiposity.

MEASURES OTHER THAN BODY MASS INDEX

Understanding the pathophysiology of excess adipose tissue changes the framing of the desire for BMI as a proxy. The goal is finding a proxy that best represents disease states and differentiates between states of health. Given this goal, several more direct measures of adiposity are available. Of note, most of these measures are used in research settings due to their high cost or lack of clinical feasibility. Importantly, none of these measures directly assesses the disease state of excess adiposity; further they cannot discriminate between normally functioning adipose tissue physiology from pathologic adipose tissue.

Available Measures of Adiposity

The measurement of adiposity has long been considered difficult in humans, especially children, given the various spaces that adipose tissue develops and deposits across the body.[8,9] Adipose tissue functions as energy storage, physical protection, and metabolic signaling, among other functions, complicating associations between structure and function, particularly in the developing child.[10,11] Measuring adiposity has been attempted for many centuries; however, most measures that have been developed to date still only function as a proxy for adipose volume, not function. Additionally, adipose tissue can be quantified with imaging, but the proportion quantified as adipose tissue does not represent total body fat, and these proportions vary with age and between genders.[12]

Measures of adiposity other than BMI are listed in **Table 1** and described as follows.

Research measures

Hydrodensitometer. Hydrodensitometry (HD), once the gold-standard for body composition assessment, is a measurement of weight underwater.[13] HD uses principles from Archimedes noting that higher fat-free mass will weigh more in water.[14,15] HD is fairly accurate; a major limitation is cost. In addition, the individual needs to be healthy, ambulatory, and able to follow very precise instructions, which limits its use in children. Second, formulae were created based on non-Hispanic white, male cadavers,[15] potentially misclassifying body composition in women and those from other races and ethnic groups.[8]

Air displacement plethysmography. Air displacement plethysmography (ADP), uses pressures and volume relationships to measure body density.[16–19] ADP was originally developed by measuring the density of inanimate objects. After recent technology allowed for the adjustment for body temperature and humidity in skin and hair,[20] several studies have shown good agreement between ADP and HD in certain populations but not in others.[19] While options exist for young infants,[21] ADP cannot be measured for most children between the ages of 6 months and 3 years.[22]

Doubly labeled water (isotope dilution methods). Isotope dilution uses a stable isotope deuterium oxide (^2H_2O) or oxygen-18 (^{18}O) labeled in water ($H_2[^{18}O]$) to measure energy expenditure. A small, concentrated dose of the isotope is administered and allowed to mix effectively with the total body water pool (~ 4 hours). The rise in isotopic concentration is measured (through expired carbon dioxide [CO_2] or excretion in the urine) which estimates total body water, from which fat-free mass is calculated.[23] This method has been validated in all ages and is accurate within 5%.[24] Isotopes are safe and provide an option for non-invasive measures of a child's total body water.[23] While it is a gold standard for body composition for children across the age range,[25–27] it is not often used as it requires proper sampling, dosing, and storage of the isotopes.

MRI. MRI uses magnetic fields to detect radiofrequency energy emitted by hydrogen atoms from the nuclei of cells to generate images of the target organ or tissue.[28] MRI creates a three-dimensional image, allowing for volumetric measurements of adipose tissue. It is highly accurate and reliable and can measure small changes over time, but use is limited in children due to sensitivity to movement and cost.[29]

Dual-energy X-ray absorptiometry. Dual-energy x-ray absorptiometry (DEXA), projects 2 beams of different energy x-rays through different body tissues to estimate the amount of density in tissues.[30] DEXA is highly correlated to MRI and computed tomography (CT) measures of adiposity ($r = 0.83 - 0.90$)[31] and is preferred given the ease of use, lower cost, and relatively lower dose of radiation than CT. A major limitation is that it does not discriminate between visceral and subcutaneous fat and overestimates fat mass when body dimensions, mostly in severe obesity, violate the assumption of independence from anteroposterior depth.[32]

Clinical measures

Waist circumference. Waist circumference (WC) is an individual's measure of their waist at the level of the umbilicus or top of the iliac crest and is the preferred method of measuring central obesity. WC is age- and sex- dependent and is highly correlated to BMI[33] and to cardiovascular disease risk and type 2 diabetes.[34] It is also better correlated with fat mass than BMI.[35] Limitations include a lack of consensus on

Table 1
Measures of adiposity and their characteristics

Measure	Brief Summary of How It Measures Adiposity	Strengths	Limitations	Age Limitation	Cost
Research Measures					
Hydrodensitometer	• Estimates fat-free and fat body densities through measurement of body weight when submerged underwater and compares to body weight in air	• Was previously considered gold standard for body composition • Fairly accurate	• Densitometry equations were developed from direct analysis of white cadavers and systematically underestimates relative fatness in other races and biologic sex[15]	8 y or older (due to compliance)	$$$$
Air Displacement Plethysmorgraphy (ADP)	• Uses pressure/volume relationships to estimate body density	• Several studies that support validity and reliability	• Validity testing shows ADP less accurate in younger children	Birth and older	$$$
Doubly Labeled Water (Isotope Dilution Methods)	• Uses stable isotopes (deuterium oxide (^2H_2O) or oxygen-18 (^{18}O) labeled in water (H2 [18O]) to estimate total body water (and thus fat mass)	• Also considered gold standard for measurement of body composition in children • Fairly accurate • Isotopes are safe for children all ages (including pre-term infants)	• Is fairly labor intensive • Often difficult to administer isotope solution orally in younger children	Birth and older	$$$
MRI	• Uses magnetic fields to detect radiofrequency energy emitted by hydrogen atoms from nuclei of cells	• Creates a 3-dimensional image from which volumetric measurements of adipose tissue can be taken • Highly accurate and reliable	• High-cost • Difficulty getting children to lay still (thus may require anesthesia for younger children)	Birth and older	$$$

	Description	Advantages	Disadvantages	Age Range	Cost
DEXA	• Uses x-ray beams of different energy levels to pass through different body tissues • Estimates amount of density in tissues transmitted in low vs high energy x-ray	• Highly correlated to MRI measures of adiposity • Easier to use compared to other research methods	• Limited availability • Uses radiation, which can have health sequelae	Birth and older (although used in older children given radiation)	$$
Clinical Measures					
Waist Circumference	• Measures individual waist at level of umbilicus or top of iliac crest	• Low cost • Ease of use • Favorable safety profile • Can assess all body shapes/sizes	• Cutoff points vary with sex and ethnic groups. • No consensus on the best anatomic location	Birth and older	$
Waist to Hip Ratio	• Ratio of waist circumference to hip ratio (widest part of the hips and buttocks) measured in the standing position	• Low cost • Ease of use • Favorable safety profile	• Measurements may be similar across body mass index (BMI) ranges due to changes in pelvic size • Unable to accurate measure change in distribution of adipose tissue	2 y and older	$
Skinfold Thickness	• Measure of thickness of 2 layers of subcutaneous fat pinched together • Common locations include bicep, tricep, subscapular, and suprailiac	• Low cost • Ease of use • Favorable safety profile • Can assess all body shapes/sizes	• Fairly uncomfortable for patient • Validation data in children is limited compared to adults • Requires considerable training to achieve reliable and accurate measurements • Does not quantify visceral adiposity	2 y and older	$

(continued on next page)

Table 1
(continued)

Measure	Brief Summary of How It Measures Adiposity	Strengths	Limitations	Age Limitation	Cost
Bioelectrical Impedance	• Uses low-voltage alternating current to measure total body water and estimate lean and fat body mass	• Relatively low cost • Safe, non-invasive • Portable • Rapid results • Less extensive operator training	• Estimation of fat mass based on hydration status • Prediction equations not validated in all ages, sexes, or race/ethnic groups	Birth and older	$$
Body Mass Index	• Is a ratio of weight to height squared	• Relative low-cost • Easy to measure and calculate • Several studies show correlation between BMI and future cardiovascular risk	• BMI oversimplifies differences in body composition • Not well-validated in non-White children	Children 2 y and older	$

Legend: Cost is estimated. Range represented by "$", ranging from $ - $$$$.

how to best measure waist circumference. Additionally, because of its dependence on age, sex, and height, there are no standards for WC values in children. Finally, it requires training to ensure accuracy, reliability, and measured in way that avoids stigma.

Waist-to-hip ratio. Waist-to-hip (WHR) uses the ratio of WC to hip circumference, measured as the widest part of the hips and buttocks while standing. WHR is correlated with intra-abdominal adipose tissue; however, its association to morbidity and mortality is inferior to WC and waist-to-height ratio.[36–39] WHR may be similar across BMI due to changes in pelvic size (especially in females) and changes in the distribution of adipose tissue and muscle mass, thus, it should be interpreted with caution.[9]

Skinfold thickness. Skinfold thickness is the measure of thickness of 2 layers of subcutaneous fat measured between a set of calipers.[9] It is often measured at the bicep or tricep of the mid-upper arm, the mid-upper thigh, or at the midpoint between the bottom rib and top of the iliac crest (suprailiac). Skinfold thickness is relatively inexpensive and has been well-correlated with body fat percentage in adults. Although used in children,[40] validation data for skinfold thickness is limited;[41–43] it is invasive, with potential for stigma, and considerable training is required.[44] It also lags when an individual losses weight.[9,45] Finally, it does not appear to improve on BMI in predicting cardiovascular risk[46–48]

Bioelectrical impedance. Bioelectrical impedance (BIA) induces an alternating current (<0.25 V) into the body and measures electrical differences in tissue water content.[9,49–51] Lean body mass and fat mass are estimated based on several assumptions including the hydration status of the individual. BIA may involve single or multiple frequency approaches and whole-body versus segmental approaches.

BIA has several advantages: it is relatively low cost, does not require extensive training, and is instantaneously measured.[52] BIA likely overestimates body fat percentage in individuals with higher BMI[53–55] and are more inaccurate in children since current prediction equations have been developed from previous population studies.[56]

Body Mass Index

Given the complexity of the measures detailed mentioned earlier, it is understandable that a simple measure using just weight and height has attracted criticism as an oversimplification. In fact, there is considerable discussion about improving measures that are associated with health outcomes,[57] understanding more about the heterogeneity of obesity,[1] and acknowledging that BMI alone will not measure body fat nor disease risk on an individual basis. Further, none of these measures assesses physiologic function, an important factor in disease that is partially independent of volume of adipose tissue.[58–60] The American Medical Association recently passed a resolution discouraging the use of BMI alone to make medical decisions and encouraging the use of BMI "in conjunction with other valid measures of risk."[61]

Echoing the historic lack of representation, the source data with which BMI-for-age assessment is categorized will not reflect every population, and similar to many sources of pediatric health data, it tends to overemphasize white children from families with fewer resource and education limitations. Moreover, BMI oversimplifies population-specific differences in visceral fat, fat-free masses, and adipose pathophysiologies that may lead to very different health outcomes. For example, the World Health Organization (WHO) has acknowledged that Asian populations have higher risk of metabolic and cardiovascular disease at lower BMI thresholds compared to European populations.[62] Indeed, attempts have been made to refine BMI cutoffs for adults across sex, race, and ethnicity categories that better reflect risk for comorbidities such as hypertension, dyslipidemia, and diabetes.[63] Acknowledging these differences in BMI are important for pediatric care given the persistence of elevated childhood BMI into adulthood.[64–66]

The ability of BMI to reflect adiposity during childhood varies by age,[67] degree of BMI,[46] and by race and ethnicity.[68] Comparing BMI to total and percent fat mass with DEXA, BMI Z-score appears to be an excellent predictor of total fat mass in children over the age of 9, but may not predict fat mass as well under the age of 9.[67] Others looking at populations with a lower mean BMI have shown that BMI is well-correlated with total and percent fat mass in children as young as 5.[69] BMI is a worse predictor of adiposity as the degree of adiposity decreases. Especially among children with a BMI under the 85% for age, Freedman found that the sensitivity of BMI as a measure of fat mass decreases as BMI-for-age becomes lower. Particularly for children with a BMI less than 85% for age and sex, differences in BMI are more likely to be attributed to differences in fat free mass. This can be contrasted with the 70% to 80% sensitivity of BMI for adiposity in children with obesity as defined as a BMI over the 95% for age.[46]

Similar to differences seen in racial and ethnic groups in adults, BMI tends to slightly overestimate adiposity among black children and slightly underestimate adiposity among Asian children. Given a similar level of BMI-for-age, black children had approximately 3% less body fat as measured by DEXA and Asian children had 1% more body fat. These differences highlight the limitations of equating BMI with adiposity at an individual level, and suggest that BMI cutoffs for the overall population may not be suited for specific risk stratification.

A meta-analysis of the diagnostic validity of BMI for obesity in children aged between 4- and 18-years tested against an array of reference standards including skinfold thickness, BIA, DEXA, ADP, and HW, showed a pooled sensitivity of 73% and specificity of 93%.[70]

BODY MASS INDEX SCREENING

In pediatric populations, rapid changes in the development of adipose tissue in the first years of life create both a peak in adiposity during infancy and a nadir during early childhood, around the time of school entry. The corresponding peak and trough of BMI during this time, and additional rapid changes in adipose physiology during puberty, mean BMI does not increase monotonically. Public health agencies and clinical societies recommend using sex- and age-specific BMI percentiles. These BMI-for-age percentiles have been a linchpin of pediatric routine care. Screening for obesity is a Grade B recommendation from the United States (US) Preventive Services Task Force starting at age 6 years[71] and recommended by the American Academy of Pediatrics starting at age 2 years.[72]

Screening for obesity and obesity related comorbidities are a recommended part of routine preventive care for children.[72] Data from children growing prior to the increase in obesity prevalence several decades ago provides the nationally-representative growth references developed by the Centers for Disease Control and prevention (CDC).[73] These clinical growth charts represent age- and sex-specific distributions of BMI among children in the US without any specific exclusion. Data were collected through multiple waves of the National Health and Nutrition Examination Survey (NHANES) and were smoothed to create curves for practical clinical use. Given the significant rightward shift in BMI distribution since these data were collected (ie, BMIs have increased), limited data were available at the upper end of the BMI distribution, and the reliability of plotting BMI above the 97th percentile has been challenged.[74] Given this limitation, additional metrics to assess and monitor BMI status have been suggested and include: BMI Z-scores; percent above the 95th percentile; and both sex- and age-adjusted and unadjusted BMI units or percent from the median.[73] Importantly, additional data from 8777 children with BMI above the 95th percentile measured in 1999 to 2016 waves of NHANES were used to develop "extended" BMI-for-age percentile and Z-score reference curves that replaced previous curves based on statistical extrapolation. These curves, newly published at the end of 2022, should be most helpful in distinguishing changes in BMI Z-score over time and provide the ability to track percentiles and Z-scores continuously across the BMI distribution.

According to survey data, under 20% of pediatric clinicians used BMI charts for routine monitoring in the early 2000s,[75] yet BMI charts are better than separate height and weight charts for flagging obesity risk.[76] This percentage of providers who use BMI charts increased in the last 2 decades alongside the implementation of electronic health records, which hold promise to improve the routine screening and diagnosis of obesity.[77,78] Enhancements to the display of BMI that address low health literacy and numeracy and engage caregivers have been shown to improve understanding.[79] One specific adaptation of the BMI reference into a poster used in clinic examination rooms increased dialogue between caregivers and clinicians and improved caregivers understanding of BMI and healthy behaviors when tested in a randomized trial (**Fig. 1**).[80]

CONSIDERATIONS IN CHILDREN UNDER 2 YEARS OF AGE

Risk for obesity and comorbidities accumulates before the age of 2, prompting a desire to use BMI or other similar measures to provide an ability to stratify risk prior to toddlerhood.[81,82] Body composition measurement in infants has also been advancing.[21,83,84] Diagnostic validity studies comparing BMI, weight-for-length (WFL), and more direct measures of adiposity suggest that BMI performs well.[85,86] BMI has a stronger association than WFL with fat mass and percent fat mass in infants measured with ADP.[85] BMI during infancy also has a high sensitivity and specificity for predicting childhood obesity. Infants with a BMI and WFL greater than or equal to 85th percentile in the first 18 months of life have a 3-fold increased risk of being obese by age 6.[86] Both the timing and magnitude of BMI during its physiologic peak during infancy has been shown to predict obesity after age 2.[87–89]

Despite the ability of BMI to better predict fat mass than WFL, the CDC continues to promote the use of WFL as a screening tool in children less than 2 years of age. Ongoing epidemiologic surveillance reports "high WFL," and defines this as a WFL greater than the 97.7% of the WHO growth standards for age and sex.[90] There are substantial methodologic differences precluding direct comparison of BMI by WHO growth standards before age 2 years to BMI-for-age references used after age 2 years. Most importantly, while neither source data are planned for update, the NHANES-based CDC data represent the distribution of weight, length, and BMI among infants and children during specific "pre-epidemic" decades in the US. The WHO methodologies aimed to exclude restrictions on normal physiologic growth to create a globally-representative sample of ideal growth. With this goal, the WHO methodology excludes infants born prior to 37 weeks gestational age, includes only breastfed infants, and excludes infants born to mothers with significant comorbidities, who smoked, or who lived in socioeconomic settings that might limit the healthy growth potential of their children. Additional methodologic distinctions are highlighted in a report by the CDC that also notes the availability, but discourages the use, of BMI under the age of 2 years.[91]

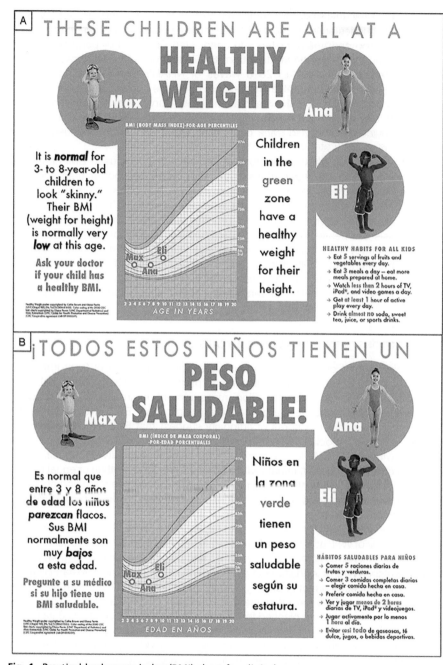

Fig. 1. Practical body mass index (BMI) chart for clinical use.

Advances Beyond Body Mass Index

The use of BMI as a screening tool has become pervasive in primary care and public health settings, and many studies have shown an association between BMI and intermediate markers of disease,[92] morbidity, and mortality.[93,94] Clinical decision support tools can improve uptake of BMI screening and linking BMI to efficient screening for comorbidities. Still, use of a given BMI in 1 individual at 1 time may not provide the information necessary to appropriately assess pathophysiology. Fortunately, there is still active and creative dialogue around the usefulness and simplicity of BMI as a proxy for body size and adiposity.[1] Although adjusting BMI based on race, ethnicity, sex, and height has been utilized,[63,73,95] newer technologies to measure body shape,[96] personalized indices,[97] and serum biomarkers of adipose pathology[98] may emerge. With advances in computer power and diagnostics, we are likely to encounter better, more personalized measures to screen for obesity in the 21st Century. While BMI remains an accurate, clinically-relevant measure, we should continue to understand the possible pitfalls of using 1 measure and the value of patient-reported outcomes related to its proper and improper use in the care of children.

CLINICS CARE POINTS

- Knowing that health care providers and health care settings are contributors to weight stigma, measurements should be performed in a way that minimizes weight stigma and centers the patient.
- BMI remains the most accurate and clinically-feasible proxy measure for adiposity.
- Routine measurement of BMI is recommended, but individualized discussion of limitations to BMI is encouraged.

DISCLOSURE

The Authors have nothing to disclose.

REFERENCES

1. Bray GA. Beyond BMI. Nutrients 2023;15(10). https://doi.org/10.3390/nu15102254.
2. Eknoyan G. Adolphe Quetelet (1796–1874)—the average man and indices of obesity. Nephrol Dial Transplant 2007;23(1):47–51.
3. Quetelet L-A-J. A Treatise on Man and the Development of His Faculties. Obes Res 1994;2(1):72–85.
4. Peterson CM, Su H, Thomas DM, et al. Tri-Ponderal Mass Index vs Body Mass Index in Estimating Body Fat During Adolescence. JAMA Pediatr 2017;171(7):629–36.
5. Keys A, Fidanza F, Karvonen MJ, et al. Indices of relative weight and obesity. J Chronic Dis 1972;25(6):329–43.
6. Whitlock G, Lewington S, Sherliker P, et al. Body-mass index and cause-specific mortality in 900 000 adults: collaborative analyses of 57 prospective studies. Lancet 2009;373(9669):1083–96.
7. Bray GA. In defense of a body mass index of 25 as the cut-off point for defining overweight. Obes Res 1998;6(6):461–2.
8. Heyward VH. Evaluation of body composition. Current issues. Sports Med 1996;22(3):146–56.
9. Horan M, Gibney E, Molloy E, et al. Methodologies to assess paediatric adiposity. Ir J Med Sci 2015;184(1):53–68.
10. Fischer-Posovszky P, Roos J, Zoller V, et al. In: White Adipose Tissue Development and Function in Children and Adolescents: Preclinical Models, In: Freemark

M.S., Pediatric obesity: etiology, pathogenesis and treatment. Cham: Humana Press; 2018. p. 81–93. https://doi.org/10.1007/978-3-319-68192-4_5.

11. Frayn KN, Karpe F, Fielding BA, et al. Integrative physiology of human adipose tissue. Int J Obes Relat Metab Disord 2003;27(8):875–88.

12. Tanamas SK, Lean MEJ, Combet E, et al. Changing guards: time to move beyond body mass index for population monitoring of excess adiposity. QJM 2016; 109(7):443–6.

13. Lohman T, Milliken LA, Medicine AcoS. ACSM's body composition assessment. Champaign, IL: Human Kinetics; 2019.

14. Brozek J, Grande F, Anderson JT, et al. DENSITOMETRIC ANALYSIS OF BODY COMPOSITION: REVISION OF SOME QUANTITATIVE ASSUMPTIONS. Ann N Y Acad Sci 1963;110:113–40.

15. Siri WE. The gross composition of the body. Adv Biol Med Phys 1956;4:239–80.

16. Gnaedinger RH, Reineke EP, Pearson AM, et al. DETERMINATION OF BODY DENSITY BY AIR DISPLACEMENT, HELIUM DILUTION, AND UNDERWATER WEIGHING. Ann N Y Acad Sci 1963;110:96–108.

17. Taylor A, Aksoy Y, Scopes JW, et al. Development of an air displacement method for whole body volume measurement of infants. J Biomed Eng 1985;7(1):9–17.

18. Fomon SJ, Jensen RL, Owen GM. DETERMINATION OF BODY VOLUME OF IN-FANTS BY A METHOD OF HELIUM DISPLACEMENT. Ann N Y Acad Sci 1963; 110:80–90.

19. Demerath EW, Guo SS, Chumlea WC, et al. Comparison of percent body fat es-timates using air displacement plethysmography and hydrodensitometry in adults and children. Int J Obes Relat Metab Disord 2002;26(3):389–97.

20. Dempster P, Aitkens S. A new air displacement method for the determination of human body composition. Med Sci Sports Exerc 1995;27(12):1692–7.

21. Demerath EW, Fields DA. Body composition assessment in the infant. Am J Hum Biol 2014;26(3):291–304.

22. Gallagher D, Andres A, Fields DA, et al. Body Composition Measurements from Birth through 5 Years: Challenges, Gaps, and Existing & Emerging Technologies-A National Institutes of Health workshop. Obes Rev 2020;21(8):e13033.

23. Zemel BS. Body composition during growth and development. Human growth and development 2022;517–45.

24. Schoeller DA, Fjeld CR. Human energy metabolism: what have we learned from the doubly labeled water method? Annu Rev Nutr 1991;11:355–73.

25. International Atomic Energy Agency. Introduction to body composition assess-ment using the deuterium dilution technique with analysis of urine samples by isotope ratio mass spectrometry. Vienna: INTERNATIONAL ATOMIC ENERGY AGENCY; 2010.

26. International Atomic Energy Agency. Body composition assessment from birth to two years of age. Vienna: INTERNATIONAL ATOMIC ENERGY AGENCY; 2013.

27. Yumani DFJ, de Jongh D, Ket JCF, et al. Body composition in preterm infants: a systematic review on measurement methods. Pediatr Res 2023;93(5):1120–40.

28. Alcantara JMA, Idoate F, Labayen I. Medical imaging in the assessment of car-diovascular disease risk. Curr Opin Clin Nutr Metab Care 2023;26(5):440–6.

29. Cadenas-Sanchez C, Idoate F, Cabeza R, et al. Effect of a Multicomponent Inter-vention on Hepatic Steatosis Is Partially Mediated by the Reduction of Intermus-cular Abdominal Adipose Tissue in Children With Overweight or Obesity: The EFIGRO Project. Diabetes Care 2022;45(9):1953–60.

30. Cullum ID, Ell PJ, Ryder JP. X-ray dual-photon absorptiometry: a new method for the measurement of bone density. Br J Radiol 1989;62(739):587–92.

31. Kohrt WM. Preliminary evidence that DEXA provides an accurate assessment of body composition. J Appl Physiol 1998;84(1):372–7.

32. Laskey MA, Lyttle KD, Flaxman ME, et al. The influence of tissue depth and composition on the performance of the Lunar dual-energy X-ray absorptiometer whole-body scanning mode. Eur J Clin Nutr 1992;46(1):39–45.

33. Glässer N, Zellner K, Kromeyer-Hauschild K. Validity of body mass index and waist circumference to detect excess fat mass in children aged 7-14 years. Eur J Clin Nutr 2011;65(2):151–9.

34. Balkau B, Deanfield JE, Després JP, et al. International Day for the Evaluation of Abdominal Obesity (IDEA): a study of waist circumference, cardiovascular disease, and diabetes mellitus in 168,000 primary care patients in 63 countries. Circulation 2007;116(17):1942–51.

35. Agbaje AO. Waist-circumference-to-height-ratio had better longitudinal agreement with DEXA-measured fat mass than BMI in 7237 children. Pediatr Res 2024. https://doi.org/10.1038/s41390-024-03112-8.

36. de Ridder CM, de Boer RW, Seidell JC, et al. Body fat distribution in pubertal girls quantified by magnetic resonance imaging. Int J Obes Relat Metab Disord 1992; 16(6):443–9.

37. Fredriks AM, van Buuren S, Fekkes M, et al. Are age references for waist circumference, hip circumference and waist-hip ratio in Dutch children useful in clinical practice? Eur J Pediatr 2005;164(4):216–22.

38. Neovius M, Linné Y, Rossner S. BMI, waist-circumference and waist-hip-ratio as diagnostic tests for fatness in adolescents. Int J Obes 2005;29(2):163–9.

39. Taylor RW, Jones IE, Williams SM, et al. Evaluation of waist circumference, waist-to-hip ratio, and the conicity index as screening tools for high trunk fat mass, as measured by dual-energy X-ray absorptiometry, in children aged 3-19 y. Am J Clin Nutr 2000;72(2):490–5.

40. Bray GA, DeLany JP, Volaufova J, et al. Prediction of body fat in 12-y-old African American and white children: evaluation of methods. Am J Clin Nutr 2002;76(5): 980–90.

41. Reilly JJ, Wilson J, Durnin JV. Determination of body composition from skinfold thickness: a validation study. Arch Dis Child 1995;73(4):305–10.

42. Moreno LA, Fleta J, Mur L, et al. Indices of body fat distribution in Spanish children aged 4.0 to 14.9 years. J Pediatr Gastroenterol Nutr 1997;25(2):175–81.

43. Moreno LA, Rodríguez G, Guillén J, et al. Anthropometric measurements in both sides of the body in the assessment of nutritional status in prepubertal children. Eur J Clin Nutr 2002;56(12):1208–15.

44. Oppliger RA, Clark RR, Kuta JM. Efficacy of skinfold training clinics: a comparison between clinic trained and experienced testers. Res Q Exerc Sport 1992; 63(4):438–43.

45. Caprio S, Hyman LD, McCarthy S, et al. Fat distribution and cardiovascular risk factors in obese adolescent girls: importance of the intraabdominal fat depot. Am J Clin Nutr 1996;64(1):12–7.

46. Freedman DS, Sherry B. The validity of BMI as an indicator of body fatness and risk among children. Pediatrics 2009;124(Suppl 1):S23–34.

47. Steinberger J, Jacobs DR, Raatz S, et al. Comparison of body fatness measurements by BMI and skinfolds vs dual energy X-ray absorptiometry and their relation to cardiovascular risk factors in adolescents. Int J Obes 2005;29(11): 1346–52.

48. Geiss HC, Parhofer KG, Schwandt P. Parameters of childhood obesity and their relationship to cardiovascular risk factors in healthy prepubescent children. Int J Obes Relat Metab Disord 2001;25(6):830–7.

49. Boulier A, Fricker J, Thomasset AL, et al. Fat-free mass estimation by the two-electrode impedance method. Am J Clin Nutr 1990;52(4):581–5.

50. Lukaski HC, Bolonchuk WW. Estimation of body fluid volumes using tetrapolar bioelectrical impedance measurements. Aviat Space Environ Med 1988;59(12):1163–9.

51. Lukaski HC, Johnson PE, Bolonchuk WW, et al. Assessment of fat-free mass using bioelectrical impedance measurements of the human body. Am J Clin Nutr 1985;41(4):810–7.

52. Lyons-Reid J, Derraik JGB, Ward LC, et al. Bioelectrical impedance analysis for assessment of body composition in infants and young children-A systematic literature review. Clin Obes 2021;11(3):e12441.

53. Shafer KJ, Siders WA, Johnson LK, et al. Validity of segmental multiple-frequency bioelectrical impedance analysis to estimate body composition of adults across a range of body mass indexes. Nutrition 2009;25(1):25–32.

54. Talma H, Chinapaw MJ, Bakker B, et al. Bioelectrical impedance analysis to estimate body composition in children and adolescents: a systematic review and evidence appraisal of validity, responsiveness, reliability and measurement error. Obes Rev 2013;14(11):895–905.

55. De Beer M, Timmers T, Weijs PJ, et al. Validation of total body water analysis by bioelectrical impedance analysis with deuterium dilution in (pre) school children. E Spen Eur E J Clin Nutr Metab. 2011;6(5):e223–6.

56. Kyle UG, Bosaeus I, De Lorenzo AD, et al. Bioelectrical impedance analysis–part I: review of principles and methods. Clin Nutr 2004;23(5):1226–43.

57. Watanabe K, Wilmanski T, Diener C, et al. Multiomic signatures of body mass index identify heterogeneous health phenotypes and responses to a lifestyle intervention. Nat Med 2023;29(4):996–1008.

58. Chait A, den Hartigh LJ. Adipose Tissue Distribution, Inflammation and Its Metabolic Consequences, Including Diabetes and Cardiovascular Disease. Front Cardiovasc Med 2020;7:22.

59. Choe SS, Huh JY, Hwang IJ, et al. Adipose Tissue Remodeling: Its Role in Energy Metabolism and Metabolic Disorders. Front Endocrinol 2016;7:30.

60. Saxton SN, Clark BJ, Withers SB, et al. Mechanistic Links Between Obesity, Diabetes, and Blood Pressure: Role of Perivascular Adipose Tissue. Physiol Rev 2019;99(4):1701–63.

61. Association AM. AMA adopts new policy clarifying role of BMI as a measure in medicine. Available at: https://www.ama-assn.org/press-center/press-releases/ama-adopts-new-policy-clarifying-role-bmi-measure-medicine. [Accessed 8 February 2024].

62. Barba C, Cavalli-Sforza T, Cutter J, et al. Appropriate body-mass index for Asian populations and its implications for policy and intervention strategies. Lancet 2004;363(9403):157–63.

63. Stanford FC, Lee M, Hur C. Race, Ethnicity, Sex, and Obesity: Is It Time to Personalize the Scale? Mayo Clin Proc 2019;94(2):362–3.

64. Simmonds M, Llewellyn A, Owen CG, et al. Predicting adult obesity from childhood obesity: a systematic review and meta-analysis. Obes Rev 2016;17(2):95–107.

65. Singh AS, Mulder C, Twisk JW, et al. Tracking of childhood overweight into adulthood: a systematic review of the literature. Obes Rev 2008;9(5):474–88.

66. Whitaker RC, Wright JA, Pepe MS, et al. Predicting obesity in young adulthood from childhood and parental obesity. N Engl J Med 1997;337(13):869–73.
67. Vanderwall C, Randall Clark R, Eickhoff J, et al. BMI is a poor predictor of adiposity in young overweight and obese children. BMC Pediatr 2017;17(1):135.
68. Freedman DS, Wang J, Thornton JC, et al. Racial/ethnic differences in body fatness among children and adolescents. Obesity 2008;16(5):1105–11.
69. Pietrobelli A, Faith MS, Allison DB, et al. Body mass index as a measure of adiposity among children and adolescents: a validation study. J Pediatr 1998; 132(2):204–10.
70. Javed A, Jumean M, Murad MH, et al. Diagnostic performance of body mass index to identify obesity as defined by body adiposity in children and adolescents: a systematic review and meta-analysis. Pediatr Obes 2015;10(3):234–44.
71. O'Connor EA, Evans CV, Burda BU, et al. Screening for Obesity and Intervention for Weight Management in Children and Adolescents: Evidence Report and Systematic Review for the US Preventive Services Task Force. JAMA 2017;317(23): 2427–44.
72. Hampl SE, Hassink SG, Skinner AC, et al. Clinical Practice Guideline for the Evaluation and Treatment of Children and Adolescents With Obesity. Pediatrics 2023;(2):151.
73. Hales CM, Freedman DS, Akinbami L, et al. Evaluation of Alternative Body Mass Index (BMI) Metrics to Monitor Weight Status in Children and Adolescents With Extremely High BMI Using CDC BMI-for-age Growth Charts. Vital Health Stat 2022;197:1–42.
74. Woo JG. Using body mass index Z-score among severely obese adolescents: a cautionary note. Int J Pediatr Obes 2009;4(4):405–10.
75. Barlow SE, Dietz WH, Klish WJ, et al. Medical Evaluation of Overweight Children and Adolescents: Reports From Pediatricians, Pediatric Nurse Practitioners, and Registered Dietitians. Pediatrics 2002;110(Supplement_1):222–8.
76. Perrin EM, Flower KB, Ammerman AS. Body mass index charts: useful yet underused. J Pediatr 2004;144(4):455–60.
77. Baer HJ, Cho I, Walmer RA, et al. Using Electronic Health Records to Address Overweight and Obesity A Systematic Review. Review. Am J Prev Med 2013; 45(4):494–500.
78. Wethington HR, Sherry B, Polhamus B. Physician practices related to use of BMI-for-age and counseling for childhood obesity prevention: A cross-sectional study. Article. BMC Fam Pract 2011;12(9):80.
79. Oettinger MD, Finkle JP, Esserman D, et al. Color-coding improves parental understanding of body mass index charting. Acad Pediatr 2009;9(5):330–8.
80. Brown CL, Howard JB, Perrin EM. A randomized controlled trial examining an exam room poster to prompt communication about weight. Pediatr Obes 2020; 15(7):e12625.
81. Lumeng JC, Taveras EM, Birch L, et al. Prevention of obesity in infancy and early childhood: a National Institutes of Health workshop. JAMA Pediatr 2015;169(5): 484–90.
82. Woo JG, Daniels SR. Assessment of Body Mass Index in Infancy: It Is Time to Revise Our Guidelines. J Pediatr 2019;204:10–1.
83. Jerome ML, Valcarce V, Lach L, et al. Infant body composition: A comprehensive overview of assessment techniques, nutrition factors, and health outcomes. Nutr Clin Pract 2023;38(Suppl 2):S7–s27.
84. Butte NF, Hopkinson JM, Wong WW, et al. Body composition during the first 2 years of life: an updated reference. Pediatr Res 2000;47(5):578–85.

85. Roy SM, Fields DA, Mitchell JA, et al. Body Mass Index Is a Better Indicator of Body Composition than Weight-for-Length at Age 1 Month. J Pediatr 2019;204: 77–83.e1.

86. Smego A, Woo JG, Klein J, et al. High Body Mass Index in Infancy May Predict Severe Obesity in Early Childhood. J Pediatr 2017;183:87–93 e1.

87. Aris IM, Rifas-Shiman SL, Li LJ, et al. Pre-, Perinatal, and Parental Predictors of Body Mass Index Trajectory Milestones. J Pediatr 2018;201:69–77.e8.

88. Roy SM, Chesi A, Mentch F, et al. Body mass index (BMI) trajectories in infancy differ by population ancestry and may presage disparities in early childhood obesity. J Clin Endocrinol Metab 2015;100(4):1551–60.

89. Wood CT, Truong T, Skinner AC, et al. Timing and Magnitude of Peak Body Mass Index and Peak Weight Velocity in Infancy Predict Body Mass Index at 2 Years in a Retrospective Cohort of Electronic Health Record Data. J Pediatr 2023;257: 113356.

90. Ogden CL, Fryar CD, Martin CB, et al. Trends in Obesity Prevalence by Race and Hispanic Origin-1999-2000 to 2017-2018. JAMA 2020;324(12):1208–10.

91. Grummer-Strawn LM, Reinold C, Krebs NF. Use of World Health Organization and CDC growth charts for children aged 0-59 months in the United States. MMWR Recomm Rep (Morb Mortal Wkly Rep) 2010;59(Rr-9):1–15.

92. Skinner AC, Perrin EM, Moss LA, et al. Cardiometabolic Risks and Severity of Obesity in Children and Young Adults. N Engl J Med 2015;373(14):1307–17.

93. Twig G, Yaniv G, Levine H, et al. Body-Mass Index in 2.3 Million Adolescents and Cardiovascular Death in Adulthood. Article. N Engl J Med 2016;374(25):2430–40.

94. Horesh A, Tsur AM, Bardugo A, et al. Adolescent and Childhood Obesity and Excess Morbidity and Mortality in Young Adulthood-a Systematic Review. Current obesity reports 2021;10(3):301–10.

95. Heymsfield SB, Peterson CM, Thomas DM, et al. Why are there race/ethnic differences in adult body mass index-adiposity relationships? A quantitative critical review. Obes Rev 2016;17(3):262–75.

96. Ashby N, Jake LaPorte G, Richardson D, et al. Translating digital anthropometry measurements obtained from different 3D body image scanners. Eur J Clin Nutr 2023;77(9):872–80.

97. Trefethen N. BMI (Body Mass Index). Available at: https://people.maths.ox.ac.uk/trefethen/bmi.html. [Accessed 14 February 2024]

98. Tans R, van Diepen JA, Bijlsma S, et al. Evaluation of chitotriosidase as a biomarker for adipose tissue inflammation in overweight individuals and type 2 diabetic patients. Int J Obes 2019/09/01 2019;43(9):1712–23.

Promoting Healthy Eating and Activity from the Start

Early Obesity Prevention

Kori B. Flower, MD, MS, MPH[a],*, Jessica Hart, MD[a],
Heather Wright Williams, MD[a], Rebecca Chasnovitz, MD[a]

KEYWORDS

• Obesity • Prevention • Infancy • Weight gain

KEY POINTS

• Excess weight gain can begin in infancy and is associated with avoidable long-term health problems.
• Pediatric clinicians can intervene during frequent well visits in infancy to promote healthy weight gain.
• Counseling in primary care settings can focus on known risk factors including lack of breastfeeding, large bottle size, early introduction of solid foods, juice and sugar-sweetened beverages, screen time, lack of active time, and insufficient sleep.

BACKGROUND
The Role of Office-Based Individual Counseling in Early Obesity Prevention

A healthy start to early childhood eating and activity patterns is shaped by factors at multiple levels, including household composition and culture, childcare and early education settings, and neighborhood and community opportunities. These factors, in turn, are influenced by local, state, and federal programs and policies that impact families' economic circumstances and opportunities for healthy eating and activity. Acknowledging the importance of these contextual and societal influences, pediatric clinicians have important opportunities with individual families to promote healthy eating and activity from the start. Frequent well child visits in early childhood provide pediatric clinicians with multiple time points for counseling about early eating and activity. Further, children's caregivers frequently bring questions about growth, nutrition, and physical activity to pediatric clinicians. This article describes how

[a] General Pediatrics and Adolescent Medicine, University of North Carolina at Chapel Hill, 231 MacNider CB 7220, Chapel Hill, NC 27599, USA
* Corresponding author. University of North Carolina at Chapel Hill, 231 MacNider CB 7220, Chapel Hill, NC 27599.
E-mail address: kflower@unc.edu

Pediatr Clin N Am 71 (2024) 797–804
https://doi.org/10.1016/j.pcl.2024.06.002   **pediatric.theclinics.com**

individual-level counseling on healthful eating and physical activity can make the most of pediatric clinicians' frequent contact and relationships with families in the early childhood years.

Prevention Begins Prenatally

Ideally, obesity prevention begins before birth. During pregnancy, the in utero environment affects future risk for diseases including hypertension,[1] obesity,[2] and diabetes.[3,4] Healthy weight gain during pregnancy is highly beneficial, as this impacts both maternal health and infant birthweight, which then affect long-term cardiovascular disease risk. For example, maternal weight gain can increase the risk of infants being either small or large for gestational age, which increases the long-term risk of cardiovascular disease.[5] Infants of mothers with gestational diabetes have an increased risk of obesity in childhood and long-term higher risk of cardiovascular disease.[6] Healthy nutrition during pregnancy is, therefore, essential to prevent transgenerational cycles of obesity and cardiovascular disease.

Importance of Prevention in Early Childhood

Preventing unhealthy weight gain early is important because early childhood weight is predictive of weight later in childhood, adolescence, and even adulthood.[5,7–9] Rapid weight gain in infancy has been defined as crossing at least one percentile line on standard growth charts, which typically depict percentile lines at the 2nd, 10th, 25th, 50th, 75th, 90th, and 98th percentiles, and equates to a change in weight standard deviation score greater than 0.67.[10] Importantly, rapid weight gain in infancy is associated with later obesity.[2,10,11] Therefore, limiting rapid weight gain in infancy can help to prevent later obesity. In infancy, parents and other caregivers play a central role in shaping the feeding and activity behaviors that influence weight gain. Engaging parents and other caregivers in family-centered approaches is critical in early childhood.[12–15] Studies show that behavior changes that engage parents are among the most effective.[14,15]

Preventing Early Rapid Weight Gain

Since preventing early rapid weight gain in infancy can reduce the later risk of obesity and its sequelae, it is important to address eating and activity behaviors that are modifiable and can contribute to excess weight gain. Modifiable factors are shown in **Box 1**, and actions that can be taken to address them are described in later section. Research has demonstrated that these high-risk behaviors for obesity are frequently present by 2 months of age; therefore, early counseling is essential.[16]

Box 1
Risk behaviors for early rapid weight gain

Lack of exclusive breastfeeding

Bottle feeding and bottle size

Solid food introduction before age 4 months

Drinking sugar-sweetened beverages

Screen time

Sleep

DISCUSSION: PROMOTING HEALTHY BEHAVIORS AND PREVENTING EARLY OBESITY IN THE OFFICE SETTING

The following sections review the evidence for modifiable behaviors and steps that can be taken to reduce early obesity risk in pediatric primary care office settings:

Breastfeeding

Exclusive breastfeeding has many benefits, including protective effects against childhood obesity, and should be recommended through 6 months of age.[17,18] Pediatric clinicians play a key role in providing support to mother–infant dyads establishing breastfeeding. Education regarding the benefits of exclusive breastfeeding should begin at first contact with the family, either at prenatal visits or in the newborn nursery, and continue in the outpatient setting. Recommendations for encouraging exclusive breastfeeding include:

- Emphasizing the importance of skin-to-skin contact, breastfeeding within the first hour after birth, and rooming in during the baby's nursery stay.[19]
- Lactation consultant support in the hospital and embedded in the pediatric clinic.[19] If needed, but unavailable in the clinic, the clinician should assist with referring the family to a lactation consultant and take steps to make this as convenient and timely as possible.
- Recommending the use of formula supplementation only when medically necessary.[19]
- Advocacy efforts to create societal changes that will continue to normalize breast milk as the ideal infant nutrition.[20]

Bottle Feeding

Exclusive breastfeeding may not always be possible, and some families may choose to provide their infants with nutrition through formula. Additionally, even those infants receiving exclusive breastmilk may sometimes be fed from a bottle. The use of large bottle sizes (>6 oz/180 ml) has been associated with increased formula intake and excessive weight gain during infancy,[21,22] both of which are risk factors for childhood obesity.[23] Therefore, in these instances, clinicians should counsel families regarding responsive feeding practices and the use of appropriate bottle size, including discouraging the use of large bottles throughout infancy.

Introduction of Solid Foods

Anticipatory guidance during infant preventive care visits should include counseling regarding recommended practices around solid food introduction. Early introduction (before 4 months old) of solids has been associated with rapid weight gain in the first year of life[21] and with later overweight and obesity.[17] This includes introducing solids such as rice cereal through the bottle, which parents sometimes do as early as 2 months of age.[16] Therefore, infants should receive exclusive breastmilk and/or formula until 6 months of age,[24] at minimum postponing all solids, including rice cereal in the bottle, until the 4 month mark.[21] Upon introduction of solids, it should be emphasized that breastmilk or formula remains the main source of nutrition for infants until around 12 months of age. No specific volume of solids daily is needed or required, and parents should be educated regarding infants' hunger cues at mealtimes.

Sugar-Sweetened Beverages

Consumption of fruit juice has been associated with an increase in body mass index (BMI) in children.[25] Fruit juice and other sugar sweetened beverages are high in sugar content and low in fiber and protein, which can lead to the intake of excess calories without the feeling of satiety.[25,26] Unfortunately, juice has been marketed toward well-meaning parents as a nutritious source of vitamins and minerals, or as an alternative to whole fruit.[25] Higher quantities of juice intake early in life have been associated with more juice intake into toddlerhood and mid-childhood.[27,28] Further, the increase in BMI associated with juice intake has been shown to be even higher for every 8 oz/ 240 ml serving of 100% fruit juice for younger children than for older children.[25] Juice intake has been shown to be higher in socioeconomically vulnerable populations,[29] which may leave some children more susceptible to the sequela of excessive juice intake compared to others.

Pediatric clinicians must play an active role in discouraging intake of juice and other sugar-sweetened beverages in order to promote healthy habits and prevent excess weight gain in infants and young children. Strategies for counseling regarding healthy juice consumption are shown in **Box 2**.

Promoting Physical Activity/Tummy Time

Routine exercise is associated with many beneficial health outcomes in early childhood, including a lower risk of excessive weight gain and adiposity.[30] Discussions promoting the importance of exercise should begin in the clinical setting in early infancy, as tummy time has been associated with improved gross motor development and may be associated with decreased BMI.[31] The World Health Organization recommends that infants get at least 30 minutes of tummy time per day.[32] Throughout infancy, physical activity can be achieved by interactive floor play.[31,32] In young children, higher amounts of exercise have been associated with decreased adiposity.[30] In accordance with American Academy of Pediatrics guidelines (2018), pediatric clinicians should recommend that children from 3 to 5 years old aim for a goal of 3 or more hours of daily exercise of varying intensity. Children from age 6 to 17 years need at least 1 hour of moderate-to-vigorous activity each day, and physical activities should include bone and muscle-strengthening activities, as well as aerobic activities.[33] This guidance is especially important for children with special health care needs, who have been shown to have higher rates of physical inactivity.[30]

Special attention should be paid to encouraging joyful movement in children who experience barriers to physical activity, children with special health and/or developmental needs, and children from minoritized or low-income households.[30] Pediatric clinicians can advocate for families to overcome these barriers by becoming familiar with and referring to community-based activity programs.[30] Additionally, different physical activity opportunities are sometimes provided to girls compared with boys; as a result, girls may benefit from active encouragement to engage in physically active play beginning in early childhood and continuing with encouragement

---

Box 2
Counseling about healthy juice consumption[26]

Delay the introduction of juice, with strict avoidance until 1 year of age.

Recommend intake of whole fruit instead of juice.

Recommend intake of water and milk over juice or other sugar-sweetened beverages.

If 100% juice is given after 1 year of age, limit to 4 oz (120 ml) per day.

Recommend elimination of juice for children with excess weight gain.

Advocate for policies that decrease juice intake and increase access to whole fruit.

Box 3
Anticipatory guidance about sleep[43]

Set a regular bedtime.

Keep bedtime routines less than 30 to 45 minutes and separate from feeding.

Allow time for babies and toddlers to self-soothe before sleep.

Create a comfortable and calm sleep environment with no screens present.

Include exposure to early morning sunlight and daytime physical activity in routines.

---

and opportunities for active play and sports participation outside the home.[30] Early promotion of *physical literacy*, described as the, "ability, confidence and desire to be physically active for life," may help set the stage for a lifetime of health benefit from the earliest stages of development through adulthood.[30,34]

Screen Time

Screen media exposure is strongly linked to excess weight gain and obesity in children, and the more hours viewed, the higher the prevalence of overweight.[35] This link becomes stronger as babies age from infancy to toddlerhood to the preschool years.[36] The most likely mediator is the consumption of more energy-dense foods and drinks, particularly when eating occurs in front of the screen, where feelings of hunger and fullness can be dulled.[35] As early as toddlerhood, screen time has been associated with greater consumption of sugar-sweetened beverages, fast food, and junk food, particularly when the screens are on during mealtimes.[37] Unfortunately, many infants begin both passive and active television watching by 2 months of age,[16] with earlier introduction predicting more daily TV watching at older ages.[38] Thus, counseling on the risks of screen exposure even during early infancy visits may be an important opportunity for intervention. These discussions can be linked to conversations around responsive feeding. However, longer term community-based interventions are likely the most effective approach to reducing screen time in this young age group.[39]

Addressing Sleep

Shorter sleep duration and poor sleep quality increase the risk of obesity in children and adolescents.[40] Growing evidence suggests that this association extends into infancy[41] and that counseling on sleep may be one of the more effective ways for pediatric clinicians to help prevent obesity. The Prevention of Overweight in Infancy randomized controlled trial found that a brief, early infancy office-based intervention focused on preventing sleep problems decreased the risk of obesity at 2 years, with the effect sustained at 3.5 and 5 years. Interestingly, the complementary intervention group promoting breastfeeding, healthy eating, and physical activity had higher BMI z scores at 2 and 5 years compared to the control group.[42] Anticipatory guidance to promote healthful sleep is shown in **Box 3**.

SUMMARY

Pediatric clinicians have many opportunities to intervene and promote healthful diet and activity patterns in the first years of life because of frequent contact with young children and longitudinal relationships with families. By focusing counseling on known behaviors that are associated with obesity risk, pediatric clinicians can play an important role in preventing obesity at the individual and population levels. Parents expect to receive information about their child's growth during well visits; discussion of the growth chart during early childhood provides a natural opportunity to provide counseling to optimize nutrition and activity. Effective preventive counseling to promote healthful weight gain can begin at the earliest newborn visits and include promotion of breastfeeding, discussion of correct bottle size if bottles are used, delaying solid foods and juice, promoting active play, developing healthy sleep patterns, and avoiding electronic screens.

CLINICS CARE POINTS

- Promote exclusive breastfeeding beginning in the newborn period, as this is associated with healthful weight gain.

- Parents often use a bottle size that is larger than needed for the infant's nutritional needs, and this can lead to overfeeding and early excess weight gain. Counsel parents to use the best bottle size for the infant's age and size as well as teach hunger and satiety cues.[22]

- Counsel caregivers to postpone introducing solid foods until at least 4 months (preferably 6 months) to limit early rapid weight gain.[21]

- Encourage caregivers to avoid exposing infants to screens, as this is associated with worse dietary habits, more screen time as toddlers, and there is good evidence about the relationship of screen time and obesity.[38]

- Counsel caregivers early in infancy about avoiding juice and sugar-sweetened beverages.[27,28]

- Encourage physical activity from infancy throughout adolescence. Children aged younger than 6 years old need at least 3 hours of activity of varying intensity per day and children aged 6 years and older need at least 1 hour of moderate-to-vigorous physical activity daily.[33]

DISCLOSURE

Dr H.W. Williams discloses receiving food and beverages totaling US$15.08 from Glaxo Smith Kline in 2019. Otherwise, the authors have nothing to disclose.

REFERENCES

1. Paauw ND, van Rijn BB, Lely AT, et al. Pregnancy as a critical window for blood pressure regulation in mother and child: programming and reprogramming. Acta Physiol 2017;219(1):241–59.
2. Baird J, Fisher D, Lucas P, et al. Being big or growing fast: systematic review of size and growth in infancy and later obesity. BMJ 2005;331(7522):929.
3. Boney CM, Verma A, Tucker R, et al. Metabolic syndrome in childhood: association with birth weight, maternal obesity, and gestational diabetes mellitus. An Pediatr 2005;115(3):e290–6.
4. Domanski G, Lange AE, Ittermann T, et al. Evaluation of neonatal and maternal morbidity in mothers with gestational diabetes: a population-based study. BMC Pregnancy Childb 2018;18(1):367.
5. Leunissen RW, Kerkhof GF, Stijnen T, et al. Timing and tempo of first-year rapid growth in relation to cardiovascular and metabolic risk profile in early adulthood. JAMA 2009;301(21):2234–42.
6. Alexander BT, Dasinger JH, Intapad S. Fetal programming and cardiovascular pathology. Compr Physiol 2015;5(2):997–1025.
7. Taveras EM, Rifas-Shiman SL, Belfort MB, et al. Weight status in the first 6 months of life and obesity at 3 years of age. An Pediatr 2009;123(4):1177–83.

8. Smego A, Woo JG, Klein J, et al. High Body Mass Index in Infancy May Predict Severe Obesity in Early Childhood. J Pediatr 2017;183:87–93 e1.

9. Nader PR, O'Brien M, Houts R, et al. Identifying risk for obesity in early childhood. An Pediatr 2006;118(3):e594–601.

10. Ong KK, Loos RJ. Rapid infancy weight gain and subsequent obesity: systematic reviews and hopeful suggestions. Acta Paediatr 2006;95(8):904–8.

11. Feldman-Winter L, Burnham L, Grossman X, et al. Weight gain in the first week of life predicts overweight at 2 years: A prospective cohort study. Matern Child Nutr 2018;14(1). https://doi.org/10.1111/mcn.12472.

12. Golan M. Parents as agents of change in childhood obesity–from research to practice. Int J Pediatr Obes 2006;1(2):66–76.

13. Golan M, Crow S. Targeting parents exclusively in the treatment of childhood obesity: long-term results. Obes Res 2004;12(2):357–61.

14. Golan M, Kaufman V, Shahar DR. Childhood obesity treatment: targeting parents exclusively v. parents and children. Br J Nutr 2006;95(5):1008–15.

15. Redsell SA, Edmonds B, Swift JA, et al. Systematic review of randomised controlled trials of interventions that aim to reduce the risk, either directly or indirectly, of overweight and obesity in infancy and early childhood. Matern Child Nutr 2016;12(1):24–38.

16. Perrin EM, Rothman RL, Sanders LM, et al. Racial and ethnic differences associated with feeding- and activity-related behaviors in infants. An Pediatr 2014; 133(4):e857–67.

17. Sirkka O, Vrijkotte T, Halberstadt J, et al. Prospective associations of age at complementary feeding and exclusive breastfeeding duration with body mass index at 5-6 years within different risk groups. Pediatr Obes 2018;13(8):522–9.

18. Yan J, Liu L, Zhu Y, et al. The association between breastfeeding and childhood obesity: a meta-analysis. BMC Public Heal 2014/12/13 2014;14(1):1267.

19. Meek JY, Noble L, Section on B. Policy Statement: Breastfeeding and the Use of Human Milk. An Pediatr 2022;150(1). https://doi.org/10.1542/peds.2022-057988.

20. Office of the Surgeon General (US); Centers for Disease Control and Prevention (US); Office on Women's Health (US). The Surgeon General's Call to Action to Support Breastfeeding. Office of the Surgeon General (US). Available at: https://www.ncbi.nlm.nih.gov/books/NBK52682/. Accessed February 9, 2024.

21. Wood CT, Witt WP, Skinner AC, et al. Effects of Breastfeeding, Formula Feeding, and Complementary Feeding on Rapid Weight Gain in the First Year of Life. Acad Pediatr 2021;21(2):288–96.

22. Wood CT, Skinner AC, Yin HS, et al. Bottle Size and Weight Gain in Formula-Fed Infants. An Pediatr 2016;138(1). https://doi.org/10.1542/peds.2015-4538.

23. Barbara AD, Lynn SE, Howard HS, et al. Rapid infant weight gain predicts childhood overweight. Obesity (Silver Spring, Md) 2006;14:491–9.

24. Papoutsou S, Savva SC, Hunsberger M, et al. Timing of solid food introduction and association with later childhood overweight and obesity: The IDEFICS study. Matern Child Nutr 2018;14(1). https://doi.org/10.1111/mcn.12471.

25. Nguyen M, Jarvis SE, Chiavaroli L, et al. Consumption of 100% Fruit Juice and Body Weight in Children and Adults: A Systematic Review and Meta-Analysis. JAMA Pediatr 2024. https://doi.org/10.1001/jamapediatrics.2023.6124.

26. Heyman MB, Abrams SA, Heitlinger LA, et al. Section On Gastroenterology H, Nutrition, Committee On N. Fruit Juice in Infants, Children, and Adolescents: Current Recommendations. An Pediatr 2017;139(6). https://doi.org/10.1542/peds. 2017-0967.

27. Sonneville KR, Long MW, Rifas-Shiman SL, et al. Juice and water intake in infancy and later beverage intake and adiposity: could juice be a gateway drink? Obesity (Silver Spring) 2015;23(1):170–6.

28. Kay MC, Pankiewicz AR, Schildcrout JS, et al. Early Sweet Tooth: Juice Introduction During Early Infancy is Related to Toddler Juice Intake. Acad Pediatr Sep-Oct 2023;23(7):1343–50.

29. Drewnowski A, Rehm CD. Socioeconomic gradient in consumption of whole fruit and 100% fruit juice among US children and adults. Nutr J 2015;14:3.

30. 2018 Physical Activity Guidelines Advisory Committee. 2018 Physical Activity Guidelines Scientific Report. Available at: https://health.gov/sites/default/files/2019-09/PAG_Advisory_Committee_Report.pdf. Accessed February 11, 2024.

31. Hewitt L, Kerr E, Stanley RM, et al. Tummy Time and Infant Health Outcomes: A Systematic Review. An Pediatr 2020;145(6). https://doi.org/10.1542/peds.2019-2168.

32. WHO. Guidelines on physical activity, sedentary behaviour and sleep for children under 5 years of age. World Health Organization 2019. Available at: https://iris.who.int/handle/10665/311664. [Accessed 9 February 2024].

33. Lobelo F, Muth ND, Hanson S, et al. Physical Activity Assessment and Counseling in Pediatric Clinical Settings. An Pediatr 2020;145(3). https://doi.org/10.1542/peds.2019-3992.

34. Aspen Institute. Physical Literacy in the United States: A Model, Strategic Plan, and Call to Action. Available at: https://www.aspeninstitute.org/publications/physical-literacy-model-strategic-plan-call-action/. [Accessed 9 February 2024].

35. Robinson TN, Banda JA, Hale L, et al. Screen Media Exposure and Obesity in Children and Adolescents. An Pediatr 2017;140(Suppl 2):S97–101.

36. LeBlanc AG, Spence JC, Carson V, et al. Systematic review of sedentary behaviour and health indicators in the early years (aged 0-4 years). Appl Physiol Nutr Metab 2012;37(4):753–72.

37. Lutz MR, Orr CJ, Shonna Yin H, et al. TV Time, Especially During Meals, is Associated with Less Healthy Dietary Practices in Toddlers. Acad Pediatr 2023. https://doi.org/10.1016/j.acap.2023.09.019.

38. Hish AJ, Wood CT, Howard JB, et al. Infant Television Watching Predicts Toddler Television Watching in a Low-Income Population Acad Pediatr 2020. https://doi.org/10.1016/j.acap.2020.11.002.

39. Downing KL, Hnatiuk JA, Hinkley T, et al. Interventions to reduce sedentary behaviour in 0-5-year-olds: a systematic review and meta-analysis of randomised controlled trials. Br J Sports Med 2018;52(5):314–21.

40. Morrissey B, Orellana L, Allender S, et al. The Sleep-Obesity Nexus: Assessment of Multiple Sleep Dimensions and Weight Status Among Victorian Primary School Children. Nat Sci Sleep 2022;14:581–91.

41. Chaput JP, Gray CE, Poitras VJ, et al. Systematic review of the relationships between sleep duration and health indicators in the early years (0-4 years). BMC Public Heal 2017;17(Suppl 5):855.

42. Taylor RW, Gray AR, Heath AM, et al. Sleep, nutrition, and physical activity interventions to prevent obesity in infancy: follow-up of the Prevention of Overweight in Infancy (POI) randomized controlled trial at ages 3.5 and 5 y. Am J Clin Nutr 2018;108(2):228–36.

43. Bathory E, Tomopoulos S. Sleep Regulation, Physiology and Development, Sleep Duration and Patterns, and Sleep Hygiene in Infants, Toddlers, and Preschool-Age Children. Curr Probl Pediatr Adolesc Health Care 2017;47(2):29–42.

Applying an Equity Lens to Pediatric Obesity
Clinical, Environmental, and Policy Considerations for Clinicians

Colin J. Orr, MD, MPH[a],*, Michelle C. Gorecki, MD, MPH[b],
Jennifer A. Woo Baidal, MD, MPH[c]

KEYWORDS

- Health equity • Pediatric obesity • Social drivers of health • Disparities

KEY POINTS

- Pediatric obesity is influenced by structural discrimination/inequities.
- The etiology of pediatric obesity is multifactorial, including intra/interpersonal, societal, and policy levels.
- Within each level, equity considerations can inform approaches to prevention, diagnosis, and treatment approaches for pediatric obesity.

INTRODUCTION

Pediatric obesity is a public health crisis that has important health equity implications for children. According to nationally representative data from the years 2017 to 2020, the prevalence of obesity among children in the United States 2 to 19 years of age was 19.7%, representing 14.7 million children.[1] This overall prevalence of obesity among children is worrisome; however, the burden of obesity is not shared equally among all communities. Disparities in pediatric obesity are seen by child race,[1] child ethnicity,[1] socioeconomic status,[1] poverty,[2] gender identity,[3] geography,[4] and exposure to discrimination.[5] Race and ethnicity are social constructs; therefore, observed disparities by race and ethnicity are driven by societal inequities as opposed to biologic or genetic factors. Given the morbidity and mortality associated with obesity

[a] University of North Carolina at Chapel Hill School of Medicine, Chapel Hill, North Carolina; [b] Department of General and Community Pediatrics, Cincinnati Children's Hospital Medical Center, Cincinnati, Ohio; [c] Department of Pediatrics, Stanford University, 750 Welch Road, Palo Alto, CA, USA
* Corresponding author. Department of Pediatrics, Vanderbilt University Medical Center, 2200 Children's Way, Suite 2404, Nashville, TN 37232.
E-mail address: colin.orr@vumc.org

Pediatr Clin N Am 71 (2024) 805–818
https://doi.org/10.1016/j.pcl.2024.07.001
0031-3955/24/© 2024 Elsevier Inc. All rights are reserved, including those for text and data mining, AI training, and similar technologies.
pediatric.theclinics.com

(See Physical Exam and Screening for Comorbidities Chapter), clinicians should understand the root origins that drive obesity inequities among children who are afflicted by pediatric obesity.

Pediatric obesity is a complex and multifactorial disease process (See Overview of Pediatric Disease Chapter). Clinical Practice Guidelines (CPG) were recently published to guide clinicians in the management and treatment of pediatric obesity (See Overview of Pediatric Obesity Treatment and the new CPG Guidelines Chapter).[6] In the CPG are discussions of the equity considerations in pediatric obesity. The authors seek to augment this work by examining pediatric obesity from a health equity perspective. Varied mechanisms for pediatric obesity operate in specific communities and contribute to inequities that result in pediatric obesity disparities. This nuanced understanding of the etiology of pediatric obesity can inform clinical practice and advocacy efforts. There are existing health equity frameworks that consider the roles of racism, discrimination, health systems access and structure, and socioenvironmental contexts in pediatric obesity (**Table 1**).

Given the complexity of pediatric obesity, we need frameworks that integrate multilevel etiologies of pediatric obesity in context and highlight the areas of opportunities for clinicians to contribute to addressing disparities in obesity (**Fig. 1**). The overarching goal of this article is to serve as a review of the mechanisms and opportunities for intervention for obesity using an equity lens for clinicians.

FACTORS FOR OBESITY: EQUITY CONSIDERATIONS

The mechanisms of pediatric obesity are present at the individual, family, community, societal, and policy levels.[12] Within each level, equity considerations can inform pediatric obesity approaches in the clinical setting.[7,8] Later, the authors will provide examples of obesity drivers at each level, with an emphasis on clinically relevant equity implications.

Individual/Intrapersonal/Clinic Level: Prenatal

Multiple individual-level factors influence a child's risk for obesity. Some of these drivers are present during the prenatal period, while others emerge at various points during childhood.[13] While not directly in scope of the clinical care provided by clinicians, knowledge of the prenatal period from an equity and obesity perspective can inform subsequent care and anticipatory guidance (see **Fig. 1**). Gestational diabetes

Table 1		
List of frameworks used to conceptualize pediatric obesity		
Framework	**Details**	**Level**
National Academies of Medicine (NAM)[7]	Explores how racism and discrimination influence health	Multi-level
National Academies of Medicine[8] and Browne et al[9]	Racism can work at multiple levels to contribute to disparities in pediatric obesity	Multi-level
Gurewich et al[10]	Proposed relationships within health systems to reduce health disparities by addressing social drivers of health to improve health outcomes	Health system
Kumanyika et al[11]	Conceptualizes how societal and environmental factors influence obesity disparities from a policy level	Societal/Policy

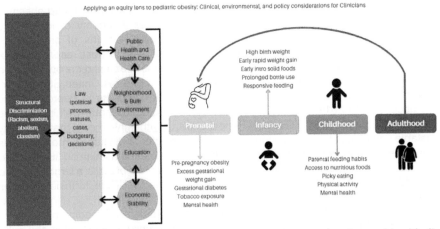

Fig. 1. Determinants of obesity (*Adapted from* Yearby R. Structural racism and health disparities: Reconfiguring the social determinants of health framework to include the root cause. Journal of Law, Medicine & Ethics. 2020;48(3), 518-526;with permission).

is a pediatric obesity risk factor that could be identified during the newborn visit and has equity implications.[14] The overall burden of gestational diabetes is increasing; however, inequities in the prevalence of gestational diabetes exist with burden differing across individuals from different racial and ethnic groups.[15] Structural discrimination and racism drive some of the racial and ethnic disparities observed in gestational diabetes rates.[16] Individuals identifying as Asian/Pacific Islander (102.7 per 1000 live births) or Hispanic (66.6 per 1000 live births) have higher incidence of gestational diabetes compared to the individuals who identified as non-Hispanic White with a rate of 55.7.5 per 1000 live births.[15] Maternal pre-pregnancy body mass index (BMI) is an additional prenatal risk factor for offspring obesity during childhood and is overly represented in certain communities.[14] Obesity is common in the adult population, with 41.9% of adults diagnosed with obesity based on nationally representative 2017 data.[17] There are notable disparities in adult obesity by sex and income, similar to disparities in childhood obesity by sex and income, which are also driven by historical disinvestment including structural discrimination, such as community opportunity and food deserts.[18,19] The role of structural discrimination will be discussed in greater detail later.

Individual/Intrapersonal/Clinic Level: Postnatal

There are several postnatal factors that operate at the individual/intrapersonal level that can modify a child's risk for obesity. The newborn and early infancy period is a critical development window where inequities in pediatric obesity can become clinically apparent. Prior work, using nationally representative data from the Early Childhood Longitudinal Study Birth Cohort, found for infants identified as Asian and Black approximately 15% and 70%, respectively, of the racial and ethnic disparities in BMI-z score at 9 months was attributed to the velocity of infant weight gain during the prior 9-month period when compared to infants identified as White.[20] In that study, socioeconomic status contributed to observed disparities in BMI-z score, especially between children identified as White compared to those with Hispanic ethnicity.[20] This suggests that the early environment, with its positive and detrimental factors, plays an important role in risk for pediatric obesity and its disparities (see **Fig. 1**, cite The Toxic Food Environment and Nutrition).

Infant nutrition is an early determinant of infant growth, development, and obesity. The World Health Organization (WHO) and the American Academy of Pediatrics (AAP) recommend exclusive breastfeeding for at least 6 months of an infant's life,[21,22] which is suggested to prevent early rapid weight gain.[23] These recommendations encourage the introduction of solid foods at 6 months of age and the opportunity for continued breastfeeding beyond 24 months if desired. In the United States, the number of infants who are exclusively breastfed until 6 months is approximately 25% according to 2019 data.[24] Overall, the breastfeeding rates are well below the goal of 42.4% established by Healthy People 2030.[25] Within the United States, there is notable variation in the prevalence of exclusive breastfeeding at age 6 months. The prevalence of exclusive breastfeeding at age 6 months can be as high as 36.5% and as low as 13.9% depending on the state a family resides.[24] As of 2022, a large majority of US states do not have legislation for paid family and medical leave, further hindering efforts to support breastfeeding.[24]

Another potential determinant of child weight status is parental feeding behaviors. Parental feeding behaviors have been associated with child weight status and risk for obesity,[26] and variations can be seen by race and ethnicity.[27] For example, a study that enrolled a low socioeconomic status and racial and ethnically diverse sample found that parents that identified as non-Hispanic Black had increased odds of putting their 2 month old child to bed with a bottle, while parents identifying as Hispanic had increased odds of encouraging their child to finish their food compared to parents identifying as non-Hispanic White.[27–29]

Essential to understanding obesity from an equity perspective is to appreciate a child and family's lived experience and values. Discrimination can work at multiple levels to alter a child's risk for obesity (see **Fig. 1**).[5] At the individual level, experience with racial discrimination can lead to higher BMI z-score as well risk factors for obesity such as increased waist circumference.[5] Cultural considerations can be important to consider in weight discussions with children and their families. Culture can influence a family's understanding of child feeding, caregiver roles, activity levels, food choices, preferred child appearance, and the overall food environment.[30] Culturally tailored messages and interventions focused on child weight and the prevention or management of overweight may benefit from consideration of these factors.[31]

Language is a social driver of health and is important to consider for pediatric obesity equity.[32] A scoping review that explored common elements of interventions to prevent obesity among children from racial or ethnic minority groups found that considering and addressing language was an important component for interventions.[33]

Community and Local Environment

A child's local and community environment can modify individual-level risk for obesity (see **Fig. 1**). At the state level, there are wide variations in the prevalence of pediatric obesity. Of the states reporting data on prevalence of adolescent obesity to the 2019 Youth Behavior Surveillance, the state-level prevalence of adolescent obesity ranged from 10% to 23%.[34] Within the states, smaller units of geography, such as rural or urban settings, can have important implications for pediatric obesity. A study using nationally representative data found that children from rural areas had 30% increased odds of being overweight compared to children from urban settings.[35]

Access to healthy and nutritious foods is a community-level driver of pediatric obesity (cite the "Role of food and beverage environments in child health and weight-related behaviors" article). Unfortunately, not all communities have ready access to nutritious food. Two distinct but interrelated concepts regarding food access and equity are food insecurity (FI) and food desert. The United States Department of

Agriculture (USDA) defines FI as "a household-level economic and social condition of limited or uncertain access to adequate food."[36] FI is common, affecting 17.3% of US households with children in 2022.[37] There are notable variations in FI by state, income, and race and ethnicity.[38] For example, individuals from the non-Hispanic Black or Hispanic community have almost twice the prevalence of FI compared to individuals from the non-Hispanic White community.[38] FI can be linked to pediatric obesity[39]; however, the potential mechanisms such as dietary quality and parental feeding behaviors can vary by demographic characteristics.[28,29,40] This highlights that within the experience of FI there are health equity considerations because not all communities may be impacted by FI in the same manner. One potential exacerbating factor of FI related to food access is food deserts. The USDA defines a food desert as "low-income [census] tracts in which a substantial number or proportion of the population has low access to supermarkets or a large grocery store."[41] Food deserts are a community-level equity issue for pediatric obesity, given the factors which place a census tract at risk for being a classified as a food desert has overlap with known inequities in pediatric obesity. For example, census tracts with a higher poverty rate, less education, and higher prevalence of individuals identifying as non-Hispanic Black or Hispanic are more likely to live in a food desert.[41]

Ability to access grocery stores relative to fast food options has important implications for equity and pediatric obesity. A review article found that populations with lower incomes had to travel greater distances to access grocery stores.[42] The review also found that predominately Black neighborhoods had fewer healthful food options and more fast food options.[42] Individuals in rural communities perceived an insufficient number of supermarkets. These structural disparities in access to healthy food options relative to unhealthy food options likely contribute to the inequities in pediatric obesity.[43]

Additional community-level measures can further our understanding of the nuance and complexity of pediatric obesity from an equity perspective. Measures such as the Childhood Opportunity Index (COI)[44] and Social Vulnerability Index (SVI)[45] are applied to census tracts to provide information on how community can influence weight outcomes.[46] One study found that children from a high COI or low SVI census tract had decreased risk for obesity. The authors found that COI and SVI at birth were an important driver for future obesity risk.[46] A separate study also found lower community-level measures of resource/opportunity were associated with nutrition and risk for obesity. Structural racism has been associated with lower COI.[47] Further, neighborhood inequities in rates of violent crimes are associated with pediatric obesity, and neighborhood-level stressors can have cumulative effects.[48] Patients live in communities with varying levels of COI and SVI, and this will have a significant impact on their obesity risk.

Policy Considerations

Several federal nutrition programs are designed to support equity in nutrition. The Special Supplemental Nutrition Program for Women, Infants, and Children (WIC) "serves to safeguard the health of low-income pregnant, postpartum, and breastfeeding women, infants, and children up to age 5 who are at nutritional risk by providing nutrition foods to supplement diets, information on healthy eating including breastfeeding promotion and support, and referrals to health care."[49] By design, WIC is intended to support nutritional equity by supporting families who are at risk for poor nutritional outcomes. Between 2010 and 2020, participation in WIC was associated with a decrease in obesity among enrolled children and improved weight-for-length measurements among infants and toddlers.[50] However, there were significant variations in reported prevalence of obesity, and not all states observed a decrease in obesity.[50] Overall, during the study years, the prevalence of obesity among children enrolled in WIC decreased from 15.9% to 14.4%; however, the prevalence of obesity ranged from 8% to 19.9% and some states observed an increase in obesity among children enrolled in WIC.[50] Additionally, children from the Hispanic or American Indian or Alaska Native communities enrolled in WIC had an increase in obesity prevalence.[50] While WIC is designed to support nutritional equity, there are clear inequities in obesity among WIC participants.

Despite the importance of WIC for supporting nutrition equity, there are a large number of children who are eligible for participation who are not enrolled. Participation in the program decreases as children age.[51] Participation of eligible families also varies by race and ethnicity. In 2020, individuals from the Hispanic community had the highest coverage rate (62%) while individuals identifying as non-Hispanic White had a coverage rate of 35%.[51] This observation highlights the importance of discussing federal nutrition benefits with all families who are eligible as there might be unexpected gaps in resource utilization. There are also important differences in coverage rates by a family's state of resident.[51] One barrier to WIC participation is the administrative burden on families.[52] As an important program in supporting health and nutritional equity, there are multiple dimensions of equity that can be considered clinically to further the equity and benefit WIC participation. A recent report found that electronic health record integration was feasible to facilitate and increase WIC referrals and enrollment.[53]

Given its implications for health equity, it is important to consider the impact of school closures early during the COVID-19 pandemic. For children most at for risk for obesity and nutritional insufficiency, the school environment can be an important opportunity to support nutrition. The closure of schools during the pandemic may have asymmetric health consequences, where children from communities most at risk incurred an elevated risk for obesity and poor nutrition in the setting of school closures.[54] As the world continues to respond and adapt to COVID-19, it will be important for clinicians to consider how to address the lack of nutritional support and the necessary purchasing decisions (such as shelf-stable, ultra-processed foods) during shelter in place orders to avoid exacerbation of inequities that existed prior to the pandemic.[54]

The advertisement of food and beverages to children is a policy-level factor that has implications for equity in pediatric obesity. Exposure to unhealthy food through advertisement online and the television contributes to pediatric obesity.[55] There is evidence that the advertisement of healthy food choices is directed to children identified as non-Hispanic Black and Spanish-speaking children.[55] Advertisement of unhealthy food options can also be directed at families of lower socioeconomic status.[56]

Promoting Pediatric Obesity Equity: Recommendations for Clinicians

Clinicians play a critical role in addressing pediatric obesity in an equitable fashion. The mechanisms of pediatric obesity are multifactorial, complex, and interdependent. Despite the magnitude and complexity of pediatric obesity, there are tangible actions that clinicians can take to promote equity in pediatric obesity. During routine clinical encounters, clinicians should provide anticipatory guidance and counseling on obesity in a culturally relevant and non-judgmental manner. Evidence suggests that unhealthy feeding behaviors can begin early infancy.[27] Early anticipatory guidance on the introduction of solid foods, optimal infant nutrition (breastmilk/formula), and satiety cues can prevent the development of behaviors potentially linked to obesity.

The Greenlight Program is 1 example of a low-health literacy primary care intervention to prevent pediatric obesity in a diverse (racial, ethnic, and socioeconomic status) cohort.[57] This program showed evidence of weight trajectory differences through 15 months for all children who received the intervention[58] but actually a heterogeneity of treatment effect analysis found that the intervention had a greater effect for those with limited health literacy and those whose caregivers spoke Spanish.[59] The Greenlight Program uses a literacy-sensitive and culturally and linguistically-tailored approach to obesity prevention by helping parents set and achieve healthy feeding and activity-related goals.

Promoting healthy physical activity and dietary behaviors are the foundational factors in the prevention and management of pediatric obesity. The US Food and Drug Administration has approved medications for the treatment of pediatric obesity (cite Pharmacotherapy in Treatment of Obesity in Pediatric Patients).[6] Overall, these drugs are underutilized in primary care settings. The AAP clinical practice guidelines note that pharmacotherapy may be offered to children 12 years of age with obesity[6]; however, all children who may benefit from these medications may not have equal access to these drugs due to insurance coverage, or access to referral centers/clinics with expertise in the management of medications to treat obesity. Most US state Medicaid plans exclude anti-obesity medication (AOM) coverage.[60] Likely owing to their recent recommendation, few studies have examined disparities in access and use among pediatric patients. One study found lower prescription rates among Hispanic/Latino youth than White, non-Hispanic youth and that use of an interpreter increased the likelihood of prescribing AOMs among non-English-speaking patients/families.[61] Equity interventions to increase access to AOMs and stop widening of disparities include expanding insurance coverage of AOMs, offering AOMs to all qualifying patients, and using linguistically-appropriate means to discuss AOMs. Improving access and clinician comfort, awareness of these medications, and discussing them with patients and their families in an unbiased, equitable fashion can reduce disparities in medication management of pediatric obesity. In situations where there are barriers to medication management in the primary care setting, systems can be developed to ensure that all families who are eligible are referred to centers with expertise in obesity in an unbiased fashion.

In addition to lifestyle and medical management options for pediatric obesity, surgical options such as bariatric surgery (see "Metabolic and bariatric surgery for adolescents" chapter) also exist. Evidence-based guidelines recommend that clinicians discuss bariatric surgery evaluation with adolescents who have "$\geq$class 2 obesity; BMI $\geq$ 35 kg/m^2, or 120% of the 95th percentile for age and sex, whichever is lower,"[6] Early recognition and referral of patients to centers with expertise in these surgeries is critical as evidence suggests that health benefits are optimized with earlier surgical management. There are multiple barriers for patients accessing surgical management options including a paucity of centers that perform surgeries for pediatric obesity. A recent study demonstrated the equity considerations in who would benefit from surgical management and who is able to access these services. This retrospective analysis using local data merged with data from the National Health and Nutrition Survey (NHANES); the authors found a complex interaction between race, ethnicity, and insurance status. No differences in surgeries were identified insurance type; however, individuals identifying as Hispanic or non-Hispanic Black with public insurance had decreased odds of obtaining surgery.[62] The author speculated multiple potential etiologies for their observations including the role of unconscious bias in those who are referred and/or counseled to consider surgery.[62] Similar to the authors' recommendations to improve equity in access to AOMs, opportunities to improve surgical access include improving clinician comfort, awareness of surgical recommendations, and discussing them with patients and their families in an unbiased, equitable fashion which can reduce disparities in surgical management of pediatric obesity.

Clinicians should consider monitoring for inequities within their practice. For example, clinicians may use quality improvement methods to monitor any interventions for equity and to address inequities in their practice.

Quality improvement (QI) is an important part of all clinical care and a requirement for certification by the American Board of Pediatrics.[63] By first applying an equity lens to identify health care and health outcomes disparities that exist, meaningful benchmarks and metrics that focus on improvements for all children while also narrowing disparities can help contribute to health equity. Health Equity Assessment Toolkits exist to facilitate this process, and can be used to assess all proposed clinic policy and programs.[64] By examining overall and subgroup changes to QI interventions, clinical policies, and programs, practitioners can monitor whether new initiatives improve outcomes in an equitable manner, or modify interventions as needed to address persistent or widening disparities.[65]

Community-Level Considerations for Clinicians

An understanding of the environment that children live and grow in is essential for provide equitable care. There is evidence that approximately 16% of health is influenced by the clinical environment.[66] This suggests an understanding of the unique community barriers and facilitators for equitable pediatric obesity care. While there are many community drivers that can influence risk for pediatric obesity, the authors will focus primarily on food security, given its asymmetric burden on communities who carry a higher prevalence and morbidity from obesity and tangible steps for clinicians. The AAP published a policy statement outlining how clinics could address food insecurity by "screening and intervening."[67] Implementation of food insecurity screening must be done in a thoughtful way. Prior qualitative studies done with racially and ethnically diverse families demonstrate that food insecurity screening is overall acceptable in primary care settings; however, careful attention needs to be paid to ensure families do not feel stigmatized, targeted, or will have Child Protective Services called if a family discloses food insecurity.[68,69] The Food Research and Action Center and AAP developed a toolkit to support clinicians and clinics in the food insecurity screening process.[70]

Societal/Policy-Level Considerations for Clinicians

An important policy interaction to further equity in pediatric obesity is participation in federal nutrition assistance programs. Programs, such as WIC for example, are designed to reduce food insecurity and promote adequate nutrition and growth for young children. Federal nutrition assistance programs have been shown to mitigate pediatric obesity.[71] Despite the importance of WIC, there is underutilization. Addressing a family's WIC status in a non-judgmental, culturally relevant manner and facilitating connection to resources when appropriate are clinic-policy interactions to support nutrition equity.

An awareness of the policy environment and its movement toward health equity is important for clinicians. There has been a shift among payers to focus on addressing inequities in care. A 2022 report from the Joint Commission outlined requirements to mitigate health disparities, including screening and addressing health-related social needs.[72] Social care interventions may promote equity in pediatric obesity[73]; however, a recent study suggested that there are barriers to the implementation of social care in primary care.[74]

SUMMARY FOR CLINICIANS

Pediatric obesity is a public health emergency. The "phenotype" of pediatric obesity can appear similar; however, the mechanisms leading to pediatric obesity can vary based on multiple factors. Awareness of the complex interactions of these factors is essential to inform equitable care in the prevention and management of pediatric obesity. There are factors operating at multiple levels to influence a child's risk for obesity. Clinicians play an important role in supporting children and their families. The clinician is a trusted source of information. There are multiple opportunities for counseling and anticipatory guidance, especially during the first year of life which is a critical period for growth and nutrition and when there are multiple clinical encounters. These clinical encounters permit an opportunity to support prevention of pediatric obesity by supporting breast-feeding, recognizing of satiety cues, and screening and addressing food insecurity through referral to community and federal programs. Additionally, clinicians can be aware of treatment, medication, and surgical options for children and work to ensure equitable referral and access to these treatment options. Pediatric obesity is complex; however, clinicians can help support efforts to support equity in pediatric obesity, including through facilitating patients' connection to local and federal resources.

CLINICS CARE POINTS

- Clinicians should screen and address health-related social needs.
- An obesity-specific intervention includes connecting families to nutrition assistance programs, (such as WIC, Supplemental Nutrition Assistance Program), or community services organizations.
- The etiology of pediatric obesity is multifactorial, including intra/interpersonal, societal, and policy level. Within each level, equity considerations can inform approaches to pediatric obesity with families in the clinical setting.
- Pediatric obesity risk factors begin in the prenatal period and are influenced by structural discrimination/inequities (see **Fig. 1**).
- Consider screening for health-related social needs and develop resource lists or referral processes to address identified needs.
- Be aware of local resources to address structural barriers driving inequities (eg, connection to local food pantries, federal nutrition assistance programs).
- Use quality improvement methods to monitor any interventions for equity and to address inequities in your practice.

Suggested actions for clinicians to promote equity in pediatric obesity
- Develop clinic-based processes to connect patients to resources.
- Screen for health-related social needs (when resources exist to address positive findings).
- Use quality improvement methods to monitor interventions to promote equity (ensure equity is not worsening with use of interventions).
- Practice discussing obesity using patient-centered, non-judgmental language.

DISCLOSURE

The authors have no disclosures to report. Dr M.C. Gorecki's effort on this project was supported by the National Research Service Award in Primary Medical Care, T32HP10027, through the Health Resources and Services Administration, United States. Dr C.J. Orr work was supported by the National Institute of Diabetes and Digestive and Kidney Diseases, United States of the National Institutes of Health under Grant Number K23DK132513 (C.J. Orr). The content is solely the responsibility of the authors and does not necessarily represent the official views of the National Institutes of Health.

REFERENCES

1. Prevention C for DC and. Childhood Obesity Facts. 2019. Available at: https://www.cdc.gov/obesity/data/childhood.html.
2. Inoue K, Seeman TE, Nianogo R, et al. The effect of poverty on the relationship between household education levels and obesity in U.S. children and adolescents: an observational study. Lancet Reg Heal - Am 2023;25. https://doi.org/10.1016/j.lana.2023.100565.
3. Schvey NA, Pearlman AT, Klein DA, et al. Obesity and Eating Disorder Disparities Among Sexual and Gender Minority Youth. JAMA Pediatr 2021;175(4):412.
4. Ogden CL, Fryar CD, Hales CM, et al. Differences in obesity prevalence by demographics and urbanization in US Children and Adolescents, 2013-2016. JAMA, J Am Med Assoc 2018;319(23):2410–8.
5. Cuevas AG, Krobath DM, Rhodes-Bratton B, et al. Association of Racial Discrimination With Adiposity in Children and Adolescents. JAMA Netw Open 2023;6(7):e2322839.
6. Hampl SE, Hassink SG, Skinner AC, et al. Clinical Practice Guideline for the Evaluation and Treatment of Children and Adolescents With Obesity. Pediatrics 2023;151(2). https://doi.org/10.1542/peds.2022-060640.
7. Thompson D, editor. Framing the dialogue on race and ethnicity to advance health equity. Washington, D.C.: National Academies Press; 2016. https://doi.org/10.17226/23576.
8. Callahan EA, editor. A health equity approach to obesity efforts. Washington, D.C.: National Academies Press; 2019. https://doi.org/10.17226/25409.
9. Browne NT, Hodges EA, Small L, et al. Childhood Obesity within the Lens of Racism. Pediatr Obes 2022;17(5). https://doi.org/10.1111/ijpo.12878.
10. Gurewich D, Garg A, Kressin NR. Addressing Social Determinants of Health Within Healthcare Delivery Systems: a Framework to Ground and Inform Health Outcomes. J Gen Intern Med 2020;35(5):1571–5.
11. Kumanyika SK. Advancing Health Equity Efforts to Reduce Obesity: Changing the Course. Annu Rev Nutr 2022;42:453–80.
12. Campbell MK. Biological, Environmental, and Social Influences on Childhood Obesity. Pediatr Res 2016;79(1–2):205–11.
13. Hu J, Aris IM, Lin PID, et al. Longitudinal associations of modifiable risk factors in the first 1000 days with weight status and metabolic risk in early adolescence. Am J Clin Nutr 2021;113(1):113–22.
14. Woo Baidal JA, Locks LM, Cheng ER, et al. Risk Factors for Childhood Obesity in the First 1,000 Days: A Systematic Review. Am J Prev Med 2016;50(6):761–79.
15. Shah NS, Wang MC, Freaney PM, et al. Trends in Gestational Diabetes at First Live Birth by Race and Ethnicity in the US, 2011-2019. JAMA, J Am Med Assoc 2021;326(7):660–9.
16. Agarwal S, Wade AN, Mbanya JC, et al. The role of structural racism and geographical inequity in diabetes outcomes. Lancet 2023;402(10397):235–49.
17. Centers for Disease Control and Prevention. Adult Obesity. 2022. Available at: https://www.cdc.gov/obesity/data/adult.html. [Accessed 8 January 2024].
18. Ogden CL, Fakhouri TH, Carroll MD, et al. Prevalence of Obesity Among Adults, by Household Income and Education — United States, 2011–2014. MMWR Morb Mortal Wkly Rep 2017;66(50):1369–73.
19. Ogden CL, Carroll MD, Fakhouri TH, et al. Prevalence of Obesity Among Youths by Household Income and Education Level of Head of Household — United States 2011–2014. MMWR Morb Mortal Wkly Rep 2018;67(6):186–9.

20. Isong IA, Rao SR, Bind MA, et al. Racial and ethnic disparities in early childhood obesity. Pediatrics 2018;141(1):e20170865.

21. World Health Organization. Breastfeeding and Complementary Feeding. Available at: https://www.paho.org/en/topics/breastfeeding-and-complementary-feeding#:~:text=The World Health Organization recommends,two years old or beyond. Accessed January 10, 2024.

22. Meek JY, Noble L. Policy Statement: Breastfeeding and the Use of Human Milk. Pediatrics 2022;150(1). https://doi.org/10.1542/peds.2022-057988.

23. Wood CT, Witt WP, Skinner AC, et al. Effects of Breastfeeding, Formula Feeding, and Complementary Feeding on Rapid Weight Gain in the First Year of Life. Acad Pediatr 2021;21(2):288–96.

24. Centers for Disease Control and Prevention. Breastfeeding Report Card. 2022. Available at: https://www.cdc.gov/breastfeeding/data/reportcard.htm. [Accessed 10 January 2024].

25. Health People 2030. Increase the Proportion of Infants Who Are Breastfed Exclusively through Age 6 Months — MICH-15. Available at: https://health.gov/healthypeople/objectives-and-data/browse-objectives/infants/increase-proportion-infants-who-are-breastfed-exclusively-through-age-6-months-mich-15. [Accessed 10 January 2024].

26. Hurley KM, Cross MB, Hughes SO. A Systematic Review of Responsive Feeding and Child Obesity in High-Income Countries. In: Journal of nutrition. 2011. p. 495–501. https://doi.org/10.3945/jn.110.130047.

27. Perrin EM, Rothman RL, Sanders LM, et al. Racial and ethnic differences associated with feeding- and activity-related behaviors in infants. Pediatrics 2014;133(4):e857–67.

28. Orr CJ, Ben-Davies M, Ravanbakht SN, et al. Parental Feeding Beliefs and Practices and Household Food Insecurity in Infancy. Acad Pediatr 2019;19(1):80–9.

29. Orr CJ, Ravanbakht S, Flower KB, et al. Associations Between Food Insecurity and Parental Feeding Behaviors of Toddlers. Acad Pediatr 2020. https://doi.org/10.1016/j.acap.2020.05.020.

30. Chatham RE, Mixer SJ. Cultural Influences on Childhood Obesity in Ethnic Minorities: A Qualitative Systematic Review. J Transcult Nurs 2020;31(1):87–99.

31. Okoniewski W, Sundaram M, Chaves-Gnecco D, et al. Culturally Sensitive Interventions in Pediatric Primary Care Settings: A Systematic Review. Pediatrics 2022;149(2). https://doi.org/10.1542/peds.2021-052162.

32. Ortega P, Vela M, Jacobs EA. Raising the Bar for Language Equity Health Care Research. JAMA Netw Open 2023;6(7):e2324485. https://doi.org/10.1001/jamanetworkopen.2023.24485.

33. Wang X, Ammerman A, Orr CJ. Family-based interventions for preventing overweight or obesity among preschoolers from racial/ethnic minority groups: A scoping review. Obes Sci Pract 2021. https://doi.org/10.1002/osp4.578.

34. Division of Population Health NC for CDP and HP. Adolescent Obesity Prevalence: Trends Over Time (2003-2019). 2021. Available at: https://www.cdc.gov/healthyschools/obesity/obesity-youth.htm. [Accessed 22 January 2024].

35. Crouch E, Abshire DA, Wirth MD, et al. Rural–Urban Differences in Overweight and Obesity, Physical Activity, and Food Security Among Children and Adolescents. Prev Chronic Dis 2023;20:1–10.

36. Agriculture USD of. Definitions of Food Security. on-line. 2019. Available at: https://www.ers.usda.gov/topics/food-nutrition-assistance/food-security-in-the-us/definitions-of-food-security.aspx.

37. United States Department of Agriculture. Food Security and Nutrition Assistance. 2023. Available at: https://www.ers.usda.gov/data-products/ag-and-food-statistics-charting-the-essentials/food-security-and-nutrition-assistance/: ~ :text=In 2022%2C 17.3 percent of households with children were food insecure. [Accessed 2 August 2024].

38. Rabbit MP, Hales LJ, Burke MP, et al. Household food security in the United States in 2022 2023.

39. Kaur J, Lamb MM, Ogden CL. The Association between Food Insecurity and Obesity in Children-The National Health and Nutrition Examination Survey. J Acad Nutr Diet 2015;115(5):751–8.

40. Liu J, Rehm CD, Onopa J, et al. Trends in Diet Quality among Youth in the United States, 1999-2016. JAMA, J Am Med Assoc 2020;323(12):1161–74.

41. Dutko P, Ver Ploeg M, Farrigan T. Characteristics and influential factors of food deserts, ERR-140. U.S. Department of Agriculture: Economic Research Service; 2012.

42. Walker RE, Keane CR, Burke JG. Disparities and access to healthy food in the United States: A review of food deserts literature. Health Place 2010;16(5):876–84.

43. Larson NI, Story MT, Nelson MC. Neighborhood Environments. Am J Prev Med 2009;36(1):74–81.e10.

44. Institute for Child, Youth, and Family Policy at the Heller School for Social Policy and Management at Brandeis University. Child Opportunity Index (COI). Available at: https://www.diversitydatakids.org/child-opportunity-indexdiversitydatakids.org. (Accessed July 31, 2024).

45. Agency for Toxic Substances and Disease Registry. CDC/ATSDR Social Vulnerability Index. For Toxic Substances and Disease Registry. CDC/ATSDR Social Vulnerability Index. 2024. Available at: https://www.atsdr.cdc.gov/placeandhealth/svi/index.htmlAgency (Accessed July 31, 2024).

46. Aris IM, Perng W, Dabelea D, et al. Associations of Neighborhood Opportunity and Social Vulnerability with Trajectories of Childhood Body Mass Index and Obesity among US Children. JAMA Netw Open 2022;5(12):E2247957. https://doi.org/10.1001/jamanetworkopen.2022.47957.

47. Blatt LR, Sadler RC, Jones EJ, et al. Historical Structural Racism in the Built Environment and Contemporary Children's Opportunities. Pediatrics 2024;153(2). https://doi.org/10.1542/peds.2023-063230.

48. Theall KP, Chaparro MP, Denstel K, et al. Childhood obesity and the associated roles of neighborhood and biologic stress. Prev Med Reports 2019;14. https://doi.org/10.1016/j.pmedr.2019.100849.

49. United States Department of Agriculture. About WIC. 2022. Available at: https://www.fns.usda.gov/wic/about-wic. [Accessed 2 January 2024].

50. Centers of Disease Control and Prevention. Obesity Among Young Children Enrolled in WIC. 2022. Available at: https://www.cdc.gov/obesity/data/obesity-among-WIC-enrolled-young-children.html. [Accessed 2 January 2024].

51. United States Department of Agriculture. National and State Level Estimates of WIC Eligibility and Program Reach in 2020. 2023. Available at: https://www.fns.usda.gov/research/wic/eligibility-and-program-reach-estimates-2020. [Accessed 2 January 2024].

52. Agyapong E, Vasan A, Anyigbo C. Reducing WIC Administrative Burdens to Promote Health Equity. JAMA Pediatr 2024. https://doi.org/10.1001/jamapediatrics.2023.6504.

53. Monroe BS, Rengifo LM, Wingler MR, et al. Assessing and Improving WIC Enrollment in the Primary Care Setting: A Quality Initiative. Pediatrics 2023;152(2). https://doi.org/10.1542/peds.2022-057613.

54. Rundle AG, Park Y, Herbstman JB, et al. COVID-19–Related School Closings and Risk of Weight Gain Among Children. Obesity 2020;28(6):1008–9.

55. Coleman PC, Hanson P, van Rens T, et al. A rapid review of the evidence for children's TV and online advertisement restrictions to fight obesity. Prev Med Reports 2022;26:101717. https://doi.org/10.1016/j.pmedr.2022.101717.

56. Powell LM, Wada R, Kumanyika SK. Racial/ethnic and income disparities in child and adolescent exposure to food and beverage television ads across the U.S. media markets. Health Place 2014;29:124–31.

57. Sanders LM, Perrin EM, Yin HS, et al. "Greenlight study": a controlled trial of low-literacy, early childhood obesity prevention. Pediatrics 2014;133(6):e1724–37.

58. Sanders LM, Perrin EM, Yin HS, et al. A health-literacy intervention for early childhood obesity prevention: A cluster-randomized controlled trial. Pediatrics 2021; 147(5). https://doi.org/10.1542/peds.2020-049866.

59. Heerman WJ, Yin HS, Schildcrout JS, et al. The Effect of an Obesity Prevention Intervention Among Specific Subpopulations: A Heterogeneity of Treatment Effect Analysis of the Greenlight Trial. Child Obes 2024. https://doi.org/10.1089/chi.2023.0171.

60. Liu BY, Rome BN. State Coverage and Reimbursement of Antiobesity Medications in Medicaid. JAMA 2024;331(14):1230.

61. Bomberg EM, Palzer EF, Rudser KD, et al. Anti-obesity medication prescriptions by race/ethnicity and use of an interpreter in a pediatric weight management clinic. Ther Adv Endocrinol Metab 2022;13:20420188221090010. https://doi.org/10.1177/20420188221090009.

62. Perez NP, Westfal ML, Stapleton SM, et al. Beyond insurance: race-based disparities in the use of metabolic and bariatric surgery for the management of severe pediatric obesity. Surg Obes Relat Dis 2020;16(3):414–9.

63. The American Board of Pediatrics. Improving Health and Health Care. 2024. Available at: https://www.abp.org/content/improving-health-and-health-care-part-4. [Accessed 5 July 2024].

64. World Health Organization. Health Equity Assessment Toolkit. Available at: https://www.who.int/data/inequality-monitor/assessment_toolkit. [Accessed 5 July 2024].

65. Lion KC, Faro EZ, Coker TR. All Quality Improvement Is Health Equity Work: Designing Improvement to Reduce Disparities. Pediatrics 2022;149(Supplement 3). https://doi.org/10.1542/peds.2020-045948E.

66. Hood CM, Gennuso KP, Swain GR, et al. County Health Rankings. Am J Prev Med 2016;50(2):129–35.

67. Anonymous. Promoting Food Security for All Children. Pediatrics 2015;136(5): e1431–8. https://doi.org/10.1542/peds.2015-3301.

68. Orr CJ, Chauvenet C, Ozgun H, et al. Caregivers' Experiences With Food Insecurity Screening and Impact of Food Insecurity Resources. Clin Pediatr 2019; 58(14):1484–92.

69. Palakshappa D, Vasan A, Khan S, et al. Clinicians' perceptions of screening for food insecurity in suburban pediatric practice. Pediatrics 2017;140(1): e20170319.

70. Ashbrook A., Essel K., Montez M., Bennett-Tejes D., *Screen and Intervene: A Toolkit for Pediatricians to Address Food Insecurity.* Available at: https://frac.org/aaptoolkit. (Accessed July 31, 2024).

71. Heerman WJ, Kenney E, Block JP, et al. A Narrative Review of Public Health Interventions for Childhood Obesity. Curr Obes Rep 2024. https://doi.org/10.1007/s13679-023-00550-z.

72. The Joint Commission. *National Patient Safety Goal to Improve Health Care Equity.*; 2022. Available at: https://www.jointcommission.org/standards/r3-report/r3-report-issue-38-national-patient-safety-goal-to-improve-health-care-equity/. (Accessed July 31, 2024).

73. Cruz Herrera E, Figueroa-Nieves AI, Woo Baidal JA. The potential role of social care in reducing childhood obesity. Curr Opin Pediatr 2023. https://doi.org/10.1097/mop.0000000000001309.

74. Garg A, Brochier A, Tripodis Y, et al. A Social Care System Implemented in Pediatric Primary Care: A Cluster RCT. Pediatrics 2023;152(2). https://doi.org/10.1542/peds.2023-061513.

Weight Bias and Stigma in Pediatric Obesity

Brooke E. Wagner, PhD[a], Stephen Cook, MD, MPH[b],*

KEYWORDS

- Weight bias • Obesity • Stigma • Provider behavior • Patient-centered care
- Pediatrics

KEY POINTS

- Obesity is one of the most common chronic diseases in pediatrics whose complexity involves many social, environmental, and biologic contributing factors.
- Despite this growing science, many misperceptions still perpetuate views that obesity is a result of personal weakness, or in the case of children, poor parenting.
- Weight or obesity stigma is experienced in childhood and adolescence in many settings, such as schools, family interaction, and the health care setting.
- Pediatric clinicians and health care systems for children need to be aware of these biases.
- System-level and individual-level strategies are developing to address weight bias.

INTRODUCTION

Stigma of individuals or groups leads to various discriminations that reduce social acceptance, reduce opportunities, and worsen social inequities for these individuals or groups.[1] Weight stigma refers to the social devaluation of a person based on body weight, and it commonly leads to teasing, rejection, and bullying among youth.[2] Stigmatizing behaviors are a result of weight-related biases and stereotypes or negative beliefs that people of higher weight status are lazy or lack willpower.[2] Weight stigma is pervasive during childhood and adolescent years, with as many as 50% of all youth, and 78% of youth seeking weight treatment having been bullied because of their weight.[3] Well-established physical and psychosocial health consequences of weight stigma make it especially harmful during a critical period of development and relationship building for youth. Lasting negative health impacts of these experiences highlight the importance of addressing weight stigma early on. The pediatric health care setting can be one of many sources of weight-stigmatizing experiences

[a] Department of Population Health Sciences, Duke Center for Childhood Obesity Research, Duke University School of Medicine, 215 Morris Street, Durham, NC, USA; [b] Nationwide Children's Hospital, 700 Children's Drive, LA 5F, Columbus, OH, USA
* Corresponding author.
E-mail address: Stephen.cook@osumc.edu

Pediatr Clin N Am 71 (2024) 819–830
https://doi.org/10.1016/j.pcl.2024.07.005
0031-3955/24/© 2024 Elsevier Inc. All rights reserved, including those for text and data mining, AI training, and similar technologies.

for youth and can create barriers to health-seeking behaviors and engagement in care for many health conditions.[4–6] This has prompted calls to action for health care settings to reduce weight biases and stigmatizing behavior among pediatric providers.[2,7] The American Academy of Pediatrics recently released an evidence-based, Clinical Practice Guideline for obesity care for children and youth,[8] which harnessed an important opportunity to raise awareness of harmful individual-level and institutional-level weight biases in health care settings. This overview focuses on the complexity and pervasiveness of weight stigma experienced by youth and their families. This discussion highlights the pediatric health care setting and providers and their role in weight bias.

COMMON SOURCES OF WEIGHT STIGMA

Youth are subject to weight stigma from many different people and settings. Most commonly, children experience weight stigma from peers, educators, family members, and media. In school settings, teachers and parents have viewed weight-related bullying as the most common type of bullying in schools,[9,10] and it was reported by adolescents as the most prevalent form of verbal harassment at school from both peers and friends.[11,12] Unfortunately, youth are not exempt from negative experiences from educators and parents either. For example, teachers have had lower expectations of students with obesity, both physically and academically,[13] and assigned lower grades to students with overweight.[14] Parents have been identified among youth as additional sources of comments and teasing about their weight.[3]

Media platforms also promote baseless societal standards for acceptable body shapes and sizes, exacerbating the problem of weight biases and stigma that youth face. Increases in electronic and Internet usage in recent years make youth particularly vulnerable to stigmatizing messages and experiences through media sources. Television shows and movies have perpetuated stigmatizing content through stereotypical and negative portrayals of characters with larger body sizes as unhealthy and the targets of ridicule.[15,16] More recent literature has begun to examine personally targeted electronic forms of weight-based stigma or victimization in youth (ie, cyberbullying or cybervictimization); social media, online, and text are common sources of teasing and name calling due to weight.[11,17]

HEALTH IMPLICATIONS OF WEIGHT STIGMA EXPERIENCED DURING CHILDHOOD

Childhood and adolescence are important formative years for identity, self-concept, and relationship building, which make them especially vulnerable to social influences. In the case of overweight and obesity, weight stigma is particularly widespread,[18] and those with overweight experience greater levels of rejection and bullying than their peers with normal weight.[19]

Social-emotional Health

Judgments and stigmatizing experiences because of weight are particularly damaging to emotional and psychological health during these formative years. Studies show that youth that are teased or bullied because of their weight have an increase in depressive symptoms, anxiety, and body dissatisfaction, as well as lower levels of self-esteem and overall quality of life.[3,20,21] Some youth have reported that they would go as far as to seek weight loss treatment in order to avoid continued bullying and improve social interactions.[21] Youth may also face academic challenges as a result of stigma, including lower academic performance and avoiding certain classes or even school altogether.[22] More extreme consequences, like self-harm and suicidality, are also of significant concern as a result of any form of victimization; recent evidence suggests that adolescents experiencing negative treatment based on weight have nearly double the odds of engaging in physical self-harm.[23]

Physical Health

Youth that experience teasing or victimization because of their weight are also at an increased risk for engaging in negative health behaviors, especially related to disordered eating and low engagement in physical activity. Dieting, unhealthy weight control behaviors, overeating, and loss of control eating have been found to be significantly more prevalent among adolescents that had been previously teased about weight.[24] Among younger students (8–12 years), weight teasing mediated the relationship between body mass index (BMI) and disordered eating behaviors,[25] which suggests that negative experiences associated with weight play a significant role in how youth cope with these experiences through behaviors. Less literature exists around physical activity outcomes among youth. Still, some have demonstrated lower levels of confidence engaging in physical activity, overall lower levels of physical activity, less participation in sports, and specifically avoiding school activities that include physical activity (ie, PE classes, afterschool activities).[3,7]

Weight Bias Internalization

Acknowledging and accepting weight-based stereotypes about oneself is termed weight bias internalization (WBI).[26] WBI is associated with negative physical health and behaviors (ie, low physical activity and maladaptive eating behaviors), as well as negative mental health outcomes (ie, low self-esteem, quality of life, depression, and anxiety).[27,28] Importantly, strong positive associations were found between experiences of weight stigma and WBI.[28] Since WBI occurs as a result of known biases or stigmatizing events, the psychological and physical health consequences as a result of weight stigma experiences may be driven, in part, by WBI. For example, in a sample of treatment seeking adolescents, WBI mediated the relationship between weight-based teasing and disordered eating behaviors.[29] More research is needed to better understand the specific role that WBI plays between experiences of stigma and other health outcomes among youth.

Longitudinal Consequences and the Cycle of Obesity

Negative implications resulting from weight stigma that occurred during childhood may persist over time and even into adulthood. Adults who experienced weight-based teasing early in childhood were found to use eating as a way to cope and unhealthy weight control behaviors many years later.[24,30] Psychosocial consequences, such as low levels of self-esteem, decreased body satisfaction, and higher levels of depression, were reported in adults 5 to 15 years after experiences of weight teasing.[30–32] Although scarce, weight-based teasing has also been linked to substance use up to 10 years later, including increased alcohol consumption and binge-drinking frequency, marijuana use, and cigarette use.[3]

Psychological distress and maladaptive health behaviors because of weight stigma may contribute to additional weight gain among children and adolescents. Weight-based victimization and teasing during childhood were found to be predictive of a higher BMI and fat mass and a greater risk of having obesity in adulthood.[30,33] Additional weight gain may perpetuate weight-stigmatizing experiences in adulthood and continue the promotion of a weight stigma-obesity feedback loop (**Fig. 1**).[34] It is clear that consequences of weight stigma begin early and may be long-lasting, which

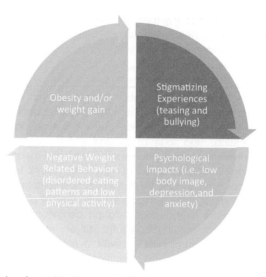

Fig. 1. Negative cycle of weight stigma and obesity.

emphasizes the importance of early intervention to reduce weight biases and stigmatizing behaviors.

WEIGHT BIAS AND STIGMA IN HEALTH CARE

Weight biases are also pervasive among both medical trainees and health care professionals toward patients with obesity.[35–38] Recent literature indicates that these biases exist across multiple health care occupations (ie, medical doctors, dietitians, psychologists, and even exercise physiologists)[36] and medical specialties (ie, urology, anesthesiology, and orthopedic surgery).[38] While a substantial amount of current literature pertains to the care specifically of adult populations,[39,40] more recent evidence has confirmed that these biases also exist among a range of providers treating pediatric patients.[41] In a study of US pediatric health care providers (mostly nurses), participants expressed strong implicit and explicit weight biases, and agreed that, in general, health care providers have some level of bias against patients of higher weight.[42] In inpatient settings, strong implicit weight biases were prevalent among advanced practice providers and nurses, which were even acknowledged by providers during qualitative interviews.[37] Age and years of practice have also been positively associated with implicit biases about weight.[42] Similar findings extend globally, where multiple pediatric disciplines in the Netherlands expressed negative attitudes and frustrations toward patients with obesity.[41] For example, pediatricians and general practitioners reported the highest number of negative weight-biased attitudes and, especially, felt that children with obesity were noncompliant with treatment recommendations and that they were difficult.[41]

Impact on Patient Communication and Quality of Care

The impact of weight bias can influence the way providers talk with patients and the quality of care delivered. In one study, adolescent patient perceptions of their relationship with providers (ie, feelings of trust, perception of providers' positive regard) were negatively associated with BMI z-score. Patients also reported being less comfortable talking with doctors about their weight compared to others in their life.[43] Weight biases among providers may also result in the use of stigmatizing language with patients when discussing excess body weight. For example, providers in a pediatric inpatient care setting reported often using the medical definitions and growth curves during weight-related conversations so as not to "sugarcoat" the discussion or allow the message of importance to be lost on the patient.[37] However, a recent exploration of adolescent-preferred weight terminology found that "obese" and "extremely obese" were two of the least preferred words used during provider interactions.[44] Parents seem to agree that such terms were among the most stigmatizing and least preferred terms to be used during clinical interactions between providers and their child.[45] Thus, nuanced preferences for terminology may result in unintended feelings of shame or stigma among patients. Beyond the use of stigmatizing terminology, parents have also felt stigmatized and blamed for their child's weight status.[37,46] Pediatric providers with higher levels of weight bias have shared greater concerns about the role of parents not only in their child's weight status but also the in impacting the likelihood for treatment compliance.[37] Parents often feel stigmatized by association[37] and have reported feelings of blame and embarrassment during interactions with their child's clinician.[47] During appointments, clinicians have made negative comments about their child's nutrition or weight and have made parents fear future appointments and additional comments by providers.[47]

Beyond patient–provider communication, weight biases may also result in poorer quality care for pediatric patients with obesity through the promotion of stigmatizing environments. In a study of different types of Dutch health care professionals, over 60% of both general practitioners and pediatricians reported having heard or witnessed other professionals make negative comments about patients with obesity,[41] which not only creates a stigmatizing environment among providers but also for all patients who may have heard these comments. The office environment itself might further risk the quality of care if patients are being weighed and spoken to about the reason for their visit in public spaces.[43] Although the literature is minimal among pediatric providers, recent qualitative data have found that providers also often believe that weight impacts specifically inpatient care, from deciding on a course of treatment to general difficulties in providing care.[37] Ultimately, weight biases among pediatric providers often lead to stigmatizing encounters between providers and patients and negatively impacting the quality of both communication and care that patients with a higher body weight receive.

Avoidance in Health Care

In addition to negative health outcomes mentioned previously, experiencing weight stigma specifically within health care settings may also lead to avoiding or delaying health care altogether. In a nationwide survey, some parents reported that they would seek a new provider or would avoid future appointments altogether if they perceived stigmatizing behavior toward their child during visits.[45] Although much of the current literature is based on parent perspectives, their reactions are important as the caretakers often schedule appointments and make sure their child gets to them. Adult literature also indicates that stigmatizing situations and lower patient-centered communication mediate the relationship between BMI and delaying care and attempting to switch doctors.[39] A greater understanding of how child and adolescent patients perceive stigmatizing situations from health care providers is still needed.

TOWARD STIGMA-FREE PEDIATRIC CARE

Providers have a unique opportunity to be role models in providing nonbiased stigma-free care and creating a space in which youth can develop trust and are empowered to improve their health. As a result, a 2020 joint international consensus statement made a call to action to take a pledge to eliminate weight bias and support initiatives aimed at preventing weight discrimination (**Box 1**).[2] Encouraging findings among pediatric clinicians revealed that most providers agree that patients with obesity deserve compassion and respect,[41] weight stigma is harmful to patients, and providers have a responsibility to address weight biases that they hold.[42] Some providers even felt that improving their care around weight-related discussions (ie, language used and a health focus) could play a role in mitigating potential harms that may result from talking about weight with pediatric patients.[48] A 2017 policy statement on pediatric weight stigma provides specific and foundational clinical practice and advocacy recommendations for pediatricians,[7] alongside more broad recommendations from the 2020 consensus statement to include researchers, media, and even policymakers.[2] There are additional online resources provided at the end of this article.

THE ROLE OF PEDIATRIC CLINICIANS IN REDUCING WEIGHT BIAS AND STIGMA

To expand on the 2017 policy statement, as well as recent literature on approaches for stigma reduction in health care, we have provided a list of settings and opportunities for positive impact and is described in more detail in later discussion.

1. *Personal awareness and assessment.*[3,7,49] By acknowledging that weight stigma exists within pediatric health care, and that pediatric clinicians are not resistant to weight biases, we can begin to work toward stigma-free pediatric care. This can start with the assessment of personal biases about weight, using measures such as the Weight Implicit Association Test, to increase self-awareness.[50]
2. *Training and continuing education.*[7,49,51,52] A position statement by The Obesity Society in 2018 called for reframing the narrative of obesity from lifestyle choices

---

Box 1
The pledge included in the 2020 International Consensus Statement to end weight stigma and bias[2]

The pledge to eliminate weight bias and stigma of obesity
  We recognize that
  • Individuals affected by overweight and obesity face a pervasive form of social stigma based on the typically unproven assumption that their body weight derives primarily from a lack self-discipline and personal responsibility.
  • Such portrayal is inconsistent with current scientific evidence demonstrating that body-weight regulation is not entirely under volitional control, and that biological, genetic, and environmental factors critically contribute to obesity.
  • Weight bias and stigma can result in discrimination and undermine human rights, social rights, and the health of afflicted individuals.
  • Weight stigma and discrimination cannot be tolerated in modern societies.
  We condemn
  • The use of stigmatizing language, images, attitudes, policies, and weight-based discrimination, wherever they occur.
  We pledge
  • To treat individuals with overweight and obesity with dignity and respect.
  • To refrain from using stereotypical language, images, and narratives that unfairly and inaccurately depict individuals with overweight and obesity as lazy, gluttonous, and lacking willpower or self-discipline.
  • To encourage and support educational initiatives aimed at eradicating weight bias through dissemination of current knowledge of obesity and body-weight regulation.
  • To encourage and support initiatives aimed at preventing weight discrimination in the workplace, education, and health care settings.

or behavioral issues as a cause to treating obesity as the complex chronic disease that it is. By increasing the understanding of the complexity of obesity, from noncontrollable factors like genetic and environmental factors[53] to social determinants of health and previous trauma,[54] level of weight bias may be reduced[52] and higher quality care can be provided. While medical school and residency programs should implement training on obesity as a disease, providers should seek out additional training throughout their professional career. Training should also include cross-cultural competencies to address the intersection of weight bias and racial disparities, as well as "allyship" training to better support inclusivity and reduce discrimination.[55] Specific points to address weight bias in medical training are highlighted in **Box 2**.

3. *Clinical environment.*[7,49,51] Waiting rooms and examination rooms in a clinical practice should be home to furniture that is comfortable for people of larger body sizes, printed materials that are weight inclusive, appropriate size physical examination materials (ie, gowns and robes, blood pressure cuffs), and allow for privacy when taking weight measurements. Role modeling professional behavior and nonstigmatizing care should also occur at all levels, from faculty to trainee. This can be achieved through the use of kind and preferred language and terminology including "people first" language ("child with overweight" rather than "overweight child"), as well as supportive and motivating care. Demonstrating positive behavior between providers and colleagues fosters an environment in which nonstigmatizing behavior and communication becomes common practice.

4. *Language and communication.*[7,44,45,49,56–59] Communication is a key component to effectively address stigma and bias. Although previously acknowledged as a standard of practice and a first step in reducing stigmatizing language,[60,61] 2023 joint international statement to support and encourage the use of people-first language aimed to continue these efforts and highlight its importance.[59] It is also important to ask permission to talk about weight and utilize preferred terms when talking about weight. Weight-related terminology preferences, on the other hand, tend to be much more nuanced and person specific. Parents and adolescents reported similar preference for the use of terms like "weight" and "plus size," while "extremely obese," "obese," and "fat" were least desirable.[44,45,58] However, preferences differed across adolescent gender, weight status, and level of internalized weight stigma.[44] Starting the conversation by asking permission to discuss weight. This should occur with the parent of preadolescent patients as well

---

Box 2
Summarized strategies for reducing bias in pediatric health care settings

Steps to reduce bias in medical training
1. Recognize complexity of obesity as a disease, not a personal failure.
2. Focus on health, and not weight, as the primary goal.
3. Provide experiential learning from patients with obesity.
4. Use tools to increase professional and personal awareness of weight bias.
5. Offer training to clinicians and staff to counteract their weight bias.
6. Respect patients' autonomy for their preference to engage with obesity treatment.
7. Use people-first language.
8. Provide health care settings that accommodate patients of different body size.
9. Offer nonstigmatizing images of people with obesity in public health, clinical and marketing materials.
10. Advocate for students, clinicians, and staff to take the pledge of the international joint statement to eliminate weight stigma.

as asking the adolescent patient's permission to discuss weight with them is a neutral way to approach weight-related discussions, which can lead to questions about preferred terminology. Accordingly, providers should ask patients what terms they are most comfortable with using.

5. *Health-focused and patient-centered approach to treatment.*[7,34,49,62] When approaching the topic of weight with pediatric patients and their parent/caregiver/family, clinicians should acknowledge the complexity of obesity and discuss the range of contributors. With this, all treatment options that align with the patient's medical history should be reviewed to find a best fit for the patient and their family.

SUMMARY

The pervasiveness of weight bias and stigma is still very prevalent in many aspects of our society. Unfortunately, youth are not sheltered from the harmful effects of weight stigma. Health care has taken many steps to raise awareness of, and address, the negative biases patients experience relative to physical, developmental, and intellectual disabilities, as well as many chronic conditions. The research on the negative impacts of weight bias and stigma has been around for nearly as long as it has for other chronic conditions. Yet, when it comes to raising awareness and taking steps to address these factors, the health care system has been very slow to respond. The slow response, in and of itself, could be viewed as a type of institutional weight bias. Pediatric clinicians have always been strong advocates for the health of children and their families. The policy statements and clinical guidelines by leading pediatric professional groups might be the early sign of a turning tide. These steps are greatly needed now as health care is experiencing rapid advances to address obesity and unhealthy weight.

POINTS FOR HEALTH CARE AND EDUCATION OF HEALTH CARE PROVIDERS

For additional resources, pediatric health care providers should examine these sites:

1. Supportive Obesity Care (Sponsored by the Rudd Center): https://supportiveobesity care.rudd.center.uconn.edu/.
2. Rudd Center Research: https://uconnruddcenter.org/research/weight biasstigma/.
3. The Obesity Action Coalition Advocacy page: https://www.obesityaction.org/advocacy/what-we-fight-for/weight-bias.
4. Balanced View: Addressing Weight Bias and Stigma in Health Care https://balancedviewbc.ca (5 Module course).

CLINICS CARE POINTS

- Academic institutions, professional bodies, and regulatory agencies must ensure that formal teaching on the causes, mechanisms, and treatments of obesity are incorporated into standard curricula for medical trainees and other health care providers.

- Health care providers specialized in treating obesity should provide evidence of stigma-free practice skills. Professional bodies should encourage, facilitate, and develop methods to certify knowledge of stigma and its effects, along with stigma-free skills and practices.

- Given the prevalence of obesity and obesity-related diseases, appropriate infrastructure for the care and management of people with obesity, including severe obesity, must be the standard of care for accreditation of medical facilities and hospitals.

DISCLOSURE

The authors have no commercial or financial conflicts of interest to disclose.

REFERENCES

1. Stangl AL, Earnshaw VA, Logie CH, et al. The Health Stigma and Discrimination Framework: a global, crosscutting framework to inform research, intervention development, and policy on health-related stigmas. BMC Med 2019;17(1):31.
2. Rubino F, Puhl RM, Cummings DE, et al. Joint international consensus statement for ending stigma of obesity. Nat Med 2020;26(4):485–97.
3. Puhl RM, Lessard LM. Weight Stigma in Youth: Prevalence, Consequences, and Considerations for Clinical Practice. Curr Obes Rep 2020;9(4):402–11.
4. Phelan SM, Burgess DJ, Yeazel MW, et al. Impact of weight bias and stigma on quality of care and outcomes for patients with obesity. Obes Rev 2015;16(4): 319–26.
5. Puhl RM, Brownell KD. Confronting and coping with weight stigma: An investigation of overweight and obese adults. Obesity 2006;14(10):1802–15.
6. Puhl RM, Heuer CA. The stigma of obesity: a review and update. Obesity 2009; 17(5):941–64.
7. Pont SJ, Puhl R, Cook SR, et al. Stigma Experienced by Children and Adolescents With Obesity. Pediatrics 2017;140(6). https://doi.org/10.1542/peds.2017-3034.
8. Hampl SE, Hassink SG, Skinner AC, et al. Executive Summary: Clinical Practice Guideline for the Evaluation and Treatment of Children and Adolescents With Obesity. Pediatrics 2023;151(2). https://doi.org/10.1542/peds.2022-060641.
9. Bradshaw CP, Waasdorp TE, O'Brennan LM, et al. Teachers' and Education Support Professionals' Perspectives on Bullying and Prevention: Findings From a National Education Association Study. School Psych Rev 2013;42(3):280–97.
10. Puhl RM, Latner JD, O'Brien K, et al. Cross-national perspectives about weight-based bullying in youth: nature, extent and remedies. Pediatr Obes 2016;11(4): 241–50.
11. Puhl RM, Peterson JL, Luedicke J. Weight-based victimization: bullying experiences of weight loss treatment-seeking youth. Pediatrics 2013;131(1):e1–9.
12. Himmelstein MS, Puhl RM. Weight-based victimization from friends and family: implications for how adolescents cope with weight stigma. Pediatric Obesity 2019;14(1):e12453. https://doi.org/10.1111/ijpo.12453.
13. Nutter S, Ireland A, Alberga AS, et al. Weight Bias in Educational Settings: a Systematic Review. Current Obesity Reports 2019;8(2):185–200.
14. Finn KE, Seymour CM, Phillips AE. Weight bias and grading among middle and high school teachers. Br J Educ Psychol 2020;90(3):635–47.
15. Howard JB, Skinner AC, Ravanbakht SN, et al. Obesogenic Behavior and Weight-Based Stigma in Popular Children's Movies, 2012 to 2015. Pediatrics 2017; 140(6). https://doi.org/10.1542/peds.2017-2126.
16. Eisenberg ME, Carlson-McGuire A, Gollust SE, et al. A content analysis of weight stigmatization in popular television programming for adolescents. Int J Eat Disord 2015;48(6):759–66.
17. Lessard LM, Puhl RM. <scp>Weight-based</scp> cybervictimization: Implications for adolescent health. Pediatric Obesity 2022;17(6). https://doi.org/10.1111/ijpo.12888.
18. Puhl RM, Latner JD. Stigma, obesity, and the health of the nation's children. Psychol Bull 2007;133(4):557–80.

19. Morales DX, Prieto N, Grineski SE, et al. Race/Ethnicity, Obesity, and the Risk of Being Verbally Bullied: a National Multilevel Study. Journal of Racial and Ethnic Health Disparities 2019;6(2):245–53.

20. Warnick JL, Darling KE, West CE, et al. Weight Stigma and Mental Health in Youth: A Systematic Review and Meta-Analysis. J Pediatr Psychol 2022;47(3):237–55.

21. Reece LJ, Bissell P, Copeland RJ. I just don't want to get bullied anymore, then I can lead a normal life'; Insights into life as an obese adolescent and their views on obesity treatment. Health Expect 2016;19(4):897–907.

22. Puhl RM, Luedicke J. Weight-based victimization among adolescents in the school setting: emotional reactions and coping behaviors. J Youth Adolesc 2012;41(1):27–40.

23. Sutin AR, Robinson E, Daly M, et al. Perceived Body Discrimination and Intentional Self-Harm and Suicidal Behavior in Adolescence. Child Obes 2018;14(8):528–36.

24. Hooper L, Puhl R, Eisenberg ME, et al. Weight teasing experienced during adolescence and young adulthood: Cross-sectional and longitudinal associations with disordered eating behaviors in an ethnically/racially and socioeconomically diverse sample. Int J Eat Disord 2021;54(8):1449–62.

25. Côté M, Legendre M, Aimé A, et al. The paths to children's disordered eating: The implications of BMI, weight-related victimization, body dissatisfaction and parents' disordered eating. Clinical Psychology in Europe 2020;2(1). https://doi.org/10.32872/cpe.v2i1.2689.

26. Durso LE, Latner JD. Understanding self-directed stigma: development of the weight bias internalization scale. Obesity 2008;16(Suppl 2):S80–6.

27. Butt M, Harvey A, Khesroh E, et al. Assessment and impact of paediatric internalized weight bias: A systematic review. Pediatr Obes 2023;18(7):e13040. https://doi.org/10.1111/ijpo.13040.

28. Foster T, Eaton M, Probst Y. The relationship between internalised weight bias and biopsychosocial outcomes in children and youth: a systematic review. J Eat Disord 2024;12(1):38.

29. Zuba A, Warschburger P. The role of weight teasing and weight bias internalization in psychological functioning; a prospective study among school-aged children. Eur Child Adolesc Psychiatr 2017;26(10):1245–55.

30. Puhl RM, Wall MM, Chen C, et al. Experiences of weight teasing in adolescence and weight-related outcomes in adulthood: A 15-year longitudinal study. Prev Med 2017;100:173–9.

31. Eisenberg ME, Neumark-Sztainer D, Paxton SJ. Five-year change in body satisfaction among adolescents. J Psychosom Res 2006;61(4):521–7.

32. Eisenberg ME, Neumark-Sztainer D, Haines J, et al. Weight-teasing and emotional well-being in adolescents: longitudinal findings from Project EAT. J Adolesc Health 2006;38(6):675–83.

33. Schvey NA, Marwitz SE, Mi SJ, et al. Weight-based teasing is associated with gain in BMI and fat mass among children and adolescents at-risk for obesity: A longitudinal study. Pediatric Obesity 2019;14(10):e12538. https://doi.org/10.1111/ijpo.12538.

34. Haqq AM, Kebbe M, Tan Q, et al. Complexity and Stigma of Pediatric Obesity. Child Obes 2021;17(4):229–40.

35. Phelan SM, Dovidio JF, Puhl RM, et al. Implicit and explicit weight bias in a national sample of 4,732 medical students: the medical student CHANGES study. Obesity 2014;22(4):1201–8.

36. Lawrence BJ, Kerr D, Pollard CM, et al. Weight bias among health care professionals: A systematic review and meta-analysis. Obesity 2021;29(11):1802–12.
37. Halvorson EE, Curley T, Wright M, et al. Weight Bias in Pediatric Inpatient Care. Acad Pediatr Sep-Oct 2019;19(7):780–6.
38. Philip SR, Fields SA, Van Ryn M, et al. Comparisons of Explicit Weight Bias Across Common Clinical Specialties of US Resident Physicians. J Gen Intern Med 2023. https://doi.org/10.1007/s11606-023-08433-8.
39. Phelan SM, Bauer KW, Bradley D, et al. A model of weight-based stigma in health care and utilization outcomes: Evidence from the learning health systems network. Obes Sci Pract 2022;8(2):139–46.
40. Gudzune KA, Bennett WL, Cooper LA, et al. Perceived judgment about weight can negatively influence weight loss: a cross-sectional study of overweight and obese patients. Prev Med 2014;62:103–7.
41. van der Voorn B, Camfferman R, Seidell JC, et al. Weight-biased attitudes about pediatric patients with obesity in Dutch healthcare professionals from seven different professions. J Child Health Care 2023. https://doi.org/10.1177/13674935221133953. 13674935221133953.
42. Turner SL. Pediatric healthcare professionals' attitudes and beliefs about weight stigma: A descriptive study. J Pediatr Nurs 2023;75:64–71.
43. Cohen ML, Tanofsky-Kraff M, Young-Hyman D, et al. Weight and its relationship to adolescent perceptions of their providers (WRAP): A qualitative and quantitative assessment of teen weight-related preferences and concerns. J Adolesc Health 2005;37(2):163.
44. Puhl RM, Himmelstein MS. Adolescent preferences for weight terminology used by health care providers. Pediatr Obes 2018;13(9):533–40.
45. Puhl RM, Peterson JL, Luedicke J. Parental perceptions of weight terminology that providers use with youth. Pediatrics 2011;128(4):e786–93.
46. Edmunds LD. Parents' perceptions of health professionals' responses when seeking help for their overweight children. Fam Pract 2005;22(3):287–92.
47. Gorlick JC, Gorman CV, Weeks HM, et al. I Feel Like Less of a Mom": Experiences of Weight Stigma by Association among Mothers of Children with Overweight and Obesity. Child Obes 2021;17(1):68–75.
48. Loth KA, Lebow J, Uy MJA, et al. First, Do No Harm: Understanding Primary Care Providers' Perception of Risks Associated With Discussing Weight With Pediatric Patients. Glob Pediatr Health 2021;8. https://doi.org/10.1177/2333794X211040979. 2333794X211040979.
49. Braddock A, Browne NT, Houser M, et al. Weight stigma and bias: A guide for pediatric clinicians. Obes Pillars 2023;6:100058. https://doi.org/10.1016/j.obpill.2023.100058.
50. Greenwald AG, Nosek BA, Banaji MR. Understanding and using the implicit association test: I. An improved scoring algorithm. J Pers Soc Psychol 2003;85(2):197–216.
51. Talumaa B, Brown A, Batterham RL, et al. Effective strategies in ending weight stigma in healthcare. Obes Rev 2022;23(10). https://doi.org/10.1111/obr.13494.
52. Watowicz RP, Ramesh H. Short-term improvement in self-perceived knowledge and weight bias following a 15-week course on pediatric obesity. Journal of Dietetic Education 2023;1(2).
53. Dietz WH, Baur LA, Hall K, et al. Management of obesity: improvement of healthcare training and systems for prevention and care. Lancet 2015;385(9986):2521–33.

54. Williams DR, Braddock A, Houser M, et al. Review of upstream social factors contributing to childhood obesity. Obes Pillars 2022;4:100040. https://doi.org/10.1016/j.obpill.2022.100040.
55. Waldrop SW, Wang D, Kancherla D, et al. Current status of weight bias and stigma in pediatrics and the need for greater focus on populations at risk. Curr Opin Pediatr 2024;36(1):42–8.
56. Provvidenza CF, Hartman LR, McPherson AC. Fostering positive weight-related conversations between health care professionals, children, and families: Development of a knowledge translation Casebook and evaluation protocol. Child Care Health Dev 2019;45(1):138–45.
57. Puhl RM. What words should we use to talk about weight? A systematic review of quantitative and qualitative studies examining preferences for weight-related terminology. Obes Rev 2020;21(6):e13008. https://doi.org/10.1111/obr.13008.
58. Puhl RM, Himmelstein MS, Armstrong SC, et al. Adolescent preferences and reactions to language about body weight. Int J Obes 2017;41(7):1062–5.
59. Weghuber D, Khandpur N, Boyland E, et al. Championing the use of people-first language in childhood overweight and obesity to address weight bias and stigma: A joint statement from theEuropean-Childhood-Obesity-Group(ECOG), the<scp>European-Coalition-for-People-Living-with-O. Pediatric Obesity 2023;18(6). https://doi.org/10.1111/ijpo.13024.
60. Palad CJ, Yarlagadda S, Stanford FC. Weight stigma and its impact on paediatric care. Curr Opin Endocrinol Diabetes Obes 2019;26(1):19–24.
61. Kyle TK, Puhl RM. Putting people first in obesity. Obesity 2014;22(5):1211.
62. Cardel MI, Newsome FA, Pearl RL, et al. Patient-Centered Care for Obesity: How Health Care Providers Can Treat Obesity While Actively Addressing Weight Stigma and Eating Disorder Risk. J Acad Nutr Diet 2022;122(6):1089–98.

The Built Environment and Childhood Obesity

Maida P. Galvez, MD, MPH[a,b,*], Katharine McCarthy, PhD, MPH[c,d],
Chethan Sarabu, MD[e], Alison Mears, AIA LEED AP[f]

KEYWORDS

- Childhood obesity • Built environment • Ecological systems theory
- Physical activity • Children and nature • Obesogens

KEY POINTS

- The built environment includes physical structures where children live, learn, eat, sleep, and play.
- Features of the built environment (eg, availability of parks and playgrounds) can influence children's physical activity (PA) levels, diet, sleep, stress, and overall health including risk for obesity.
- Neighborhood level disparities in the built environment contribute to disparities in PA levels and risk for obesity seen in low-income communities and communities of color.
- To combat the childhood obesity epidemic, consideration of environmental public health prevention strategies and policies that promote healthy behaviors and healthy communities is required.

DEFINITIONS
Built Environment

This includes the physical features of neighborhoods including homes, schools, workplaces, neighborhood walkability/density, green spaces, transportation networks, and more that can influence overall community health.[1]

[a] Department of Environmental Medicine & Climate Science, Icahn School of Medicine at Mount Sinai, Gustave Levy Place Box 1057, New York, NY 10029, USA; [b] Department of Pediatrics, Icahn School of Medicine at Mount Sinai, Gustave Levy Place Box 1057, New York, NY 10029, USA; [c] Department of Population Health Science & Policy, Blavatnik Family Women's Health Research Institute, Icahn School of Medicine at Mount Sinai, 1770 Madison Avenue, Floor 2, New York, NY, USA; [d] Department of Obstetrics, Gynecology & Reproductive Science, Blavatnik Family Women's Health Research Institute, Icahn School of Medicine at Mount Sinai, 1770 Madison Avenue, Floor 2, New York, NY, USA; [e] Cornell Tech, 2 West Loop Road, New York, NY 10044, USA; [f] Healthy Materials Lab, Parsons School of Design, 2 West 13th Street Room 310
* Corresponding author. Icahn School of Medicine, 1 Gustave L. Levy Place Box 1057, New York, NY 10029.
E-mail address: maida.galvez@mssm.edu

Pediatr Clin N Am 71 (2024) 831–843
https://doi.org/10.1016/j.pcl.2024.06.004
0031-3955/24/© 2024 Elsevier Inc. All rights reserved, including those for text and data mining, AI training, and similar technologies.
pediatric.theclinics.com

Ecological Systems Theory

Framework for understanding how a child's growth and development can be influenced by the child's micro and macro environments (home, school, community, and society), as well as by social interactions within those environments as proposed by Child Psychologist, Urie Bronfenbrenner, PhD.[2]

Obesogens

A class of environmental chemicals that disrupt metabolism (eg, through endocrine disruption) and as a result can promote weight gain.[3]

INTRODUCTION

Over the last several decades, there has been a notable shift in the general thinking about the root causes of childhood obesity. For many years, childhood obesity was considered to be a problem rooted solely in an individual's behaviors, that is, a child's caloric intake compounded by a sedentary lifestyle. With obesity rates rising rapidly across the United States (US) over the last several decades, and concerns that this disproportionately impacted low-income communities and communities of color, focus has shifted to upstream factors rooted in the ecological systems theory that can positively or negatively influence a child's diet, physical activity (PA), and risk for obesity.[4,5] Ongoing research is examining factors in the built environment, the physical spaces in which children live, learn, eat, sleep, and play, across urban, suburban, and rural settings and how these physical spaces impact children's health.[6,7] This inquiry spans children's homes, schools, communities, workplaces, and society at large. The underlying principle of this growing field of work is the recognition that the environment makes a difference and that public health interventions that foster healthy environments can promote healthy lifestyles for all children and their families.

HISTORY

The US Centers for Disease Control and Prevention (CDC) maps of adult obesity rates by state and trends over time released in the early 2000's made it easy to grasp both the alarming rise in obesity in the US and the direct link to place.[8] This period coincided with emerging research examining the built environment (the local food environment, PA environment, neighborhood walkability, neighborhood density, transportation networks, and more) and the influence on risk for obesity. Early research, for example, examined density of food and PA resources and proximity to homes and schools highlighting disparities by neighborhood and socioeconomic demographics. Not surprisingly, the very same communities with high rates of childhood obesity are the ones that also lack access to: fresh fruits and vegetables, parks and playgrounds, green spaces, organized sports, or gyms.[9] This is compounded by concerns of violence and crime, which keeps children indoors in low-income communities and communities of color.

Built Environment research has significantly advanced along with available technologies. The initial focus on objective and subjective measures of the environment has moved into direct measurement of behavior-environment interactions. Global positioning systems (GPS) tracking devices are readily available on mobile devices and when used in research studies in combination with dietary recalls, PA monitors, heart rate monitors, and more, there is now the ability to gain a much deeper understanding of environmental risk factors for obesity. Advances in environmental exposure assessment (eg, to assess indoor and outdoor air quality), devices to measure exposure to environmental exposures in the form of wearables, as well as biomonitoring (eg, blood and urine testing for environmental exposures), has further advanced the field.[10] Researchers are now able to study human exposures to obesogens, a wide range of common environmental chemicals found in consumer products that we are all exposed to in our daily lives.[11] Obesogens are chemicals that can interfere with metabolism or disrupt endocrine system function (also referred to as endocrine disruptors). These include phthalates, bisphenol A, perfluoroalkyl substances (PFAS), pesticides, indoor and outdoor air pollutants, and more. Through their hormonal effects (eg, altered thyroid function), obesogens can increase risk for obesity.

Research findings have already informed transformational change in communities across the US.[12–14] Here, we provide an overview of the built environment and impacts on PA and obesity to inform further educational efforts, clinical management, research, advocacy, and needed policy change.

BACKGROUND
Physical Activity Resources

Outdoor play in parks and playgrounds is important not only for children's physical development, but also for their social, emotional, and cognitive development. Sports fields, walking/hiking trails, and bicycle paths create additional opportunities for children to be outdoors and active. They are also effective ways to combat highly addictive screen time, which keeps children indoors, sedentary, and snacking. Children in the US typically far exceed the American Academy of Pediatrics (AAP) guidance of 2 hours per day of screen time, spending upwards of 7.5 hours per day on screens.[15] This also makes it challenging to meet the 60 minutes per day of PA recommended by the US CDC.[16] Time spent outdoors is associated with increased active time and decreased sedentary behaviors[17] and availability of parks is associated with lower rates of childhood obesity.[18] However, a number of studies have demonstrated disparities in availability of resources, access, density or proximity of resources to homes or schools, and quality (eg, # of amenities) by neighborhood race or ethnicity and income.[19,20] The importance of access and availability of such resources was underscored during the coronavirus disease 2019 (COVID-19) pandemic when families increasingly sought out outdoor spaces for children to play to promote children's mental health and wellness.[21,22] This highlights the critical role of parks, playgrounds, sports fields, and other PA resources in supporting overall community health.

Neighborhood Walkability/Density

Neighborhood's walkability, or the extent to which the neighborhood design facilitates walking, is a key to promoting PA and decreasing sedentary behavior. Walkability can be measured by neighborhood attributes including density (the number of points of interest in a given area), land use mix, street grid layout, the availability of destinations to travel (eg, stores, schools), the distance to public transportation, as well as the safety and desirability of walking routes.[23] Neighborhoods with higher residential density are associated with greater walking and biking among children and adolescents.[24,25] This may reflect the fact that areas with high residential density typically also have a greater number of destinations within walking or biking distance, which may promote PA.[26] Both residing in a neighborhood, and moving to a neighborhood with higher walkability is associated with greater PA and healthier weight status among children and adolescents.[27–30] While neighborhood walkability is beneficial across childhood and adolescence, evidence suggests that adolescents may be more likely to benefit from neighborhood features that encourage walking than younger children.[28]

Transportation

Greater access to public transportation (eg, higher density, number or proximity to bus, train, light rail, tram/metro, or ferry stops) in residential neighborhoods is generally observed as a protective factor against child obesity.[31,32] Greater access to public transportation facilitates active transport (eg, walking, cycling) and can result in higher PA and lead to lower obesity. While increasing the proportion of students who engage in active transport to school is a national health goal,[33] only 1 in 10 US students aged 5 to 17 years reported usually walking or biking to school in 2017, a modest decline from 13% in 2009 according to the National Transit Survey data. Reductions in child active transport highlight the need for continued investments in infrastructure to improve safety and walkability of school and residential neighborhoods. For example, programs such as 'walking school buses' and safe routes to school have been associated with greater PA among children.[34] Similarly, neighborhood design land use regulations coupled with strategies to promote bicycle sharing, protect bicycle facilities have shown effectiveness in encouraging active transport.[35]

Access to Nature

A range of studies have explored the relationship between access to nature and childhood obesity. A systematic review found that temperature, altitude, and air quality can impact weight-related behaviors in children.[36] Another systematic review found that access to green space was positively associated with PA and negatively associated with television-watching time, body mass index (BMI), and weight status among children. Better access to green space was significantly linked to a lower risk of overweight or obesity. The majority of the included studies found a positive association between access to green space and PA, and a negative association between access to green space and childhood weight-related behaviors or outcomes.[37]

More specifically, a study of outdoor play in a Head Start program with 2810 children found that the more children played outdoors during the school day, the greater the decrease in BMI, and these associations were also stronger in children who were less active at home.[38] Another study of school children aged 5 to 6 years found that, as time playing outdoors increased, there was a dose-dependent increase in moderate-to-vigorous PA as measured by accelerometers.[39] In a longitudinal cohort study, access to both parkland and recreation programs was associated with a reduced risk of overweight and obesity as measured by BMI at age 18 years. The effect sizes for access to recreation programming were much larger than those for parkland access, with significant gender differences in the impact of access to recreation programs.[40] Finally, a systematic review of the impact of green and blue spaces relation to childhood obesity, across 16 studies found that these spaces positively impact PA and eating behavior.[41] Another large study examining the built environment in Durham, North Carolina found park proximity to be associated with decreased BMI in a racially or ethnically socioeconomically diverse cohort of youth.[42] This finding was not consistent across all built environment features (eg, an inverse association was found with proximity to Healthy Miles Trails) suggesting family level interventions are needed.[42]

Violence and Crime

Exposure to community violence is an unfortunate reality for many children in the US, particularly those in urban areas. In 2016, over 77000 public school students were reported to live within a short distance of more than 10 violent crimes (homicides, aggravated assaults, and robberies).[43] Reduced outdoor PA[44] and increased stress[45,46] are 2 pathways by which neighborhood violence may influence childhood obesity.

Systematic review evidence from prospective studies demonstrated that neighborhood crime and low-perceived safety were risk factors for increased weight in childhood, but that evidence was at times inconsistent.[47] More recently, a study using public school student physical fitness measures in New York City found that adolescent girls exposed to violent crime in their neighborhood had meaningful gains in BMI and an increased probability of being overweight than those not exposed to crime but who lived in the same neighborhood.[43] The finding was specific to violence, rather than property crime, and no evidence of association was documented among boys.[43] Results suggest that efforts to curb exposure to neighborhood violence and increase perceptions of safety may be important levers to prevent child obesity and associated adverse consequences.

Air and Noise Pollution

A growing evidence base has documented the association between traffic-related effects, most notably air and noise pollution, on children health, including the endocrine system, sleeping habits, and PA.[48–50] Multiple studies have documented a link between air pollution (nitrogen dioxide and nitrogen oxides) exposure and childhood obesity.[18,51,52] For example, a study of children and adolescents who moved to more polluted areas, compared to the same or less polluted areas, had higher age- and sex-adjusted BMI in the 6 months following moving, adjusting for factors including neighborhood socioeconomic conditions.[51] Some evidence has also documented lower PA behaviors, including active transport, in areas with higher noise pollution. However, the association between noise pollution and child obesity is inconclusive, with the exception of evidence from a longitudinal cohort study, which found higher noise pollution exposure in pregnancy, but not in childhood, was associated with increased BMI trajectories.[52] Evidence from adult cohorts; however, have found road traffic noise is significantly related to increased waist circumference, waist-hip ratio, and central obesity. Those with combined exposure to multiple sources of noise (road, railway, and aircraft) may have particularly high risk.[53] Taken together, data suggest that environmental policies to reduce emissions, promote public transit, and limit high pollution traffic such as diesel trucks, from areas with populated housing, schools, and parks or playgrounds, may reduce the risk of obesity in children.

Obesogens in Building Materials

Many building products and other common consumer products contain endocrine disrupting chemicals called environmental obesogens.[54] Obesogens include bisphenol A, phthalates, parabens, polybrominated diphenyl ethers (or flame retardants), polychlorinated biphenyls, PFAS, pesticides, indoor and outdoor air pollutants, and more. They are found in a range of consumer products (**Fig. 1**). Through their hormonal effects (eg, altered thyroid function) obesogens can increase risk for obesity.

Upwards of 90% of time is spent indoors, and the materials that make up the indoor environment, and the chemicals used to make them, can impact human health. Building products are not inert and their chemical ingredients can be released as the building materials and other consumer products degrade. Exposure to the chemicals that are shed from materials and products used to construct buildings and create indoor environments contributes to indoor air that is typically 2 to 5 times worse than outdoor air quality.

Young children, babies, and pregnant people and their fetuses are most at risk of exposure to these chemicals, in part due to their developing organ systems. Young children and crawling babies also spend larger periods of time closer to the floor where airborne chemicals attach to dust and are either suspended in the air or fall

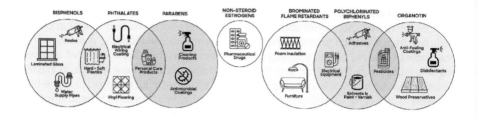

Fig. 1. Sources of obesogens: common building and consumer products. (*Courtesy of* Parsons Healthy Materials Lab.)

to the ground. They also have age-appropriate hand-to-mouth behaviors that place them at increased risk for exposure. Children can be exposed to these chemicals through inhalation, dermal absorption, or ingestion.

Environmental advocates, consumers, architects, designers, researchers, clinicians, and more are demanding increased transparency from manufacturers to more readily identify potential environmental hazards. There are over 85000 chemicals in common usage in the US. The chemicals that provide the ingredient contents of building products are rarely regulated[55] with only 5 partially regulated chemicals, including asbestos and lead. Moreover, there is an absence of adequate chemical testing before a chemical is released onto the market. Often manufacturers do not know all the additives in their products, neither the potential harm that these chemicals can cause nor the impact of the chemicals on the performance of their products. In many cases, chemicals can be simply eliminated or replaced with a safer alternative.

Obesogen Case Example: Perfluoroalkyl and Polyfluoroalkyl Substances

PFASs are highly fluorinated chemicals referred to as forever chemicals due to their persistence in the environment. These chemicals are found in many consumer products including cookware and are also common additives in a range of building products from roofing to paints and upholstery. Due to the otain and water resistance proportioo of highly fluorinated chemicals, they can be found as finishes in carpets, wall coverings, furniture upholstery, as well as in clothing. They are also additives in products like acrylic paints, which coat up to 5 surfaces in every home. Given widespread use, PFASs are found in water, food, air, and indoor dust. Human exposure occurs throughout the life cycle of the chemicals from production, use to disposal, and as a consequence PFASs are now universally detected in the population.[56,57] Children are most exposed inside their homes and at school as the interior products can shed fine dust (particulate matter) where children can inhale, ingest, or absorb these chemicals. Adverse health effects include preeclampsia, low birth-weight, elevated cholesterol, altered liver function, decreased immune response to some vaccines, and kidney and testicular cancer.[58] They have also been associated with obesity.[59,60]

Built Environment and Climate Change

Climate change is already directly impacting children's daily lives. High heat days, extreme weather events, and wildfires are now causing school physical education, sports practices, games, and class cancellations across the US[61,62]. Air pollution, a by-product of climate change, has been linked to childhood obesity.[63] Studies have shown the complex and multifaceted in which environmental factors, including climate change, can contribute to the obesity epidemic in children.[61,64,65] The use of fossil fuels, a major contributor to climate change, has been associated with both global warming and the obesity epidemic.[66] Further research is needed to fully understand the full extent of ways in which climate change may influence obesity. The AAP proposes child-centered climate solutions in the 2024 Policy Statement "Climate Change and Children's Health: Building a Healthy Future for Every Child".[67]

Healthy building materials and climate change

Recent studies have explored the intersection of chemicals, indoor air quality (IAQ), rising temperatures caused by climate change, and human health impacts.[68] Changes to our outdoor environments impact the way human-made materials perform indoors. Studies are beginning to show a clear link between rising global temperatures and deteriorating IAQ. According to a report in the International Journal of Environmental Research and Public Health, "The increase in temperature may lead to higher indoor concentrations of airborne pollutants causing higher risks of allergy, cancer, and endocrine disruption."[69] Given associations between IAQ and obesity, climate change has multiple potential pathways for which it can contribute to rising rates of obesity globally.[70,71]

Tools to model *IAQ Climate Change* impacts can help identify factors that can be exacerbated by climate change.[72] Importantly, climate impacts are not experienced equally. Globally, urban areas face higher temperatures and residents of areas with less resources and less green space will continue to suffer disproportionately as temperatures rise. In the US, neighborhoods across the country that were redlined in the early 20th century are typically the hottest in their respective regions. According to the New York Times, "neighborhoods that are poorer and have more residents of color can be 5 to 20° Fahrenheit hotter in summer than wealthier, whiter parts of the same city".[73] Localized areas of higher temperatures may lead to higher indoor concentrations of endocrine disrupting chemicals disproportionately impacting poor communities. Creating healthy indoor environments through use of healthy building materials can reduce climate-related health outcomes in children. Reducing the impacts of climate change will take a global effort and cooperation.

SUMMARY

While childhood obesity has long been recognized as multifactorial, only more recently has the medical literature experienced a paradigm shift to recognize the built environment as a key determinant of these outcomes. A growing evidence base demonstrates the promise of policy and neighborhood interventions to modify upstream features of the built environment on improving childhood obesity outcomes. These range from healthy neighborhood design that promotes walkability and access to parks and green spaces to environmental regulations aimed at curbing air and noise pollution in residential areas and in restricting the use of obesogens in building environments. To disrupt life course trajectories that lead to adverse health outcomes like obesity in midlife and beyond, the adoption of multiple strategies and a focus on translation of research evidence to clinical practice, is paramount.

CLINICS CARE POINTS

As per the Community Preventive Services Task Force (CPSTF), there is sufficient evidence base to recommend the following interventions to support PA in combination with behavioral, social, and educational approaches[74].

- *Individual:* Classroom-based PA breaks and lessons, enhanced physical education, promotion of healthy behavior change along with social supports
- *Family:* whole family PA interventions
- *Community:* community wide PA educational campaigns, creating or improving places for physical activity, increasing opportunities for active transport to school (eg, walking school bus), and healthy community design including combined efforts to integrate transportation networks, parks, trails, greenways, physical activity promoting land use, and environmental design.[74]

These recommendations can be shared in multiple settings including at well-child visits. In keeping with Ecological Systems Theory, broad consideration of public health policies that support and promote PA across children's micro and macro environments is needed to implement these CPSTF recommendations. Given extreme heat and weather-related events due to climate change and their resulting impacts on PA and outdoor time, promotion of climate resilient communities can further support these efforts. Additionally, interventions can be targeted to communities, where interventions are needed most, which includes high poverty communities, and communities of color (also referred to as Environmental Justice communities) given disproportionate environmental burdens, high rates of obesity and related co-morbidities, and potential for greater health impacts.

For Obesogens

- The national network of CDC/US EPA funded Pediatric Environmental Health Specialty Units[75] is a go-to resource for clinicians, public health professionals, and families for evidence-based information on a range of priority environmental health concerns. For example, Prescriptions for Prevention[76] are readily available in English and Spanish. These can be tailored to geographic regions to provide clinicians and families with actionable messages to prevent and reduce environmental exposures and connect families to needed community resources.
- Families can look to consumer guides for safer products, including from Environmental Working Group[77] and Green Science Policy Institute.[56]
- Many non-chemical alternatives to finishes, adhesives, and sealants can be adopted. The use of non-synthetic fabrics also called "natural" materials have inherent properties that can make a product naturally stain resistant or washable to remove stains-eliminating the need for the addition of forever chemicals. For example, mineral-based paints do not contain PFAS.
- Materials guidance can offer homeowners, architects, designers, and builders the tools to immediately avoid the worst in class chemicals and identify healthy building products. Look to existing resources that can provide independently vetted better building materials such as on the Healthy Materials Lab website[78] which points to additional reliable, independent sources of information.
- Decision-makers and companies can evaluate the manufacturing process, purchase, use, and regulations to reduce and remove PFAS wherever possible.[56]
- Reconsideration of our regulatory framework is needed to ensure products are fully studied for their environmental and human health impacts before they are widely available on the market. Advocate for increased chemical oversight and restriction of the use of synthetic chemicals in consumer and building products.

DISCLOSURE

Dr. M.P. Galvez is supported by grant UL1TR004419 from the National Center for Advancing Translational Sciences, United States, National Institutes of Health, United States, grants P30ESO23515 and K12ES033594 from the National Institute of Environmental Health Sciences, United States, and grant DOH01-C32994GG-3450000 from the New York State Department of Health, United States (New York State Children's Environmental Health Centers). Dr.M.P. Galvez is also supported in part by cooperative agreement FAIN: NU61TS000296 from the CDC and Prevention, United States/Agency for Toxic Substances and Disease Registry (CDC/ATSDR). The U.S. Environmental Protection Agency (EPA) provided support through Inter-Agency Agreement DW-75 to 95877701 with CDC/ATSDR. The AAP supports the Pediatric Environmental Health Specialty Units as the National Program Office. The findings and conclusions presented have not been formally disseminated by CDC/ATSDR or EPA and should not be construed to represent any agency determination or policy. Use of trade names that may be mentioned is for identification only and does not imply endorsement by the CDC/ATSDR or EPA. A. Mears, AIA and Parsons Healthy Materials Lab is supported by a grant from The JPB Foundation, United States. A. Mears is Director of Parsons Healthy Materials Lab. Dr K. McCarthy is supported by grants UL1TR004419 and R01DK134725 funded by the National Institutes of Health.

REFERENCES

1. Centers for Disease Control and Prevention. The Built Environment Assessment Tool Manual. 2023. Available at: https://www.cdc.gov/physicalactivity/resources/built-environment-assessment/index.htm. [Accessed 21 March 2024].
2. Cornell Human Ecology; Bronfenbrenner Center for Translational Research. Available at: https://bctr.cornell.edu/about-us/urie-bronfenbrenner. [Accessed 21 March 2024].
3. National Institute of Environmental Health Sciences. Obesity, Diabetes, and Other Metabolic Disorders. Available at: https://www.niehs.nih.gov/research/supported/health/obesity. [Accessed 21 March 2024].
4. McLeroy KR, Bibeau D, Steckler A, et al. An ecological perspective on health promotion programs. Health Educ Q 1988;15(4):351–77.
5. Brown CL, Halvorson EE, Cohen GM, et al. Addressing Childhood Obesity: Opportunities for Prevention. Pediatr Clin North Am 2015;62(5):1241–61.
6. Davison KK, Birch LL. Childhood overweight: a contextual model and recommendations for future research. Obes Rev 2001;2(3):159–71.
7. Galvez MP, Pearl M, Yen IH. Childhood obesity and the built environment. Curr Opin Pediatr 2010;22(2):202–7.
8. Defining Adult Overweight and Obesity | Overweight & Obesity | CDC. Available at: https://www.cdc.gov/obesity/adult/defining.html. [Accessed 10 February 2021].
9. Bole A, Bernstein A, White MJ, et al. The Built Environment and Pediatric Health. Pediatrics 2024;153(1). https://doi.org/10.1542/peds.2023-064773.
10. Vrijheid M, Fossati S, Maitre L, et al. Early-Life Environmental Exposures and Childhood Obesity: An Exposome-Wide Approach. Environ Health Perspect 2020;128(6):67009.
11. Egusquiza RJ, Blumberg B. Environmental Obesogens and Their Impact on Susceptibility to Obesity: New Mechanisms and Chemicals. Endocrinology 2020;161(3). https://doi.org/10.1210/endocr/bqaa024.

12. Southern Nevada Health District. Healthy Community Design. Available at: https://gethealthyclarkcounty.org/get-moving/healthy-community-design/. [Accessed 21 March 2024].

13. Boston Metropolitan Area Planning Council. Healthy Community Design. Available at: https://www.mapc.org/our-work/expertise/public-health/healthy-community-design/. [Accessed 21 March 2024].

14. Trust for Public Land. East Harlem Fitness Zone. Available at: https://www.tpl.org/our-work/east-harlem-fitness-zone. [Accessed 21 March 2024].

15. Centers for Disease Control and Prevention. Screen Time vs. Lean Time Infographic. 2018. Available at: https://www.cdc.gov/nccdphp/dnpao/multimedia/infographics/getmoving.html#:~:text=About%20Screen%20Time,watching%20a%20screen%20for%20fun. [Accessed 21 March 2024].

16. Centers for Disease Control and Prevention. How much physical activity do children need. 2023. Available at: https://www.cdc.gov/physicalactivity/basics/children/index.htm. [Accessed 21 March 2024].

17. Tandon PS, Saelens BE, Zhou C, et al. A Comparison of Preschoolers' Physical Activity Indoors versus Outdoors at Child Care. Int J Environ Res Public Health 2018;15(11). https://doi.org/10.3390/ijerph15112463.

18. Malacarne D, Handakas E, Robinson O, et al. The built environment as determinant of childhood obesity: A systematic literature review. Obes Rev 2022; 23(Suppl 1):e13385.

19. Watson KB, Harris CD, Carlson SA, et al. Disparities in Adolescents' Residence in Neighborhoods Supportive of Physical Activity - United States, 2011-2012. MMWR Morb Mortal Wkly Rep 2016;65(23):598–601.

20. Molina-García J, Queralt A, Adams MA, et al. Neighborhood built environment and socio-economic status in relation to multiple health outcomes in adolescents. Prev Med 2017;105:88–94.

21. Larson LR, Mullenbach LE, Browning MHEM, et al. Greenspace and park use associated with less emotional distress among college students in the United States during the COVID-19 pandemic. Environ Res 2022;204(Pt D):112367.

22. Hazlehurst MF, Muqueeth S, Wolf KL, et al. Park access and mental health among parents and children during the COVID-19 pandemic. BMC Publ Health 2022; 22(1):800.

23. Rundle AG, Chen Y, Quinn JW, et al. Development of a Neighborhood Walkability Index for Studying Neighborhood Physical Activity Contexts in Communities across the U.S. over the Past Three Decades. J Urban Health 2019;96(4):583–90.

24. Zou Y, Ma Y, Wu Z, et al. Neighbourhood residential density and childhood obesity. Obes Rev 2021;22(Suppl 1):e13037.

25. Saelens BE, Handy SL. Built environment correlates of walking: a review. Med Sci Sports Exerc 2008;40(7 Suppl):S550–66.

26. Giles-Corti B, Bull F, Knuiman M, et al. The influence of urban design on neighbourhood walking following residential relocation: longitudinal results from the RESIDE study. Soc Sci Med 2013;77:20–30.

27. Yang S, Chen X, Wang L, et al. Walkability indices and childhood obesity: A review of epidemiologic evidence. Obes Rev 2021;22(Suppl 1):e13096.

28. McGrath LJ, Hopkins WG, Hinckson EA. Associations of objectively measured built-environment attributes with youth moderate-vigorous physical activity: a systematic review and meta-analysis. Sports Med 2015;45(6):841–65.

29. Carlson JA, Saelens BE, Kerr J, et al. Association between neighborhood walkability and GPS-measured walking, bicycling and vehicle time in adolescents. Health Place 2015;32:1–7.

30. Jiang Q, Forseth B, Fitzpatrick L, et al. Prospective associations of neighborhood healthy food access and walkability with weight status in a regional pediatric health system. Int J Behav Nutr Phys Activ 2023;20(1):113.

31. Hermosillo-Gallardo ME, Jago R, Sebire SJ. Association between urbanicity and physical activity in Mexican adolescents: The use of a composite urbanicity measure. PLoS One 2018;13(9):e0204739.

32. Xu F, Jin L, Qin Z, et al. Access to public transport and childhood obesity: A systematic review. Obes Rev 2021;22(S1). https://doi.org/10.1111/obr.12987.

33. Kontou E, McDonald NC, Brookshire K, et al. active school travel in 2017: Prevalence and correlates. Prev Med Rep 2020;17:101024.

34. Boarnet MG, Anderson CL, Day K, et al. Evaluation of the California Safe Routes to School legislation: urban form changes and children's active transportation to school. Am J Prev Med 2005;28(2 Suppl 2):134–40.

35. Pucher J, Dill J, Handy S. Infrastructure, programs, and policies to increase bicycling: an international review. Prev Med 2010;50(Suppl 1):S106–25.

36. Jia P, Dai S, Rohli KE, et al. Natural environment and childhood obesity: A systematic review. Obes Rev 2021;22(Suppl 1):e13097.

37. Jia P, Cao X, Yang H, et al. Green space access in the neighbourhood and childhood obesity. Obes Rev 2021;22(S1). https://doi.org/10.1111/obr.13100.

38. Ansari A, Pettit K, Gershoff E. Combating Obesity in Head Start. J Dev Behav Pediatr 2015;36(8):605–12.

39. Larouche R, Garriguet D, Tremblay MS. Outdoor time, physical activity and sedentary time among young children: The 2012-2013 Canadian Health Measures Survey. Can J Public Health 2017;107(6):e500–6.

40. Wolch J, Jerrett M, Reynolds K, et al. Childhood obesity and proximity to urban parks and recreational resources: a longitudinal cohort study. Health Place 2011;17(1):207–14.

41. Alejandre JC, Lynch M. "Kids Get in Shape with Nature": A Systematic Review Exploring the Impact of Green Spaces on Childhood Obesity. J Nutr Sci Vitaminol (Tokyo) 2020;66(Supplement):S129–33.

42. White MJ, McClure E, Killeen J, et al. Changes in the Recreational Built Environment and Youth Body Mass Index. Acad Pediatr 2021;21(1):76–83.

43. Laurito A, Schwartz AE, Elbel B. Exposure to local violent crime and childhood obesity and fitness: Evidence from New York City public school students. Health Place 2022;78:102937.

44. An R, Yang Y, Hoschke A, et al. Influence of neighbourhood safety on childhood obesity: a systematic review and meta-analysis of longitudinal studies. Obes Rev 2017;18(11):1289–309.

45. Theall KP, Chaparro MP, Denstel K, et al. Childhood obesity and the associated roles of neighborhood and biologic stress. Prev Med Rep 2019;14:100849.

46. Sandy R, Tchernis R, Wilson J, et al. Effects of the built environment on childhood obesity: the case of urban recreational trails and crime. Econ Hum Biol 2013;11(1):18–29.

47. Daniels KM, Schinasi LH, Auchincloss AH, et al. The built and social neighborhood environment and child obesity: A systematic review of longitudinal studies. Prev Med 2021;153:106790.

48. Clark C, Crombie R, Head J, et al. Does traffic-related air pollution explain associations of aircraft and road traffic noise exposure on children's health and cognition? A secondary analysis of the United Kingdom sample from the RANCH project. Am J Epidemiol 2012;176(4):327–37.

49. Stansfeld S, Clark C. Health Effects of Noise Exposure in Children. Curr Environ Health Rep 2015;2(2):171–8.
50. Jerrett M, McConnell R, Wolch J, et al. Traffic-related air pollution and obesity formation in children: a longitudinal, multilevel analysis. Environ Health 2014;13:49.
51. Warkentin S, de Bont J, Abellan A, et al. Changes in air pollution exposure after residential relocation and body mass index in children and adolescents: A natural experiment study. Environ Pollut 2023;334:122217.
52. Wang Z, Zhao L, Huang Q, et al. Traffic-related environmental factors and childhood obesity: A systematic review and meta-analysis. Obes Rev 2021;22(Suppl 1):e12995.
53. Pyko A, Eriksson C, Oftedal B, et al. Exposure to traffic noise and markers of obesity. Occup Environ Med 2015;72(8):594–601.
54. Gupta R, Kumar P, Fahmi N, et al. Endocrine disruption and obesity: A current review on environmental obesogens. Current Research in Green and Sustainable Chemistry 2020;3:100009.
55. United States Environmental Protection Agency. Summary of the Toxic Substances Control Act. 2016. Available at: https://www.epa.gov/laws-regulations/summary-toxic-substances-control-act#:~:text=The%20Toxic%20Substances%20Control%20Act%20of%201976%20provides%20EPA%20with,%2C%20drugs%2C%20cosmetics%20and%20pesticides. [Accessed 21 March 2024].
56. Green Science Policy Institute. Building A Better World: Eliminating Unnecessary PFAs in Building Materials.; 2021.
57. Fenton SE, Ducatman A, Boobis A, et al. Per- and Polyfluoroalkyl Substance Toxicity and Human Health Review: Current State of Knowledge and Strategies for Informing Future Research. Environ Toxicol Chem 2021;40(3):606–30.
58. Centers for Disease Control and Prevention. What are the health effects of PFAS. 2024. Available at: https://www.atsdr.cdc.gov/pfas/health-effects/index.html. [Accessed 21 March 2024].
59. Grieger JA, Hutchesson MJ, Cooray SD, et al. A review of maternal overweight and obesity and its impact on cardiometabolic outcomes during pregnancy and postpartum. Ther Adv Reprod Health 2021;15. https://doi.org/10.1177/2633494120986544. 263349412098654.
60. Liu Y, Wosu AC, Fleisch AF, et al. Associations of Gestational Porfluoroalkyl Substances Exposure with Early Childhood BMI z-Scores and Risk of Overweight/Obesity: Results from the ECHO Cohorts. Environ Health Perspect 2023;131(6):67001.
61. Sheffield PE, Galvez MPUS. Childhood Obesity and Climate Change: Moving Toward Shared Environmental Health Solutions. Environ Justice 2009;2(4):207–14. https://doi.org/10.1089/env.2009.0027.
62. Dee SG, Nabizadeh E, Nittrouer CL, et al. Increasing Health Risks During Outdoor Sports Due To Climate Change in Texas: Projections Versus Attitudes. Geohealth 2022;6(8). https://doi.org/10.1029/2022GH000595. e2022GH000595.
63. Seo MY, Kim SH, Park MJ. Air pollution and childhood obesity. Clin Exp Pediatr 2020;63(10):382–8. https://doi.org/10.3345/cep.2020.00010.
64. Bunyavanich S, Landrigan CP, McMichael AJ, et al. The impact of climate change on child health. Ambul Pediatr 2003;3(1):44–52.
65. Iughetti L, Lucaccioni L, Predieri B. Childhood obesity and environmental pollutants: a dual relationship. Acta Biomed 2015;86(1):5–16.
66. An R, Ji M, Zhang S. Global warming and obesity: a systematic review. Obes Rev 2018;19(2):150–63.

67. Ahdoot S, Baum CR, Cataletto MB, et al. Climate Change and Children's Health: Building a Healthy Future for Every Child. Pediatrics 2024;153(3). https://doi.org/10.1542/peds.2023-065505.

68. Nazaroff WW. Exploring the consequences of climate change for indoor air quality. Environ Res Lett 2013;8(1):015022.

69. Mansouri A, Wei W, Alessandrini JM, et al. Impact of Climate Change on Indoor Air Quality: A Review. Int J Environ Res Public Health 2022;19(23):15616.

70. Lin L, Li T, Sun M, et al. Global association between atmospheric particulate matter and obesity: A systematic review and meta-analysis. Environ Res 2022;209:112785.

71. Huang C, Li C, Zhao F, et al. The Association between Childhood Exposure to Ambient Air Pollution and Obesity: A Systematic Review and Meta-Analysis. Int J Environ Res Public Health 2022;19(8). https://doi.org/10.3390/ijerph19084491.

72. Salthammer T, Zhao J, Schieweck A, et al. A holistic modeling framework for estimating the influence of climate change on indoor air quality. Indoor Air 2022;32(6):e13039.

73. Plumber BPNPB. How decades of racist housing policy left neighborhoods sweltering. New York Times; 2020.

74. The Community Guide. CPSTF Findings for Physical Activity. Available at: https://www.thecommunityguide.org/pages/task-force-findings-physical-activity.html. [Accessed 21 March 2024].

75. Pediatric Environmental Health Specialty Units. 2024. Available at: https://www.pehsu.net/index.html. [Accessed 21 March 2024].

76. New York State Children's Environmental Health Centers. PEHSU Rx for Prevention. Available at: https://nyscheck.org/pehsurx/. [Accessed 21 March 2024].

77. Environmental Working Group. Consumer Guide. Available at: https://www.ewg.org/consumer-guides. [Accessed 21 March 2024].

78. The New School Parsons. Healthy Materials Lab. Available at: https://healthymaterialslab.org/material-collections. [Accessed 21 March 2024].

The Role of Food and Beverage Environments in Child Health and Weight-Related Behaviors

Melissa N. Laska, PhD, RD[a],*, Megan R. Winkler, PhD, RN[b],
Nicole Larson, PhD, MPH, RD[a]

KEYWORDS

- Food and beverage environments • Child obesity • School food
- Retail food environments • Food assistance • Food and beverage industry marketing

KEY POINTS

- Children's eating behavior and health are influenced by multiple components of the food environment, including institutional settings like schools and child care facilities, retail stores, and digital spaces.
- Social determinants of health underscore significant disparities in health-promoting characteristics of food environments and exacerbate the adverse impact of food environments on underserved communities.
- Strategies for promoting healthier food environments include implementing comprehensive policies in child-serving institutions, improving access to nutritious foods in underserved areas, and addressing the toxic influence of food industry marketing on children and families.
- Pediatric health care providers play a crucial role in advocating for impactful policies and programs that improve equity in access to healthy foods, assessing nutritional risk, providing guidance and referrals for families to support healthy eating, and promoting media literacy skills to combat the pervasive influence of food marketing on children.

INTRODUCTION

Food and beverage environments can wield important influences on diet and health.[1] Eating behavior is strongly influenced by commercial and societal contexts to an extent that often overrides personal preferences. Understanding the dynamics of

[a] Division of Epidemiology & Community Health, School of Public Health, University of Minnesota, 1300 South 2nd Street Suite 300, Minneapolis, MN 55454, USA; [b] Department of Behavioral, Social, and Health Education Sciences, Rollins School of Public Health, Emory University, 1518 Clifton Road Northeast, Atlanta, GA 30322, USA
* Corresponding author.
E-mail address: mnlaska@umn.edu

Pediatr Clin N Am 71 (2024) 845–858
https://doi.org/10.1016/j.pcl.2024.07.003   pediatric.theclinics.com

our food environments is paramount in addressing obesity and fostering healthier eating among children and families.

Food and beverage environments (hereafter referred to as 'food environments') encompass the myriad settings in which families procure, prepare, and consume food. These environments range from school cafeterias to neighborhood grocery stores and beyond. Influential food environments in healthcare settings include hospital cafeterias, pharmacies, and clinic vending areas. In addition, now more than ever, our food environments extend into the digital realm, with industry-driven advertising and marketing of innumerable products, the majority of which are not healthy. Overall, our varied and complex food environments shape the availability, affordability, and accessibility of food and beverage options, as well as our perceptions of these products and desire for them.

Key social determinants of health, including socio-economic and racial inequities, exacerbate the impact of food and beverage environments. Underserved communities have long grappled with structural barriers like limited access to fresh, nutritious foods—along with limitations in access to health care, transportation, banking, education, and other resources—caused by a lack of community investment.[1] Instead, underserved communities are saturated with fast-food and quick-service restaurants, liquor stores, convenience stores, and dollar stores selling primarily unhealthy products. These inequities are not only important for reasons of health, but also for food justice and the premise that access to nutritious foods is a fundamental human right. (For more on food justice, see "Obesity as a Health Equity" article in this volume) Ultimately, structural factors like income inequity, urban design, and community divestment play pivotal roles in shaping environmental disparities and supporting continued cycles of poverty and poor health.[2]

Addressing social and structural determinants of health necessitates a multifaceted approach that attends to the complex influences on food access and supports environments where all people are empowered and have equitable opportunities to make healthy eating choices. The purpose of this article is to outline numerous aspects of food environments that influence eating behavior, exploring implications for public health, and underscoring the imperative of fostering equitable, health-promoting environments for all. By highlighting key empirical evidence, we aim to offer insights into effective strategies for mitigating adverse effects of unhealthy food environments and highlight opportunities for clinicians to advance public health.

FOOD ENVIRONMENTS AMONG CHILD-SERVING INSTITUTIONS
Child Care and School Settings

Child care and school settings provide environments that can influence the eating behaviors of most children and adolescents. Programs and policies at the federal, state, tribal, and local levels promote the provision of nutrient-dense food in these settings, with vast evidence that strong and comprehensive policies are effective tools for guiding the types of foods and beverages provided.[3] Federal standards require that the meals and snacks served in child care and school settings are in alignment with the *Dietary Guidelines for Americans*. Additional opportunities to promote healthy eating in these settings include expanding access to free and low-cost meals. For example, policies providing free school meals for all students have demonstrated potential to reduce stigma and increase meal program participation.[4] Universal free school meals have been implemented in several states, and ongoing efforts are monitoring the impact and reach of this policy strategy.[4] In all other states, schools provide free meals for students within low-income communities and for students with household incomes at or below 130% of the federal poverty level.

Summer Meal Programs, Recreational Facilities, and Other Institutional Settings

The Summer Food Service Program is another form of food assistance that provides funds for schools and other sponsors (eg, summer camps, community agencies) to serve meals to young people from low-income households.[5] All programs are required to include milk, fruits or vegetables, grains or breads, and meat or meat alternates. Additionally, school districts must align meal plans with federal standards for the National School Lunch Program if they utilize the Seamless Summer Option (SSO).[6] Few studies have evaluated the nutritional quality of summer meal programs[5]; however, a nationally representative study conducted by the United States (US) Department of Agriculture found these meals contribute substantially to meeting federal dietary guidance.[7] Programs utilizing the SSO provide meals with more vegetables and more often serve low-fat unflavored milk compared to other summer meal programs.[7]

Beyond studies evaluating the Summer Food Service Program, relatively little research has addressed food environments in summer camps, parks, community centers, and other recreational facilities. Research suggests that multi-component interventions have the potential to positively influence eating behaviors in recreational settings. A small number of intervention studies have evaluated the impact of modifying summer camp and park food environments (eg, replacing old water fountains, creating gardens) and demonstrated positive changes in water consumption and fruit and vegetable preferences.[8–14] Similarly, intervention research focused on recreational and sport settings has demonstrated modest success with regards to improving access to healthy snacks and beverages by developing nutrition guidelines and implementing capacity-building supports.[15,16]

Practical guidance for improving the nutritional quality of food in institutional settings outside of schools has been developed by the Centers for Disease Control and Prevention (CDC). The guidance was developed with a focus on federal facilities, but is broadly applicable to institutions providing food for children, including recreational and health care facilities.[17] In particular, there is an important opportunity to implement the CDC guidance within health care facilities, as the high availability of energy-dense and nutrient-poor foods in these environments is contradictory to the expectation of parents and the general public that health care settings promote healthy behaviors.[18] The *Food Service Guidelines for Federal Facilities* provide a set of voluntary best practices based on existing research evidence,[17] and the CDC has developed complementary action steps to guide implementation.[19]

FOOD RETAIL ENVIRONMENTS
Improving Physical Access to Retailers Selling Healthy Products

In recent years, the promotion of healthier food and beverage options in neighborhood retail stores has also been a key component of public health initiatives to combat diet-related diseases. Improving food access is a key pillar of the 2022 Biden-Harris Administration National Strategy on Hunger, Nutrition and Health in creating "healthier food environments and a healthier food supply so the healthier choice is the easier choice."[20]

In the early 2000s, a groundswell of research on "food deserts," areas lacking supermarkets or retailers providing affordable and nutritious food, shed light on pronounced inequities across the US.[21] Communities with residents who had lower incomes and identified as Black, Indigenous, or People of Color, as well as rural communities, were most likely to be food deserts. Momentum to act on these inequities led to state and local Healthy Food Financing Initiatives (HFFIs) supporting financial incentives and technical assistance to improve access to healthy food retailers, with federal funding beginning in 2011. Overall, HFFI programs have leveraged more than $320 million in grants and $1 billion in additional financing to support nearly 1000 healthy food retail projects across 48 states.[22] Many of these HFFI public-private investments have resulted in new supermarkets opening in underserved communities; however, rigorous research has yielded mixed results in terms of impacts on diet and weight-related outcomes among community residents.[23–27]

Interventions and Policies to Improve Customer Retail Environments

In addition to physical access, a range of interventions to improve the healthfulness of in-store customer retail environments and promote healthier food choices at restaurants have been tested. Typically, these interventions have been voluntary programs addressing a combination of product, promotion, placement, or pricing factors; **Table 1** highlights an array of examples of intervention strategies.

A 2022 "review of reviews" on healthy retail interventions identified 25 published systematic reviews on this topic.[28] Each review included between 12 and 125 studies, with extensive heterogeneity in inclusion criteria, measures utilized and outcomes of interest. Despite the differences in review methodology, the reviews have similarly concluded that although these interventions hold promise for improving diet and purchasing patterns, research on their effectiveness has yielded mixed results. Some studies demonstrated positive impacts on consumer preferences and purchasing behaviors, whereas others have reported negligible effects. For many interventions, multiple strategies have been employed, making it difficult to disentangle the impact of each. The variability in findings underscores the complex nature of consumer decision-making in retail environments and highlights the likely need for multicomponent interventions addressing multiple facets of the shopping experience.

Further, mixed findings to date on voluntary in-store interventions underscore the powerful external influences on retail environments, such as those of the food and beverage industry, thus, leading to increased attention to policy mechanisms that could mandate retail changes. **Table 1** also highlights complementary policy mechanisms impacting product, promotion, placement, or pricing in retail settings. Collectively, intervention and policy initiatives illustrated across **Table 1** illuminate the array of mechanisms for addressing food and beverage retail environments across numerous domains.

Improving Online Food Retail Environments

With the rise of online retail platforms, there are also emerging opportunities to promote healthier purchasing behaviors among consumers in digital spaces. Strategies like incorporating nutrition information and health-promoting cues into online product listings and leveraging algorithms to personalize recommendations hold promise for enhancing the healthfulness of online shopping. Furthermore, integration of these strategies into online platforms has implications for government assistance programs, such as the Supplemental Nutrition Assistance Program (SNAP), which has expanded to authorize online retailers in recent years.[29]

FOOD ASSISTANCE AND CHILD FOOD ENVIRONMENTS

In 2022, 17.3% of households with children were food insecure,[30] thus, making product affordability a particularly important factor shaping youth dietary practices.

Table 1
Strategies to improve in-store consumer retail food and beverage environments

Domain	Examples of Intervention approaches[28]	Examples of Policy mechanisms
Product (Stocking)	• Technical assistance: Provision of assistance in stocking healthy products, with an emphasis on perishable products. Includes support in sourcing, distribution, storage, and mitigation of spoilage. • Equipment provision: Support for refrigeration or freezer equipment to enhance stocking of healthy, perishable products.	• Federal food assistance programs: The Special Supplemental Nutrition Program for Women, Infants, and Children (WIC) requires authorized retailers to stock minimum quantities of healthy program-supported foods. The Supplemental Nutrition Assistant Program (SNAP) has much lower retailer stocking requirements. • Local Staple Foods Ordinances[67]: The City of Minneapolis, MN currently requires licensed food stores to stock minimum quantities and varieties of healthy foods and beverages.
Promotion	• Customer messaging via shelf tags, signs and promotion material identifying healthier products. Cultural tailoring of messaging may be important here. • Taste tasting, cooking demonstrations, and nutrition education focused on healthy products. • Nutrition scoring systems that rate or scale product in healthfulness.	• State and local healthy default meal policies[68]: California, Illinois, Hawaii, and Delaware, as well as numerous cities across the US require restaurants can be required to offer healthier beverages (eg, milk, 100% juice, water) as the default choice for children's meals, instead of sugary beverages. Healthy default sides, such as fruits/vegetables, can also be required. • Federal product labeling requirements, including (a) Front of Pack labeling, used to complement Nutrition Facts panel labeling, or (b) calorie labeling on chain restaurant menus.
Placement	• Featured placement on endcaps, near checkout or in other prominent locations, in addition to their primary placement area. This includes other mechanizing strategies, such as grouping complementary healthy items together (eg, carrots and hummus). • Featured placement of products at eye-level shelf locations in their primary placement area in the store.	• Healthy checkout aisles policies[69]: The City of Berkeley, CA prohibits retailers from displaying products with >5g added sugar or >200 mg sodium per serving at checkouts.

(continued on next page)

Table 1
(continued)

Domain	Examples of Intervention approaches[28]	Examples of Policy mechanisms
Pricing	• Affordable pricing for healthy foods. • Offering pricing incentives, coupons or other discounts for healthy foods.	• Gus Schumacher Nutrition Incentive Program (GusNIP),[70] a program of the USDA, provides funding for incentive programs for low-income consumers purchasing fruits and vegetables and/or participating in produce prescription programs. This includes programs like Double Up Bucks, which matches SNAP dollars spent on fresh fruits and vegetables. • Numerous jurisdictions have implemented sweetened beverage taxes, or excise taxes on sweetened drinks, such as soda, iced tea, and fruit punches.[71,72]

Compared to higher resourced households, children living at or near the federal poverty level have 2.5 times greater rates of obesity and a 6 times higher rate of food insecurity.[31]

Numerous strategies have been implemented to address child food and nutrition security. The most known programs are SNAP, the special supplemental nutrition program for women, infants and children,[32] and women, infants, and children (WIC), which serves families with children up to age 5.[33] Both programs provide key financial support to families to obtain food and require retailers to comply with stocking standards to accept federal dollars. WIC vouchers are specifically designated for purchasing nutritious foods aligned with the Dietary Guidelines for Americans, whereas SNAP benefits can be used to purchase a wide variety of food items for the household, excluding prepared hot foods. SNAP and WIC are vital programs that help families purchase food, but they do not fully eliminate experiences of food insecurity.[34–36] Thus, the emergency food system, consisting of food banks, pantries, and assembly meal sites, also has an important role. Historically, foods available in the emergency food system have been selected based on shelf stability, resulting in sub-optimal nutritional quality. In recent years, organizations have increasingly prioritized the supply of healthier foods by developing guidelines for nutrition standards for foods provided in these settings.[37,38]

A rapidly growing strategy known as "Food is Medicine" addresses concerns about nutritional quality among those with limited resources through the incorporation of nutrition assistance strategies into healthcare systems.[39] Components of the Food is Medicine strategy have been developed to target not only patients diagnosed with health conditions, but also to address nutrition and food insecurity more broadly. One example is "produce prescriptions"; programs administered by health professionals typically for 3 to 6 months and include receipt of discounted or free produce through food boxes or vouchers (eg, $30–50 per month) often for use at farmers markets.[11,40] To date, evaluations of these programs have demonstrated an impact by reducing food insecurity and improving fruit and vegetable intake among children and families,[40,41] suggesting another avenue health professionals can use to improve healthy food availability.

THE TOXIC INFLUENCE OF FOOD AND BEVERAGE INDUSTRY MARKETING ON CHILDREN, FAMILIES, AND HEALTH PROFESSIONALS

The food and beverage industry has a powerful influence in many contexts and shapes society's values and behavior for profit. A key mechanism for shaping these values has been industry's ever-present, multi-pronged marketing, advertising, and public relation campaigns—targeting both children and those responsible for protecting children, including parents, health professionals, and scientists. This powerful industry influence has been highlighted for over 2 decades,[42] and below we feature evidence showing significant work remains to curb industry influence on child health.

Industry leverages a range of marketing tactics and channels to reach young people, which are effective in adversely impacting children's dietary behavior and preferences.[43–45] Children on average see more than a dozen food and beverage advertisements daily,[46] with marketers using emotional appeals commonly with unhealthy products.[47] Some marketing has been identified as predatory, as studies demonstrate a disproportionate exposure to unhealthy food advertising among economically disadvantaged and racialized children.[48] As shown in **Table 2**, companies leverage multiple routes to reach children,[42,46,49] with significant growth among digital forms[50] as they facilitate reach to larger audiences while also being more personalized.[42,46,49] To

Table 2
Food and beverage industry's influence on media environments: selected forms of industry marketing to children

Marketing Form	Description
Traditional Media	
Print	Magazines, newspaper, flyers, including those affiliated with schools (eg, school newspapers, sports programs)
Television/movies/radio	Brand advertisements and product placements during breaks in entertainment content or within the content itself.
Out-of-home signage	Billboards, posters, and other signage in neighbourhoods, on public transportation, near schools, on scoreboards, marquees, and other locations frequented by the public.
Digital Media	
Mobile Apps	Fast food, other restaurants, and retailers have designed apps for ordering and purchasing food and beverages, with promoted products and deals embedded in the use of the application.
Emails/Search Engines	Advertisements in the returned searches, periphery of email inboxes, or sent via direct message via automated subscriptions.
Social Media	Internet-based platforms (eg, social networks) where users, including food and beverage companies and their 'influencers', can share and review others content. The industry can also purchase advertising space.
Advergaming	Commercial messages and product advertisements in digital games. Games are designed to have users return and play the game multiple times.

achieve this, industry makes considerable financial investments with approximately $2 billion spent on traditional forms of youth advertisements alone in 2009.[51] Beyond product advertisements, companies strategically tie their brands to popular youth events (eg, Olympics).[52] Key challenges to disrupting this pervasive advertising are legal barriers which protect industry's commercial speech and have led to unsuccessful reliance on industry self regulation.[53,54] In all, the current US system allows for unfettered marketing of unhealthy products and endless opportunity to normalize company brands as part of American culture.

Industry practices also have the potential to influence professionals who are otherwise dedicated to protecting children. Mounting concerns have been raised with regard to industry's influence on health and science, including: industry providing continuing education for health professionals[55]; leaders of the Academy of Nutrition and Dietetics having industry ties[56]; questionable exchanges between industry and health organizations, like CDC, about their products[57]; and insider documents disclosing industry's explicit intention to influence groups like the National Academies of Science for their benefit.[58] Infant formulas and breast milk substitutes have historically been seen as the most marketed product to child health professionals to seek their public endorsements.[59–61] When industry can connect itself to respected health and scientific organizations, it can leverage the public trust these groups have, and thus, maintain a favorable public image. While the impact of these industry strategies on health professionals is often unclear, they raise many questions about conflicts of interest, ethics, and what acceptable interactions with industry are.[62] Fortunately, clinicians and scientists are working to develop guidance to help individuals and organizations navigate controversial interactions.[63]

Recently, Gómez and colleagues[64] argued that industry is simply behaving in the regulatory policy environment the US society has allowed. While existing policy structures provide limited incentive for industry to implement changes, the industry continues to work to stabilize this status quo through their pervasive marketing and public relations and shape societal views to their benefit. We all must work together to become better equipped at consistently recognizing and questioning this influence, so as to not allow for the ultimate undermining of child health.

DISCUSSION AND SUMMARY

Pediatric health care providers can play a pivotal role in addressing the complex interplay between food environments and diet- and weight-related health among youth and families. Understanding the societal and commercial contexts that shape eating behaviors is crucial for effectively addressing obesity risk and promoting healthy lifestyles for youth and families. Providers should be aware of the social determinants of health that contribute to disparities in food environments, including institutional, retail, and marketing environments, and advocate for policies and programs that promote equitable opportunities for all children to make healthy eating choices. Additionally, health care professionals must remain vigilant against the pervasive influence of food industry marketing tactics, particularly those targeted at vulnerable populations. By integrating nutrition counseling, advocating for supportive food environments, and collaborating with community-based partners, pediatric health care providers can play a vital role in nurturing healthy environments to support the well-being of the next generation.

CLINICS CARE POINTS

- Seek to recognize and understand the social and commercial contexts that influence eating behaviors, weight and health, as well as social determinants of health that contribute to disparities in food environments. Providers should share with families that they recognize these barriers to healthy eating.

- Routinely evaluate social determinants of health to help contextualize patient needs and tailor clinical care,[65] and use non-stigmatizing approaches that acknowledge contextual challenges in many families' lives.

- Use established tools to screen for household food insecurity and connect families to food assistance resources, and support Food is Medicine programs that integrate nutrition strategies into health systems to address food insecurity and improve healthy food availability.[66]

- Screen for nutrition problems, provide basic education, and refer families for nutrition counseling as appropriate, utilizing the expertise of professionals, such as Registered Dietitians.

- Promote media literacy skills, using educational tools that can teach families to critically evaluate marketing messages and recognize persuasive tactics used by food and beverage marketers.[67]

- Collaborate with community partners to promote healthy food environments in institutional, retail, and other settings.

- Advocate for the implementation of practices within the Food Service Guidelines for Federal Facilities and the promotion of healthy foods and beverages in health care settings.[18]

- Advocate for policies and programs that promote equitable access to nutrition foods and beverages for all families.

- Remain vigilant against the influence of food industry marketing within health care settings, professional associations, and beyond. Advocate for policies to protect children from the marketing of unhealthy products and promote transparency in industry interactions in the professional health care community. Make sure waiting room environments, including available media, do not feature industry marketing of unhealthy products.

DISCLOSURE

The authors have nothing to disclose.

FUNDING

Contributions from Winkler were supported by the National Heart, Lung, and Blood Institute under Award Number R00HL144824 (PI: M. Winkler). The content is solely the responsibility of the authors and does not necessarily represent the official views of the National Institutes of Health. Funding agencies had no role in the design, analysis or writing of this article.

REFERENCES

1. Odoms-Young A, Brown AGM, Agurs-Collins T, et al. Food insecurity, neighborhood food environment, and health disparities: State of the science, research gaps and opportunities. Am J Clin Nutr 2024;119(3):850–61.
2. Weinstein JN, Geller A, Negussie Y, et al. Chapter 3: the root causes of health inequity. Communities in action: Pathways to health equity. The National Academies Press; 2017. p. 99–184.
3. Pineda E, Bascunan J, Sassi F. Improving the school food environment for the prevention of childhood obesity: What works and what doesn't. Obes Rev 2021;22(2):e13176.
4. Cohen J, Hecht A, McLoughlin G, et al. Universal school meals and associations with student participation, attendance, academic performance, diet quality, food security, and body mass index: A systematic review. Nutrients 2021; 13(3):911.
5. Turner L, Calvert H. The academic, behavioral, and health influence of summer child nutrition programs: A narrative review and proposed research and policy agenda. J Acad Nutr Diet 2019;119(6):972–83.
6. Food and Nutrition Service, U.S. Department of Agriculture, Nutrition guide. Summer food service program. 2018. FNS-GD-2018-0021, Available at: https://www.fns.usda.gov/sfsp/nutrition-guide. Accessed July 24, 2024.
7. Zimmerman T, Rothstein M, Dixit-Joshi S, et al. Usda summer meals programs: Meeting the nutritional needs of children. J Acad Nutr Diet 2024;124(3):379–86.
8. Di Noia J, Orr L, Byrd-Bredbenner C. Residential summer camp intervention improves camp food environment. Am J Health Behav 2014;38(4):631–40.
9. Heim S, Stang J, Ireland M. A garden pilot project enhances fruit and vegetable consumption among children. J Am Diet Assoc 2009;109(7):1220–6.
10. Mabary-Olsen E, Litchfield R, Foster R, et al. Can an immersion in wellness camp influence youth health behaviors? J Ext 2015;53(2).
11. Newman T, Lee JS, Thompson JJ, et al. Current landscape of produce prescription programs in the us. J Nutr Educ Behav 2022;54(6):575–81.

12. Lawman H, Lofton X, Grossman S, et al. A randomized trial of a multi-level intervention to increase water access and appeal in community recreation centers. Contemp Clin Trials 2019;79:14–20.

13. Lawman H, Grossman S, Lofton X, et al. Hydrate Philly: An intervention to increase water access and appeal in recreation centers. Prev Chronic Dis 2020; 17:E15.

14. Rosenthal M, Schmidt L, Vargas R, et al. Drink tap: A multisector program to promote water access and intake in San Francisco parks. Prev Chronic Dis 2023; 20(E74).

15. Prowse R, Lawlor N, Powell R, et al. Creating healthy food environments in recreation and sport settings using choice architecture: A scoping review. Health Promot Int 2023;38(5):1–21.

16. Riesenberg D, Blake M, Boelsen-Robinson T, et al. Policies influencing the provision of healthy food and drinks in local government-owned sport and recreation facilities in Victoria, Australia. Aust N Z J Public Health 2020;44(3):240–4.

17. Food Service Guidelines Federal Workgroup. Food Service Guidelines for Federal Facilities. Washington, DC: U.S. Department of Health and Human Services; 2017.

18. Richardson S, McSweeney L, Spence S. Availability of healthy food and beverages in hospital outlets and interventions in the UK and USA to improve the hospital food environment: A systematic narrative literature review. Nutrients 2022; 14(8):1566.

19. Centers for Disease Control and Prevention. Smart Food Choices: How to implement food service guidelines in public facilities. Atlanta, GA: Centers for Disease Control and Prevention, US Department of Health and Human Services; 2018.

20. The White House, Biden-Harris Administration National Strategy on Hunger, Nutrition and Health. 2022. Available at: https://www.whitehouse.gov/wp-content/uploads/2022/09/White-House-National-Strategy-on-Hunger-Nutrition-and-Health-FINAL.pdf. Accessed July 25, 2024.

21. Larson NI, Story MT, Nelson MC. Neighborhood environments: Disparities in access to healthy foods in the U.S. Am J Prev Med 2009;36(1):74–81.

22. About the Healthy Food Financing Initiative. America's Healthy Food Financing Initiative Reinvestment Fund. 2023. Available at: https://www.investinginfood.com/about-hffi/. [Accessed 13 March 2024].

23. Dubowitz T, Ghosh-Dastidar M, Cohen DA, et al. Diet and perceptions change with supermarket introduction in a food desert, but not because of supermarket use. Health Aff 2015;34(11):1858–68.

24. Cantor J, Beckman R, Collins RL, et al. SNAP participants improved food security and diet after a full-service supermarket opened in an urban food desert. Health Aff 2020;39(8):1386–94.

25. Rummo P, Sze J, Elbel B. Association between a policy to subsidize supermarkets in underserved areas and childhood obesity risk. JAMA Pediatr 2022; 176(7):646–53.

26. Cummins S, Flint E, Matthews SA. New neighborhood grocery store increased awareness of food access but did not alter dietary habits or obesity. Health Aff 2014;33(2):283–91.

27. Elbel B, Moran A, Dixon LB, et al. Assessment of a government-subsidized supermarket in a high-need area on household food availability and children's dietary intakes. Public Health Nutr 2015;18(15):2881–90.

28. Gupta A, Alston L, Needham C, et al. Factors influencing implementation, sustainability and scalability of healthy food retail interventions: A systematic review of reviews. Nutrients 2022;14(2).

29. Moran A., Headrick G., Khandpur N., Promoting Equitable Expansion of the SNAP Online Purchasing Pilot. Healthy Eating Research; Durham, NC: 2021. Available at: https://healthyeatingresearch.org. Accessed July 25, 2024.

30. Food security and nutrition assistance. Economic Research Service, U.S. Department of Agriculture. Updated November 29, 2023. Available at: https://www.ers.usda.gov/data-products/ag-and-food-statistics-charting-the-essentials/food-security-and-nutrition-assistance/. [Accessed 13 March 2024].

31. Food security in the U.S.: Key statistics & graphics. Economic Research Service, U.S. Department of Agriculture. Updated October 25, 2023. Available at: https://www.ers.usda.gov/topics/food-nutrition-assistance/food-security-in-the-u-s/key-statistics-graphics/. [Accessed 13 March 2024].

32. Yearly trends SNAP households by demographic and income characteristics. Food and Nutrition Service, U.S. Department of Agriculture. Updated February 28, 2024. Available at: https://www.fns.usda.gov/SNAP-household-trends. [Accessed 13 March 2024].

33. Special supplemental nutrition program for women, infants, and children (WIC) - About WIC. Food and Nutrition Service, U.S. Department of Agriculture. Updated 2022. Available at: https://www.fns.usda.gov/wic/about-wic. [Accessed 13 March 2024].

34. Carlson S, Keith-Jennings B. SNAP is linked with improved nutritional outcomes and lower health care costs. 2018. Policy Futures. January 17, 2018. Available at: https://www.cbpp.org/research/snap-is-linked-with-improved-nutritional-outcomes-and-lower-health-care-costs. [Accessed 13 March 2024].

35. Siddiqi SM, Cantor J, Dastidar MG, et al. SNAP participants and high levels of food insecurity in the early stages of the COVID-19 pandemic. Public Health Rep 2021;136(4):457–65.

36. Wilde PE. Measuring the effect of food stamps on food insecurity and hunger: Research and policy considerations. J Nutr 2007;137(2):307–10.

37. Nutrition and Obesity Policy, Research and Evaluation Network (NOPREN), Implementing and Evaluating Nutrition Policies and Standards in Food Pantries. Available at: https://nopren.ucsf.edu/sites/g/files/tkssra5936/f/Implementing%20and%20Evaluating%20Nutrition%20Policies%20and%20Standards%20in%20Food%20Pantries%20FINAL%20UPDATED.pdf. Accessed July 25, 2024.

38. Levi R, Schwartz M, Campbell E, et al. Nutrition standards for the charitable food system: Challenges and opportunities. BMC Publ Health 2022;22(1):495.

39. Mozaffarian D, Blanck HM, Garfield KM, et al. A food is medicine approach to achieve nutrition security and improve health. Nat Med 2022;28(11):2238–40.

40. Little M, Rosa E, Heasley C, et al. Promoting healthy food access and nutrition in primary care: A systematic scoping review of food prescription programs. Am J Health Promot 2022;36(3):518–36.

41. Mozaffarian D, Aspry KE, Garfield K, et al. "Food is Medicine" strategies for nutrition security and cardiometabolic health equity: JACC state-of-the-art review. J Am Coll Cardiol 2024;83(8):843–64.

42. Story M, French S. Food advertising and marketing directed at children and adolescents in the US. Int J Behav Nutr Phys Act 2004;1(1):3.

43. Norman J, Kelly B, Boyland E, et al. The impact of marketing and advertising on food behaviours: Evaluating the evidence for a causal relationship. Current Nutrition Reports 2016;5:139–49.

44. Smith R, Kelly B, Yeatman H, et al. Food marketing influences children's attitudes, preferences and consumption: A systematic critical review. Nutrients 2019; 11(4):875.

45. Brown CL, Matherne CE, Bulik CM, et al. Influence of product placement in children's movies on children's snack choices. Appetite 2017;114:118–24.

46. Powell LM, Harris JL, Fox T. Food marketing expenditures aimed at youth: Putting the numbers in context. Am J Prev Med 2013;45(4):453–61.

47. Velasquez A, Parra MF, Mora-Plazas M, et al. Food for thought or food for emotions? An analysis of marketing strategies in television food advertising seen by children in Colombia. Public Health Nutr 2023;26(11):2243–55.

48. Backholer K, Gupta A, Zorbas C, et al. Differential exposure to, and potential impact of, unhealthy advertising to children by socio-economic and ethnic groups: A systematic review of the evidence. Obes Rev 2021;22(3):e13144.

49. Mc Carthy CM, de Vries R, Mackenbach JD. The influence of unhealthy food and beverage marketing through social media and advergaming on diet-related outcomes in children-A systematic review. Obes Rev 2022;23(6):e13441.

50. Harris JLF-MF, Phaneuf L, Jensen M, et al. Fast food advertising: Billions in spending, continued high exposure by youth. 2021. Fast Food FACTS 2021: Food Advertising to Children and Teens Score. Available at: https://media. ruddcenter.uconn.edu/PDFs/FACTS2021.pdf. [Accessed 13 March 2024].

51. A review of food marketing to children and adolescents, follow-up report. 2012. Available at: https://www.ftc.gov/sites/default/files/documents/reports/review-food-marketing-children-and-adolescents-follow-report/121221foodmarketingreport. pdf. [Accessed 13 March 2024].

52. Wood B, Ruskin G, Sacks G. Targeting children and their mothers, building allies and marginalising opposition: An analysis of two Coca-Cola public relations requests for proposals. Int J Environ Res Public Health 2019;17(1):12.

53. Pomeranz JL, Mozaffarian D. Food marketing to - and research on - children: New directions for regulation in the United States. J Law Med Ethics 2022;50(3): 542–50.

54. Jensen ML, Fleming-Milici F, Harris JL. Are U.S. food and beverage companies now advertising healthy products to children on television? An evaluation of improvements in industry self-regulation, 2017-2021. Int J Behav Nutr Phys Act 2023;20(1):118.

55. Hamel VA-O, Hennessy MA-O, Mialon MA-O, et al. Interactions between nutrition professionals and industry: A scoping review. Int J Health Policy Manag 2023;12: 7626.

56. Carriedo A, Pinsky I, Crosbie E, et al. The corporate capture of the nutrition profession in the USA: The case of the Academy of Nutrition and Dietetics. Public Health Nutr 2022;25(12):1–15.

57. Maani Hessari NRG, McKee M, Stuckler D. Public meets private: Conversations between Coca-Cola and the CDC. Milbank Q 2019;97(1):74–90.

58. Sacks G, Swinburn B, Cameron A, et al. How food companies influence evidence and opinion – straight from the horse's mouth. Crit Publ Health 2017;28:1–4.

59. Brandt K.G. and da Silva G.A.P., Marketing and child feeding, J Pediatr (Rio J), 100 (Supplement 1), 2024, S57-S64.

60. Bognar Z, De Luca D, Domellöf M, et al. Promoting breastfeeding and interaction of pediatric associations with providers of nutritional products. Front Pediatr 2020;8:562870.

61. Tulleken C. Overdiagnosis and industry influence: How cow's milk protein allergy is extending the reach of infant formula manufacturers. BMJ 2018;363:k5056.

62. Cullerton K, Adams J, Forouhi N, et al. What principles should guide interactions between population health researchers and the food industry? Systematic scoping review of peer-reviewed and grey literature. Obes Rev 2019;20(8): 1073–84.
63. Cullerton KAJ, Forouhi NG, Francis O, et al. Avoiding conflicts of interest and reputational risks associated with population research on food and nutrition: The Food Research Risk (fork) Guidance and Toolkit for Researchers. BMJ 2024;384:e077908.
64. Gómez EJMN, Galea S. The pitfalls of ascribing moral agency to corporations: Public obligation and political and social contexts in the commercial determinants of health. Milbank Q 2024;102(1):28–42.
65. Hampl SE, Hassink SG, Skinner AC, et al. Clinical practice guideline for the evaluation and treatment of children and adolescents with obesity. Pediatrics 2023; 151(2). e2022060640.
66. Screen and intervene. A toolkit for pediatricians to address food insecurity. Food Research & Action Center. Updated August 11, 2022. Available at: https://frac.org/aaptoolkit. [Accessed 15 March 2024].
67. Media literacy now | Advocating for media literacy education. Media Literacy Now. Updated , 2024. Available at: https://medialiteracynow.org/. [Accessed 15 March 2024].
68. Laska MN, Caspi CE, Lenk K, et al. Evaluation of the first U.S. staple foods ordinance: Impact on nutritional quality of food store offerings, customer purchases and home food environments. Int J Behav Nutr Phys Act 2019;16(1):83.
69. Chart: State and local restaurant kids' meal policies. Center for Science in the Public Interest. Updated July 13, 2023. Available at: https://www.cspinet.org/resource/chart-state-and-local-restaurant-kids-meal-policies-2022. [Accessed 15 March 2024].
70. Berkeley Healthy Checkout. Bay Area Community Resources. Updated April 22, 2022. Available at: https://hco-berkeley.org/. [Accessed 15 March 2024].
71. Parks CA, Mitchell E, Byker Shanks C, et al. Descriptive characteristics of nutrition incentive projects across the U.S.: A comparison between farm direct and brick and mortar settings. Inquiry 2021;58:469580211064131.
72. Andreyeva T, Marple K, Marinello S, et al. Outcomes following taxation of sugar-sweetened beverages: A systematic review and meta-analysis. JAMA Netw Open 2022;5(6):e2215276-e.

Physical Examination and Evaluation for Comorbidities in Youth with Obesity

Ashley E. Weedn, MD, MPH[a], Julie Benard, MD[b],
Sarah E. Hampl, MD[c],*

KEYWORDS

- Obesity • Evaluation • Review of systems • Physical examination • Comorbidities

KEY POINTS

- Because obesity may affect every body system at different points in time, a comprehensive, longitudinal approach with evaluation and re-evaluation is needed.
- The review of systems can be approached in a head-to-toe manner and can be obtained verbally or via electronic questionnaire.
- Obtaining blood pressure with an appropriately sized blood pressure cuff and repeating manual measurements, if needed, is an important aspect of evaluation.
- The physical examination should be performed with attention to patient comfort and privacy.
- Cardiometabolic comorbidities are common in youth with obesity and their frequency increases with increasing severity of obesity.

CASE PRESENTATION

A 9 year old girl presents to her pediatric clinician with concerns about weight and health. Parents report that she has always been above the growth curve, but had a 25 pound (11.4 kg) weight gain last year. Nutrition history includes large and second portions, daily sugar-sweetened beverages, and limited fruits and vegetables. She is active in softball and sleeps 7 h/night. She had a tonsillectomy and adenoidectomy at age 2 years for noisy breathing. Her review of systems (ROS) is positive for weight gain and fatigue, congestion, coughing with activity, foot pain, snoring, headaches,

[a] Department of Pediatrics, University of Oklahoma Health Sciences Center, 1200 Children's Avenue, Suite 12400, Oklahoma City, OK 73104, USA; [b] Cape Physician Associates, Saint Francis Healthcare System, 211 Saint Francis Drive, Cape Girardeau, MO 63703, USA; [c] Children's Mercy Kansas City, Center for Children's Healthy Lifestyles & Nutrition, 2401 Gillham Road, Kansas City, MO 64108, USA
* Corresponding author.
E-mail address: shampl@cmh.edu

Pediatr Clin N Am 71 (2024) 859–878
https://doi.org/10.1016/j.pcl.2024.06.008
0031-3955/24/© 2024 Elsevier Inc. All rights reserved, including those for text and data mining, AI training, and similar technologies.

low self-esteem, and mild anxiety. Her vitals are weight: 131.1 lbs (59.5 kg) (>95 percentile), height: 56.1 inches (142.5 cm) (86 percentile), body mass index (BMI): 29.4 (130 percent of the 95th percentile [Class II]), and blood pressure (BP): 110/76 (74 percentile/91 percentile). Repeat manual BPs are normal. Physical examination is pertinent for pes planus and acanthosis nigricans in the neck and axilla.

INTRODUCTION

The disease of obesity can affect every body system at different points in time during childhood and adolescence, necessitating a comprehensive and longitudinal approach to evaluation of comorbidities. Evaluation begins with the assessment of weight and height, continues with obtaining vital signs, patient and family histories, review of systems, and performing the physical examination. Laboratory evaluation identifies "silent" cardiometabolic comorbidities that can be treated concurrently with obesity to support overall health and wellness.

Evaluation should occur in an atmosphere that is welcoming, comfortable, and private for the patient. Promoting a sensitive, nonstigmatizing experience is important in caring for patients with excess weight. Recommended accommodations include having a private area for obtaining weight and height, offering the option of a clothed physical examination, providing electronic means of completing patient questionnaires, using an appropriately sized BP cuff, and having a larger capacity examination room table and accompanying furniture.[1]

A comprehensive evaluation provides valuable information in the patient assessment and development of a treatment plan. A thorough review of systems and physical examination can point to contributing factors, identify comorbidities, and provide opportunities for an early treatment (**Fig. 1**).

Review of Systems

Beginning with a head-to-toe review of systems, asking about headaches and visual changes (double vision and blurred vision) is important as their presence raises concerns for idiopathic intracranial hypertension (IIH).[2] Frequent headaches, especially in the morning, can indicate sleep apnea or hypertension.[3] Children with obesity are also at risk for migraines through possible shared inflammatory mediators.[4]

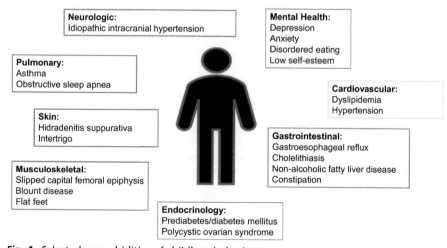

Neurologic:
Idiopathic intracranial hypertension

Mental Health:
Depression
Anxiety
Disordered eating
Low self-esteem

Pulmonary:
Asthma
Obstructive sleep apnea

Cardiovascular:
Dyslipidemia
Hypertension

Skin:
Hidradenitis suppurativa
Intertrigo

Gastrointestinal:
Gastroesophageal reflux
Cholelithiasis
Non-alcoholic fatty liver disease
Constipation

Musculoskeletal:
Slipped capital femoral epiphysis
Blount disease
Flat feet

Endocrinology:
Prediabetes/diabetes mellitus
Polycystic ovarian syndrome

Fig. 1. Selected comorbidities of childhood obesity.

Snoring or witnessed apneic episodes raise concerns for obstructive sleep apnea (OSA), as can restless sleep, daytime fatigue, behavioral concerns, and nocturnal enuresis.[3] Disordered sleep can be a consequence of obesity and contribute to weight gain as poor sleep is associated with impaired impulse control and increased sedentary behavior.[5] Asthma and obesity co-occur in many patients through various pathways, including increased occurrence of gastroesophageal reflux and OSA, and obesity may worsen severity of asthma.[6] Cough and/or shortness of breath with activity could signal exercise-induced bronchospasm or asthma with need for improved control and could also inform providers of potential discomfort during activity that may be a limiting factor, as could chest pain or tightness.

Obesity is associated with gastrointestinal disorders through several proposed mechanisms, including altered gut microflora and delayed gastrointestinal motility, in addition to shared features of suboptimal nutrition and sedentary lifestyle.[7] Location of abdominal pain suggests the type of gastrointestinal dysfunction: gastroesophageal reflux disease (epigastric pain), nonalcoholic fatty liver disease (NAFLD) and gallstones (right upper quadrant pain), or constipation (periumbilical or left lower quadrant pain).[8] Assessing for other signs of gastroesophageal reflux disease (frequent belching, nighttime coughing, or frequent emesis) and constipation (passing hard stools infrequently) in the absence of pain is also helpful.

Childhood obesity is also associated with musculoskeletal concerns, including increased pain, decreased balance and coordination, and altered gait.[9] Hip and knee pain may be signs of serious orthopedic complications like slipped capital femoral epiphysis (SCFE) and Blount disease.[10,11] Foot or ankle pain from excess weight may contribute to discomfort with activity.

Polyuria and polydipsia raise concerns for diabetes, as does nocturnal enuresis (in addition to raising concerns for sleep apnea). Reports of darkening skin especially around the neck and in the axilla signals insulin resistance. Inquiring about skin rashes in areas with increased friction suggests intertrigo, while pustules or history of abscesses may indicate hidradenitis suppurativa; both conditions are common in patients with obesity.[12] Asking about acne, male-pattern hair distribution, and history of infrequent, irregular, or absent menses in a female patient is recommended to assess for polycystic ovarian syndrome (PCOS).

Assessing for any signs of disability or developmental delay is important, as children with intellectual and physical disabilities are at higher risk for obesity.[13] Attributing factors include decreased physical activity, limited food acceptance, and a higher rate of use of weight-promoting medications.[13–15] For those undiagnosed, these symptoms signal the presence of neurodevelopmental disorders (including autism spectrum disorder) or physical disabilities.

Physical Examination

The physical examination of a child with obesity starts with the review of anthropometrics and vital signs. Reviewing weight, height, and BMI percentile is important in making the diagnosis of obesity as well as tracking changes on the growth curve over time. Children with obesity tend to be taller than average, so those with short stature warrant further evaluation for endocrine (hypothyroidism or hypercortisolism) or genetic etiologies, although endocrine disorders account for less than 1% of childhood obesity cases.[16,17]

BP is important to accurately obtain by using an appropriately fitting BP cuff. The cuff should fit so that the bladder length is 80% to 100% of the arm circumference and the cuff width should be a minimum of 40% of the arm.[18] Elevated heart rate and BP are commonly noted in patients with obesity due to increased sympathetic tone and are risk factors for future hypertension.[19]

A neurologic examination is important in the presence of headaches to determine if further evaluation is needed. In patients with persistent headaches, a retinal examination is needed to assess for IIH.[2] Sixth nerve palsy may be present, although the neurologic examination may be normal.[2] An eye examination can also identify retinitis pigmentosa, which occurs in some genetic syndromes like Bardet–Biedl syndrome.[5]

Examination of the head and face for facial dysmorphology is important for identifying genetic syndromes. An oropharyngeal examination can assess for tonsillar enlargement and/or crowding, both increase the risk for OSA.[3] Palpation for thyromegaly is also important, especially in someone with shorter stature, to evaluate for the presence of hypothyroidism.

Chest auscultation for murmurs or arrhythmias, which could limit physical activity, and palpating for chest pain are important components of the cardiac examination. Auscultation of any wheezing could signal underlying/worsening asthma that could limit physical activity and can be helpful in identifying both contributors to and consequences of obesity.

Abdominal palpation can assist in identifying complications of obesity. Epigastric pain could signal gastroesophageal reflux. Periumbilical or left lower quadrant pain raises concern for constipation. An enlarged liver size, assessed by auscultation and palpation, suggests NAFLD. Right upper quadrant pain raises concern for gallstones.

The hip and knee examination are particularly important for the musculoskeletal examination. Children with abnormal gait or any pain on rotation of the hips or limited range of motion should be evaluated for SCFE, which can be unilateral or bilateral.[10,19] Bowing of knees raises concern for Blount disease, which may lead to decreased physical activity due to pain or balance concerns.[19] Providers should also assess for abnormalities like flat feet, in-toeing, or out-toeing that may make physical activity uncomfortable. The presence of scoliosis or lordosis on the spinal examination may provide another source of pain that may limit physical activity. Neuromuscular examination assessing upper and lower extremity muscle strength and evaluation of balance and coordination, which can be decreased in patients with obesity and further contribute to decreased physical activity, are important components to recognize for treatment planning.

Examination of genitalia to determine Tanner stage aids in assessing the potential for future height attainment, keeping in mind that obesity can increase the risk of precocious puberty and, therefore, affecting adult height attainment.[19] Boys with obesity may have prominent suprapubic adipose deposition, or the phenomenon of a "vanishing or hidden penis," for which additional reassurance and hygiene advice may be needed. Additionally, while gynecomastia can be seen in any adolescent boy, those with obesity tend to have more prominent gynecomastia, which may be a source of self-consciousness. A boy with obesity along with truly small penis (micropenis) and gynecomastia could indicate hypogonadism and prompt further evaluation for genetic syndromes associated with obesity.[19]

On skin examination, noting the presence or absence of acanthosis nigricans as evidenced by thickened, dark, and velvety skin is important as it indicates insulin resistance and increased risk of diabetes development.[12] The presence of verruca or skin tags indicates more severe disease.[19] Looking for areas of friction and skin breakdown is important to screen for intertrigo, evidenced by erythematous patches and pustules that may be scaling or broken down and caused by Candida or bacterial superinfection.[12,19] Acne or increased body hair (hirsutism) may be indicative of PCOS.[20] Striae, especially those that are darker in coloration, may signal Cushing syndrome, as does shorter stature, or the presence of posterior dorsocervical prominence.

A psychiatric examination should also be done to look for indications of mental health concerns. Flat affect or tearfulness may be one of the signs of depression or anxiety. Hyperactivity or lack of focus may indicate attention deficit hyperactivity disorder. Social cues, such as lack of eye contact or impaired socialization during the visit, could indicate the presence of autism or may indicate anxiety or fear due to previous weight bias within the medical community.

Special Considerations

Examining patients with obesity may present unique challenges. Increased adipose tissue overlying the chest wall makes auscultation of the heart and lungs more difficult, and sounds may be muffled. Thicker neck tissue can make palpation for lymphadenopathy or thyromegaly more difficult. Palpation of the abdomen for hepatomegaly is also more challenging. Patients may feel embarrassed about showing skin, so sensitivity while assessing for striae or rashes is recommended. Increased subcutaneous skin overlying the spine may make visual inspection for scoliosis more difficult and may prompt more regular use of a scoliometer or radiologic studies for more accurate assessment.

The physical examination for children with obesity and disabilities can also be challenging. In particular, children with sensory concerns and autism spectrum disorder may not tolerate different components of the physical examination.[14] Repeated exposure to physical examination components, use of visual aids, and use of the patient's preferred calming/sensory aids can help facilitate the physical examination.

Children in wheelchairs may not be weighed or have height assessed as regularly as children who are ambulatory. Wheelchair scales are available allowing accurate weights to be obtained. While there have been several proposed ways to measure length, recumbent length has been shown to be a more accurate method for obtaining height in patients in wheelchairs than arm span length and self-report, with knee height being second most accurate among the options.[21] Recumbent length instructions are available.[22] There may be difficulty with transferring patients to an examination table for a complete physical examination; assistive equipment is available.[23] Patients with joint contractures or deformities, clonus, or hypertonicity may require additional support during the musculoskeletal examination. It may be more difficult to obtain accurate cardiac or pulmonary auscultation in patients with neuromuscular scoliosis or different postures. Guidance for accurate assessments in these children has been previously published.[14,24]

Physical Examinations Using Telehealth

Since the coronavirus disease 2019 pandemic, telehealth has emerged as an option to care for patients. Although in-person medical care is widely available again, telemedicine can be helpful in managing obesity, especially for follow-up visits. Telemedicine enables more frequent follow-up without barriers of additional time and transportation, especially for those in more remote locations.

Although there are benefits to utilizing telehealth in the care of patients with obesity, there are also challenges. Ensuring that parents/caregivers can accurately assess and report, the child's height and weight is an important aspect of longitudinal obesity care. The Centers for Disease Control has provided guidance on obtaining height and weight from nonclinical locations.[25] With education and resources, families may also be able to obtain and report vital signs such as BP and heart rate virtually.

Some components of the physical examination, such as auscultation of heart and lungs, are not yet widely available via telehealth appointments, but other components of the standard examination can still be obtained. Having a family member utilize a flashlight aimed at the throat can help provide a pharyngeal examination to assess for tonsillar hypertrophy. Visual inspection of the neck could potentially identify thyromegaly and acanthosis nigricans. Musculoskeletal examination can be obtained by visual inspection for varus deformity and having the patient stand, squat, and walk to determine pain or limp indicative of SCFE. Basic psychiatric examination can also be obtained by screening questionnaires, interview, and visual inspection, and aspects of the neurologic examination can be assessed during a virtual visit.[26]

EVALUATION OF COMORBIDITIES
Hypertension

Obesity is the strongest risk factor for hypertension in childhood.[27] Prevalence of hypertension ranges from 5% to 30% among youth with overweight and obesity, with higher prevalence among adolescents with increasing BMI percentile.[28] Studies have shown that hypertension is associated with increased carotid intima thickness and increased left ventricular mass during childhood.[29,30] Early evaluation is important, especially among children with obesity. The American Academy of Pediatrics (AAP) recommends the evaluation for all children beginning at the age of 3 years with repeat assessment at every clinic visit for children with overweight and obesity.[31] Diagnosis requires identification of BP percentile for children[18] (**Table 1**). Management recommendations are outlined in the AAP clinical practice guideline for screening and management of high BP in children and adolescents.[18]

Dyslipidemia

Nearly half (43%) of children and adolescents with obesity have an abnormal lipid level.[32] Excess adiposity is associated with metabolic dyslipidemia, a pattern of high triglycerides (TG) and low high-density lipoprotein (HDL) cholesterol. Youth with obesity can also have mildly elevated low-density lipoprotein (LDL) levels.[33] The AAP recommends the evaluation for dyslipidemia in children aged 2 to 9 years who have obesity and in youth aged 10 to 18 years who have overweight or obesity by obtaining a fasting lipid panel.[31] Lipid cutoff levels for children are the same across different age groups with the exception of TG[31,34] (**Table 2**). Lifestyle treatment remains the first-line treatment of children with dyslipidemia.[34]

Prediabetes and Type 2 Diabetes

Obesity is a strong risk factor for the development of type 2 diabetes (T2DM). A recent study reported that 77% of youth had obesity at the time of diagnosis of T2DM.[35] One in 5 adolescents has prediabetes.[36] Additional risk factors include maternal history of gestational diabetes, family history of diabetes, signs, or conditions associated with insulin resistance (acanthosis nigricans, hypertension, dyslipidemia, or PCOS), and the use of obesogenic psychotropic medications.[37,38] Presentation of youth-onset T2DM can vary from asymptomatic hyperglycemia to diabetic ketoacidosis in up to 25% of patients.[38]

The AAP recommends the evaluation for prediabetes and T2DM for children with obesity beginning at the age of 10 years.[31] For children with overweight, the evaluation is recommended in the presence of another risk factor for developing diabetes. Both prediabetes and T2DM can be diagnosed by hemoglobin A1c (HbA1c), oral glucose tolerance test, and/or fasting glucose in criteria established by the American Diabetes Association (ADA).[37] A second confirmatory test is recommended for diagnosis of diabetes. Lifestyle modification through diet and physical activity is recommended for both prediabetes and T2DM. Metformin currently remains the first-line medication

Table 1
Blood pressure categories by age and number of visits needed for diagnosis

BP Category	Children 1–13 y of Age	Children ≥13 y of Age	Number of Visits to Diagnosis
Normal	BP <90th percentile	BP <120/80 mm Hg	n/a
Elevated	BP ≥90th percentile to <95th percentile	120/<80–129/ <80 mm Hg	3
Stage 1	BP ≥95th percentile to <95th percentile + 12 mm Hg	130/80–139/89 mm Hg	3
Stage 2	BP ≥95th percentile + 12 mm Hg	≥140/90 mm Hg	2

From American Academy of Pediatrics[31]; with permission.

for youth with T2DM. Referral to a pediatric endocrinologist is recommended for comprehensive care.[37]

Nonalcoholic Fatty Liver Disease

NAFLD is marked by steatosis and is defined by fatty infiltration in greater than 5% of liver in the absence of any secondary causes.[39] Prevalence of NAFLD is highest among youth with obesity.[40,41] Recent data from the National Health and Nutrition Examination Survey showed that the prevalence of assumed NAFLD based on elevated alanine transaminase (ALT) levels among adolescents with overweight was 14%; the prevalence increased to 40% among adolescents with obesity.[42] NAFLD is also associated with insulin resistance.[43–45] Due to the high prevalence of associated obesity and insulin resistance, an international expert consensus statement recommended new terminology for this condition: metabolic dysfunction-associated fatty liver disease (MAFLD).[46] Diagnostic criteria for MAFLD have not yet been formally established in children. Currently, ALT remains the recommended test for evaluation; referral to a pediatric gastroenterologist is recommended for children with an ALT of 80 IU/L or greater.[39] The definitive diagnosis is by liver biopsy. Treatment is limited to lifestyle modifications, specifically eliminating sugar-sweetened beverages and increasing activity.[39,47]

Table 2
National Heart, Lung, and Blood Institute criteria for lipid testing results

Lipid Category	Low (mg/dL)	Acceptable (mg/dL)	Borderline High (mg/dL)	High (mg/dL)
Total cholesterol	—	<170	170–199	≥200
LDL cholesterol	—	<110	110–129	≥130
HDL cholesterol	<40	>45	—	—
TG				
0–9 y	—	<75	75–99	≥100
10–19 y	—	<90	90–129	≥130
Non-HDL cholesterol	—	<120	120–144	≥145

From American Academy of Pediatrics[31]; with permission.

Obstructive Sleep Apnea

Reported prevalence of OSA ranges from 24% to 61% among children with over-weight and obesity.[48] OSA is defined as a sleep disorder characterized by prolonged partial upper airway obstruction or intermittent complete obstruction that disrupts normal ventilation during sleep and normal sleep patterns.[49] Symptoms in children include snoring, night-time awakening, restless sleep, nocturnal enuresis, morning headaches, daytime sleepiness, inattention, and hyperactivity.[49,50] Diagnosis is made by night-time polysomnography, the gold standard test, with an apnea-hypopnea index greater than 1 or more episodes per hour in children.[51] First-line treatment is adenotonsillectomy if adenotonsillar hypertrophy is present; however, studies have reported that children with obesity have an increased risk for persistent OSA.[48] Additionally, obesity is a risk factor for postoperative complications; therefore, the pediatric clinician and family should weigh the risks and benefits of surgery based on the severity of OSA and obesity. Continuous positive airway pressure and weight management are recommended for those with persistent OSA or for children who do not undergo surgery.[49] If left untreated, children can have pulmonary and systemic hypertension and right-sided heart failure.[52]

Polycystic Ovarian Syndrome

PCOS is characterized by hyperandrogenism and disordered ovulatory function and is associated with obesity and insulin resistance.[53] Prevalence data for PCOS in adolescents are limited but estimates range from 3% to 11%.[54] Clinical signs and symptoms include oligomenorrhea or amenorrhea, hirsutism, acne, and/or alopecia. Diagnostic criteria have been difficult to establish because characteristic features of PCOS can be normal physiologic events during early adolescence. International specialty societies have made recommendations for diagnosis specific to adolescents: (1) evidence of clinical or biochemical hyperandrogenism and (2) persistent irregular menstrual cycles (<20 days or <45 days) at least 1 year after menarche.[55] Ultrasound imaging is no longer recommended. Excluding other medical conditions that can cause menstrual irregularities and signs of hyperandrogenism is recommended. Management is weight management and lifestyle modification to decrease cardiometabolic risk. Pharmacologic therapy is reserved for targeted treatment of PCOS symptoms, most commonly menstrual dysfunction.[56]

Idiopathic Intracranial Hypertension

IIH, previously known as pseudotumor cerebri, is a neuro-ophthalmologic condition characterized by an increased intracranial pressure in the absence of a mass or ventricular enlargement and with normal cerebrospinal fluid.[57] Obesity is a well-established risk factor among female adolescents.[58,59] The clinical presentation can vary, but typical symptoms include persistent headaches, nausea, vomiting, pulsatile tinnitus, blurred vision, and diplopia. Loss of peripheral visual fields and reduction in visual acuity may be present at diagnosis. Neck and back pain have also been reported.[60] Fundoscopic examination should assess for papilledema and neurologic examination for cranial nerve deficits. Urgent referral to a neurologist or ophthalmologist for further evaluation (including exclusion of other causes of increased intracranial pressure) and treatment is recommended if IIH is suspected. Papilledema and a lumbar puncture with an opening pressure of 28 cm H_2O or greater in youth with obesity are diagnostic.[57] Treatment of IIH includes acetazolamide and weight loss; surgery may be needed if severe and/or refractory.[60] Long-term vision loss may occur if IIH is not promptly recognized and treated.[61]

Slipped Capital Femoral Epiphysis

SCFE is characterized by the displacement of the proximal femoral epiphysis from the metaphysis.[62] Obesity is a strong risk factor for SCFE, and studies have shown increasing prevalence of SCFE with increased prevalence of obesity, with one retrospective case-control study reporting that 81% of youth who presented with SCFE had obesity.[63–66] Preadolescents with severe obesity have the highest risk of developing SCFE, with a 17 fold increased risk compared to normal-weight peers.[65] Additionally, youth with obesity are more likely to present with or develop bilateral SCFE.[67] A common symptom of SCFE is pain that is poorly localized to the hip, groin, thigh, or knee. Patients may also present with a limp. Both hips should be examined to assess for limitation of internal rotation. Pain may be elicited passively with internal rotation of the hip. Diagnosis is by bilateral anterior-posterior (AP) and lateral radiographs of the hips and pelvis. An urgent referral to a pediatric orthopedic surgeon is recommended. The surgical procedure depends on stability and severity of the slip.[68] Long-term consequences of untreated SCFE include degenerative hip disease and gait abnormalities.[69]

Blount Disease

Childhood obesity is associated with Blount disease, a disorder resulting from disruption of normal cartilage growth at the medial aspect of the proximal tibial physis.[11,70,71] The condition is characterized by tibia vara (bowing of the legs) and often accompanied by tibial torsion and procurvatum.[62] Presentation can vary depending on age. Early-onset, prior to the age of 10 years, Blount disease is typically asymmetric and often bilateral. In adolescents, presentation is typically unilateral and more frequently associated with obesity.[11] Diagnosis is made by AP and lateral radiography of the knee and lower leg. Treatment is guided by child's age and severity of the deformity and includes bracing, orthotics, surgery, and weight management.[11]

Behavioral Health

Obesity is associated with depression, anxiety, teasing, bullying, low self-esteem, decreased quality of life, and eating disorders.[72–74] Evaluation of these conditions through the use of validated pediatric questionnaires and referral to behavioral health services is discussed in subsequent articles. For instance, the AAP Clinical Practice Guideline for depression recommends evaluating for depression using a formal self-report tool, such as the patient health questionnaire-9 question (PHQ-9), for adolescents who present with symptoms of depression, as well for all adolescents, beginning at 12 years of age.[75] Recognition of these conditions is important so that pediatric clinicians can provide a safe place to discuss and provide support.

Laboratory Evaluation and Frequency of Testing

Standard laboratory evaluation for comorbidities is recommended based on BMI evaluation and age (**Table 3**). There is limited evidence on optimal age and frequency of re-evaluation of comorbidities for youth with overweight and obesity.[31] When laboratory results are normal, re-evaluation for dyslipidemia, prediabetes, and NAFLD may be considered for those with severe obesity, increasing BMI, new-onset of risk factors, and family history.[31]

Guidelines by the National Heart, Lung, and Blood Institute (NHLBI), the ADA, and the North American Society for Pediatric Gastroenterology, Hepatology, and Nutrition (NASPGHAN) provide a suggested timeframe for re-evaluation based on consensus

Table 3
Laboratory evaluation for children and adolescents with overweight and obesity by age and weight category

Age	BMI Percentile	Recommended Laboratory
<10 y	≥95th percentile	Fasting lipid panel
≥10 y	≥95th percentile	Fasting lipid panel HbA1c, fasting glucose, or oral glucose tolerance test (OGTT) ALT
≥10 y	≥85th percentile ≥85th percentile with risk factors[a]	Fasting lipid panel HbA1c, fasting glucose, or OGTT ALT

[a] T2DM risk factors: family history of T2DM, maternal gestational diabetes, signs of insulin resistance or conditions associated with insulin resistance (acanthosis nigricans, hypertension, dyslipidemia, and polycystic ovary syndrome), and obesogenic psychotropic medication. NAFLD risk factors: male sex, prediabetes/diabetes, OSA, dyslipidemia, or sibling with NAFLD.
Data from Ref.[31]

recommendations until future studies are better able to delineate how often retesting should be performed (**Tables 4–6**).

For dyslipidemia, studies that examine trajectory of weight gain and progression of abnormal lipid levels are limited. Cholesterol levels increase from birth, stabilize at around 2 years of age, reach a peak before puberty, and then decrease slightly during adolescence.[34] For children with dyslipidemia, intensive lifestyle management of obesity have shown improvements in lipid abnormalities with 6 months of treatment; therefore, repeating a lipid panel after 6 months of lifestyle treatment is recommended.[34]

For children and adolescents with obesity and prediabetes, re-evaluation is recommended.[31] One study reported that 12% of adolescents with obesity and abnormal HbA1c or impaired glucose tolerance progressed to T2DM within 1 year.[76] Frequency of repeat evaluation depends on the laboratory result and patient risk factors (see **Table 5**).

Table 4
Follow-up laboratory evaluation for dyslipidemia

Lipid Panel Components	Action
TG normal:	
<10 y: <100 mg/dL	Repeat in 1 y
≥10 y: <130 mg/dL	Repeat in 1 y
TG elevated:	
<10 y: ≥100 mg/dL	Repeat in 6 mo
≥10 y: ≥130 mg/dL	Repeat in 6 mo
TG high: ≥500 mg/dL	Referral to endocrinology
LDL	
Normal: <130 mg/dL	Repeat in 1 y
Elevated: ≥130 mg/dL	Repeat in 6 mo
High: ≥250 mg/dL	Refer to cardiology or endocrinology

Data from Ref.[34]

Table 5
Follow-up laboratory evaluation for prediabetes and type 2 diabetes

HbA1c	Action
Normal: <5.7	Repeat in 2 y
Prediabetes: 5.7–5.9 + at least one risk factor[a]	Repeat in 1 y
Prediabetes: 6–6.4	Repeat in 3–6 mo
Diabetes: ≥6.5	Refer to endocrinology

[a] Risk factors include severe obesity, weight gain, family history, acanthosis, and the use of obesogenic psychotropic medications.
  Data from Ref.[31]

The 2017 NASPGHAN guidelines recommend repeat evaluation for NAFLD if ALT levels are twice the upper limit of normal[39] (see **Table 6**). After a second abnormal ALT result, there is limited guidance on frequency of subsequent testing. Persistently elevated ALT levels and risk factors for progression of NAFLD, along with engagement of concurrent obesity treatment are all factors to consider in determining re-evaluation and referral to a gastroenterologist.[31]

SUMMARY

Detection of obesity comorbidities is aided by a head-to-toe review of systems at the initial evaluation, with the recognition that obesity can affect nearly every body system. Accurate assessment of vital signs and a thorough and sensitive physical examination should follow. Laboratory assessment directed at known comorbidities can facilitate their early identification and management. The chronic disease nature of obesity should prompt regular re-evaluation of the whole child, including physical and emotional health and laboratory reassessment at recommended intervals (**Table 7**).

CASE DISCUSSION

This 9 year old girl's laboratory evaluations showed elevated ALT at 40, fasting triglyceride level of 278, HDL of 40, and HbA1C of 5.8%. Discussion with the family led to referrals for a sleep study and orthotics, a plan for albuterol prior to activity, a goal of decreasing sugar-sweetened beverage intake to no more than one 8 oz (236 ml) beverage per week, and follow-up in 1 month.

Table 6
Follow-up evaluation for abnormal alanine transaminase level

ALT	Action
Normal: Boys <26 IU/L Girls <22 IU/L	Repeat in 2 y
Elevated: Twice the upper limit of normal Boys: ≥52 IU/L Girls: ≥44 IU/L	Repeat in 3–6 mo
≥80 IU/L	Exclude other causes of elevated liver enzymes Refer to gastroenterology

Data from Ref.[39]

Table 7
Comorbidity symptoms, signs, and evaluation

Comorbidity	Review of Systems	Physical Examination	Evaluation
IIH	Severe, recurrent headaches New-onset headaches with significant weight gain Nausea and/or vomiting Diplopia Blurred vision Pulsatile tinnitus Neck or back pain	Papilledema Cranial nerve VI palsy	Emergent referral to neurology and/or ophthalmology Lumbar puncture
OSA	Frequent snoring Gasps or labored breathing during sleep Night-time awakenings, restless sleep Inattention and/or Hyperactivity Daytime fatigue Morning headaches Nocturnal enuresis	Tonsillar hypertrophy Mallampati 3–4 Elevated BP	Polysomnogram
Asthma (or exercise-induced bronchospasm)	Cough with activity Wheezing with activity Shortness of breath Dyspnea on exertion limiting activity Chest tightness Night-time coughing	Wheezing Prolonged expiration	Clinical diagnosis Pulmonary function testing
Gastroesophageal reflux disease	Epigastric or chest pain Acid regurgitation Frequent emesis Belching Night-time cough	Epigastric tenderness	Clinical diagnosis

	History		Abdominal radiography
Constipation	Infrequent stools Hard stools Straining with defecation Periumbilical or left-lower quadrant pain Encopresis or enuresis	Tenderness to palpation in the periumbilical or left lower quadrant Palpable stool in the left lower quadrant	Abdominal radiography
NAFLD	Typically, asymptomatic vague abdominal pain	Hepatomegaly	ALT
Cholelithiasis	Right upper quadrant pain, especially postprandial	Tenderness to palpation in the right upper quadrant	Right upper quadrant ultrasound
SCFE	Altered gait Vague hip, groin, or knee pain	Altered gait Limitation on internal rotation of the hip(s) Pain with internal rotation of the hip(s) (may be bilateral or unilateral)	Emergent bilateral hip and pelvis radiography (include frog leg view if stable) Emergent referral to orthopedics
Blount disease	Leg or knee pain	Tibia vara (bowed legs)—may be unilateral or bilateral Tibial torsion	AP and lateral lower extremity radiography
T2DM/prediabetes	Polyuria Polydipsia Polyphagia Nocturia Weight change	Acanthosis nigricans Skin tags or verruca within acanthosis	HbA1c or fasting glucose level, or oral glucose tolerance test
Intertrigo	Difficult to heal skin rashes or skin breakdown	Erythematous, macerated patches	Clinical diagnosis
Hidradenitis suppurativa	Axillary or groin pain Nodules that may drain	Nodules in axilla or groin, with or without draining	Clinical diagnosis

(continued on next page)

Table 7
(continued)

Comorbidity	Review of Systems	Physical Examination	Evaluation
PCOS	Irregular menses Primary amenorrhea	Acne Hirsutism Alopecia	Free and total testosterone SHBG DHEAS Androstenedione 17-hydoxyprogesterone FSH, LH levels Estradiol Prolactin TSH and free T4
Cushing syndrome	Height concerns	Short stature Dorsocervical prominence Rounded facies Violaceous striae	24 h urinary cortisol levels
Genetic syndromes associated with obesity	Developmental delay Learning disabilities Hyperphagia	Early onset severe obesity <5 y of age Short stature Dysmorphic features* Small hands/feet	Genetic testing Referral to genetics
Hypertension	Typically, asymptomatic Headaches Blurred vision (in severe cases)	Elevated systolic and diastolic BP (ensure proper cuff size)	Manual repeat BPs
Dyslipidemia	Asymptomatic	None	Fasting lipid panel
Depression	Sadness Apathy Irritability Increased sleeping Insomnia Social withdrawal School avoidance	Flat affect	PHQ-9 or PHQ-2

Anxiety	Constant worry Social concerns Irritability Inability to relax	Typically none Fidgety Pressured speech	GAD-7, SCARED
ADHD	Inattention Impulsivity Learning or behavioral concerns at school	Fidgeting or constantly moving Poor impulse control	Vanderbilt or Connors scales
Binge eating/bulimia	Eating large portions of food in a short time Loss of control in eating Vomiting after eating (if purging)	Swollen parotid glands Calloused, scarred knuckles Enamel breakdown	BED-7 or ADO-BED
Male hypogonadism	Breast development Small penis	Tanner 2+ breast development	Testosterone levels

Abbreviations: ADHD, attention deficit hyperactivity disorder; ADO-BED, adolescent binge eating disorder measure; BED-7, binge eating disorder screener–7 question; DHEAS, dehydroepiandrosterone sulfate; GAD-7, general anxiety disorder–7 question; FSH, follicle stimulating hormone; LH, luteinizing hormone; SCARED, screen for child anxiety related disorders; SHBG, sex hormone binding globulin

Data from Refs.[2,10–12,19,74,75]

CLINICS CARE POINTS

- The MD Calc Web site has a BP calculator that converts BP measurements to BP percentiles to aid diagnosis of elevated BP and hypertension: https://www.mdcalc.com/calc/4052/aap-pediatric-hypertension-guidelines.
- A thorough ROS and PE are important components of evaluation to assess potential underlying causes of obesity and identification of common and emergent comorbidities.
- Laboratory evaluation, based on age and weight category, identifies cardiometabolic comorbidities that can be concurrently treated with obesity.
- Guidance for coding and billing for obesity evaluation can be found on the AAP obesity clinical practice guideline (CPG) Web site: www.aap.org/obesitycpg.

DISCLOSURE

Drs A.E. Weedn, J. Benard, and S.E. Hampl have no financial conflicts of interest relevant to the article to disclose.

REFERENCES

1. Pont SJ, Puhl R, Cook SR, et al. Section on obesity; obesity society. stigma experienced by children and adolescents with obesity. Pediatrics 2017;140(6): e20173034.
2. Bashiri FA, Al Abdulsalam HK, Hassan SM, et al. Pediatric intracranial hypertension. Experience from 2 Tertiary Centers. Neurosciences (Riyadh) 2019;24(4): 257–63.
3. Narang I, Mathew JL. Childhood obesity and obstructive sleep apnea. J Nutr Metab 2012;2012:134202.
4. Farello G, Ferrara P, Antenucci A, et al. The link between obesity and migraine in childhood: a systematic review. Ital J Pediatr 2017;43(1):27.
5. Krebs NF, Himes JH, Jacobson D, et al. Assessment of child and adolescent overweight and obesity. Pediatrics 2007;120(Suppl 4):S193–228.
6. Averill SH, Forno E. Management of the pediatric patient with asthma and obesity. Ann Allergy Asthma Immunol 2024;132(1):30–9.
7. Galai T, Moran-Lev H, Cohen S, et al. Higher prevalence of obesity among children with functional abdominal pain disorders. BMC Pediatr 2020;20(1):193.
8. Phatak UP& Pashankar DS, Pashankar DS. Obesity and gastrointestinal disorders in children. J Pediatr Gastroenterol Nutr 2015;60(4):441–5.
9. O'Malley GC, Shultz SP, Thivel D, et al. Neuromusculoskeletal health in pediatric obesity: incorporating evidence into clinical examination. Curr Obes Rep 2021; 10(4):467–77.
10. Peck DM, Voss LM, Voss TT. Slipped capital femoral epiphysis: diagnosis and management. Am Fam Physician 2017;95(12):779–84.
11. Janoyer M. Blount disease. Orthop Traumatol Surg Res 2019;105(1S):S111–21.
12. Darlenski R, Mihaylova V, Handjieva-Darlenska T. The link between obesity and the skin. Front Nutr 2022;9:855573.
13. Fox MH, Witten MH, Lullo C. Reducing obesity among people with disabilities. J Disabil Pol Stud 2014;25(3):175–85.
14. Curtin C, Hyman SL, Boas DD, et al. Weight management in primary care for children with autism: expert recommendations. Pediatrics 2020;145(Suppl 1): S126–39.

15. Schenkelberg MA, Mciver KL, Brown WH, et al. Preschool environmental influences on physical activity in children with disabilities. Med Sci Sports Exerc 2020;52(12):2682–9.

16. Speiser PW, Rudolf MCJ, Anhalt H, et al. Consensus statement: childhood obesity. J Clin Endocrinol Metab 2005;90(3):1871–87.

17. Kumar S, Kelly AS. Review of childhood obesity: from epidemiology, etiology, and comorbidities to clinical assessment and treatment. Mayo Clin Proc 2017;92(2): 251–65.

18. Flynn JT, Kaelber DC, Baker-Smith CM, et al. Clinical practice guideline for screening and management of high blood pressure in children and adolescents. Pediatrics 2017;140(3):e20171904.

19. Armstrong S, Lazorick S, Hampl S, et al. Physical examination findings among children and adolescents with obesity: an evidence-based review. Pediatrics 2016;137(2):e20151766.

20. Hirschler V. Skin and obesity in childhood: an update. AIMS Medical Science 2021;8(4):311–23.

21. Froehlich-Grobe K, Nary DE, Van Sciver A, et al. Measuring height without a stadiometer: empirical investigation of four height estimates among wheelchair users. Am J Phys Med Rehabil 2011;90(8):658–66.

22. Haapala H, Peterson MD, Daunter A, et al. Agreement between actual height and estimated height using segmental limb lengths for individuals with cerebral palsy. Am J Phys Med Rehabil 2015;94(7):539–46.

23. Agaronnik ND, Lagu T, DeJong C, et al. Accommodating patients with obesity and mobility difficulties: observations from physicians. Disabil Health J 2021; 14(1):100951.

24. Sarathy K, Doshi C, Aroojis A. Clinical examination of children with cerebral palsy. Indian J Orthop 2019;53(1):35–44.

25. Centers for Disease Control and Prevention. Measuring children's height and weight accurately at home. Available at: https://www.cdc.gov/healthyweight/ assessing/hmi/childrens bmi/measuring_children.html. [Accessed 12 February 2024].

26. Yao P, Adam M, Clark S, et al. A scoping review of the unassisted physical exam conducted over synchronous audio-video telemedicine. Syst Rev 2022;11(1): 219–36.

27. Flynn J. The changing face of pediatric hypertension in the era of the childhood obesity epidemic. Pediatr Nephrol 2013;28:1059–66.

28. Skinner AC, Staiano AE, Armstrong SC, et al. AAP appraisal of clinical care practices for child obesity treatment. part II: comorbidities. Pediatrics 2023;151(2): e202206064.

29. Köchli S, Endes K, Steiner R, et al. Obesity, high blood pressure, and physical activity determine vascular phenotype in young children. Hypertension 2019; 73(1):153–61.

30. Zhang T, Li S, Bazzano L, et al. Trajectories of childhood blood pressure and adult left ventricular hypertrophy: the bogalusa heart study. Hypertension 2018; 72(1):93–101.

31. Hampl SE, Hassink SG, Skinner AC, et al. Clinical practice guideline for the evaluation and treatment of children and adolescents with obesity. Pediatrics 2023; 151(2). e2022060640.

32. Nguyen D, Kit B, Carroll M. Abnormal cholesterol among children and adolescents in the united states, 2011-2014. NCHS Data Brief 2015;228:1–8.

33. Kwiterovich PO. Jr Recognition and management of dyslipidemia in children and adolescents. J Clin Endocrinol Metab 2008;93(11):4200–9.

34. EXPERT PANEL ON INTEGRATED GUIDELINES FOR CARDIOVASCULAR HEALTH AND RISK REDUCTION IN CHILDREN AND ADOLESCENTS. Expert panel on integrated guidelines for cardiovascular health and risk reduction in children and adolescents; national heart, lung, and blood institute. Expert panel on integrated guidelines for cardiovascular health and risk reduction in children and adolescents: summary report. Pediatrics 2011;128(Suppl 5):S213–56.

35. Cioana M, Deng J, Nadarajah A, et al. The prevalence of obesity among children with type 2 diabetes: a systematic review and meta-analysis. JAMA Netw Open 2022;5(12):e2247186.

36. Andes LJ, Cheng YJ, Rolka DB, et al. Prevalence of prediabetes among adolescents and young adults in the United States, 2005-2016. JAMA Pediatr 2020; 174(2):e194498.

37. American Diabetes Association. 2. Classification and diagnosis of diabetes: standards of medical care in diabetes-2021. Diabetes Care 2021;44(Suppl 1): S15–33.

38. Shah AS, Zeitler PS, Wong J, et al. ISPAD clinical practice consensus guidelines 2022: type 2 diabetes in children and adolescents. Pediatr Diabetes 2022;23(7): 872–902.

39. Vos MB, Abrams SH, Barlow SE, et al. NASPGHAN clinical practice guideline for the diagnosis and treatment of nonalcoholic fatty liver disease in children: recommendations from the expert committee on NAFLD (ECON) and the North American Society of Pediatric Gastroenterology, Hepatology and Nutrition (NASPGHAN). J Pediatr Gastroenterol Nutr 2017;64(2):319–34.

40. Welsh JA, Karpen S, Vos MB. Increasing prevalence of nonalcoholic fatty liver disease among United States adolescents, 1988-1994 to 2007-2010. J Pediatr 2013;162(3):496–500.

41. Anderson EL, Howe LD, Jones HE, et al. The prevalence of non-alcoholic fatty liver disease in children and adolescents: a systematic review and meta-analysis. PLoS One 2015;10(10):e0140908.

42. Mischel AK, Liao Z, Cao F, et al. Prevalence of elevated ALT in adolescents in the US 2011-2018. J Pediatr Gastroenterol Nutr 2023;77(1):103–9.

43. Ahmed MH, Barakat S, Almobarak AO. Nonalcoholic fatty liver disease and cardiovascular disease: has the time come for cardiologists to be hepatologists? J Obes 2012;2012:483135.

44. Ballestri S, Zona S, Targher G, et al. Nonalcoholic fatty liver disease is associated with an almost twofold increased risk of incident type 2 diabetes and metabolic syndrome. Evidence from a systematic review and meta-analysis. J Gastroenterol Hepatol 2016;31(5):936–44.

45. Watt MJ, Miotto PM, De Nardo W, et al. The liver as an endocrine organ-linking NAFLD and insulin resistance. Endocr Rev 2019;40(5):1367–93.

46. Eslam M, Alkhouri N, Vajro P, et al. Defining paediatric metabolic (dysfunction)-associated fatty liver disease: an international expert consensus statement. Lancet Gastroenterol Hepatol 2021;6(10):864–73.

47. Schwimmer JB, Ugalde-Nicalo P, Welsh JA, et al. Effect of a low free sugar diet vs usual diet on nonalcoholic fatty liver disease in adolescent boys: a randomized clinical trial. JAMA 2019;321(3):256–65.

48. Andersen IG, Holm JC, Homøe P. Impact of weight-loss management on children and adolescents with obesity and obstructive sleep apnea. Int J Pediatr Otorhinolaryngol 2019;123:57–62.

49. Marcus CL, Brooks LJ, Draper KA, et al. Diagnosis and management of childhood obstructive sleep apnea syndrome. Pediatrics 2012;130(3):576–84.
50. Bitners AC, Arens R. Evaluation and management of children with obstructive sleep apnea syndrome. Lung 2020;198(2):257–70.
51. American Academy of Sleep Medicine. International classification of sleep disorders. 3rd ed. Darien, IL: American Academy of Sleep Medicine; 2014.
52. Alexander NS, Schroeder JW Jr. Pediatric obstructive sleep apnea syndrome. Pediatr Clin 2013;60(4):827–40.
53. Anderson AD, Solorzano CM, McCartney CR. Childhood obesity and its impact on the development of adolescent PCOS. Semin Reprod Med 2014;32(3):202–13.
54. Naz MSG, Tehrani FR, Majd HA, et al. The prevalence of polycystic ovary syndrome in adolescents: a systematic review and meta-analysis. Int J Reprod Biomed 2019;17(8):533–42.
55. Witchel SF, Burghard AC, Tao RH, et al. The diagnosis and treatment of PCOS in adolescents: an update. Curr Opin Pediatr 2019;31(4):562–9.
56. Legro RS, Arslanian SA, Ehrmann DA, et al. Diagnosis and treatment of polycystic ovary syndrome: an Endocrine Society clinical practice guideline. J Clin Endocrinol Metab 2013;98(12):4565–92.
57. Friedman DI, Liu GT, Digre KB. Revised diagnostic criteria for the pseudotumor cerebri syndrome in adults and children. Neurology 2013;81(13):1159–65.
58. Brara SM, Koebnick C, Porter AH, et al. Pediatric idiopathic intracranial hypertension and extreme childhood obesity. J Pediatr 2012;161(4):602–7.
59. Kilgore KP, Lee MS, Leavitt JA, et al. Re-evaluating the incidence of idiopathic intracranial hypertension in an era of increasing obesity. Ophthalmology 2017;124(5):697–700.
60. Wang MTM, Bhatti MT, Danesh-Meyer HV. Idiopathic intracranial hypertension: pathophysiology, diagnosis and management. J Clin Neurosci 2022;95:172–9.
61. Wall M. Update on idiopathic intracranial hypertension. Neurol Clin 2017;35(1):45–57.
62. Chan G, Chen CT. Musculoskeletal effects of obesity. Curr Opin Pediatr 2009;21(1):65–70.
63. Manoff EM, Banffy MB, Winell JJ. Relationship between body mass index and slipped capital femoral epiphysis. J Pediatr Orthop 2005;25(6):744–6.
64. Murray AW, Wilson NI. Changing incidence of slipped capital femoral epiphysis: a relationship with obesity? J Bone Joint Surg Br 2008;90(1):92–4.
65. Perry DC, Metcalfe D, Lane S, et al. Childhood obesity and slipped capital femoral epiphysis. Pediatrics 2018;142(5):e20181067.
66. Bhatia NN, Pirpiris M, Otsuka NY. Body mass index in patients with slipped capital femoral epiphysis. J Pediatr Orthop 2006-Apr;26(2):197–9.
67. Aversano MW, Moazzaz P, Scaduto AA, et al. Association between body mass index-for-age and slipped capital femoral epiphysis: the long-term risk for subsequent slip in patients followed until physeal closure. J Child Orthop 2016;10(3):209–13.
68. Otani T, Kawaguchi Y, Marumo K. Diagnosis and treatment of slipped capital femoral epiphysis: Recent trends to note. J Orthop Sci 2018;23(2):220–8.
69. Kocher MS, Bishop JA, Weed B, et al. Delay in diagnosis of slipped capital femoral epiphysis. Pediatrics 2004;113(4):e322–5.
70. Dietz WH Jr, Gross WL, Kirkpatrick JA Jr. Blount disease (tibia vara): another skeletal disorder associated with childhood obesity. J Pediatr 1982;101(5):735–7.

71. Pirpiris M, Jackson KR, Farng E, et al. Body mass index and blount disease. J Pediatr Orthop 2006;26(5):659–63.
72. Latzer Y, Stein D. A review of the psychological and familial perspectives of childhood obesity. J Eat Disord 2013;1:7.
73. Rao WW, Zong QQ, Zhang JW, et al. Obesity increases the risk of depression in children and adolescents: results from a systematic review and meta-analysis. J Affect Disord 2020;267:78–85.
74. Jebeile H, Lister NB, Baur LA, et al. Eating disorder risk in adolescents with obesity. Obes Rev 2021;22(5):e13173.
75. Zuckerbrot RA, Cheung A, Jensen MS, et al. Guidelines for adolescent depression in primary care (glad-pc): part i. practice preparation, identification, assessment, and initial management. Pediatrics 2018;141(3):e20174081.
76. Magge SN, Silverstein J, Elder D, et al. Evaluation and treatment of prediabetes in youth. J Pediatr 2020;219:11–22.

Disordered Eating in Pediatric Obesity

Eileen Chaves, PhD, MSc[a,b,c,1,*], Angel DiPangrazio, RD[b,2],
Matthew Paponetti, PT, DPT[b,d,3], Griffin Stout, MD[c,e,4]

KEYWORDS

- Disordered eating • Eating disorders • Childhood obesity • Nutrition
- Physical activity • Binge eating disorder • Bulimia nervosa
- Disordered eating behaviors

KEY POINTS

- Disordered eating is prevalent in children and youth with obesity.
- It is important to screen for and treat disordered eating in this population.
- Treatment of disordered eating in children and youth with obesity should be multidisciplinary and include psychological, medical, nutrition, and physical activity care.

INTRODUCTION

Individuals with overweight and obesity are at an increased risk of developing an eating disorder (ED), across all genders and ethnicities.[1-3] For those seeking weight loss treatment, the prevalence of binge eating is reported to be between 9% and 29%.[4-6] In individuals diagnosed with binge eating disorder (BED) or bulimia nervosa (BN), developing either overweight or obesity is common. Individuals in larger bodies are half as likely as those with average or below average body mass indices (BMIs) to be diagnosed with an ED.[7]

The terms disordered eating (DE) and EDs are often used interchangeably, though they refer to different constructs. Disordered eating behaviors (DEBs) are similar to ED

---

[a] Division of Neuropsychology and Pediatric Psychology; [b] Center for Healthy Weight and Nutrition, Nationwide Children's Hospital, 380 Butterfly Gardens Drive, LAC, Suite 5F, Columbus, OH 43215, USA; [c] The Ohio State University, College of Medicine; [d] Sports and Orthopedic Therapies; [e] Division of Child and Adolescent Psychiatry, Nationwide Children's Hospital, 444 Butterfly Gardens Drive, Columbus, OH 43215, USA
[1] Present address: 96 Howard Avenue, Worthington, OH 43085.
[2] Present address: 18 W Beaumont Road, Columbus, OH 43214.
[3] Present address: 1651-B Wyandotte Road, Columbus, OH 43212.
[4] Present address: 6342 Memorial Drive, Dublin, OH 43017.
* Corresponding author. Nationwide Children's Hospital, 380 Butterfly Gardens Drive, LAC, Suite 5F, Columbus, OH 43215.
E-mail address: Eileen.Chaves@nationwidechildrens.org

Pediatr Clin N Am 71 (2024) 879–896
https://doi.org/10.1016/j.pcl.2024.06.009
pediatric.theclinics.com

behaviors, though they vary in frequency and severity. Both DEBs and diagnosable ED, that is, anorexia nervosa (AN), BN, BED, other eating and feeding disorders, including atypical AN, are common in children and youth with obesity. Both girls (at 76%) and boys (at 55%) with obesity endorse unhealthy weight control behaviors, such as food restriction, "dieting," irregular or inflexible eating patterns, or compulsive eating.[8] The prevalence of DEBs is difficult to ascertain as most current screeners detect formal ED and have no specific cutoffs for subclinical ED behaviors or DE. For the purpose of this article, we will use the term DEBs, which is inclusive of both DE and ED, as individuals with obesity present with both subclinical ED behaviors and ED (**Fig. 1**).

The gold standard treatment of pediatric obesity is multidisciplinary, including medical, psychological, nutrition, and physical activity (PA) care.[9] The treatment of children and youth with obesity and DEBs should also be multidisciplinary, encompassing all of the disciplines needed to effectively treat pediatric obesity and DEB. Multidisciplinary care provides holistic treatment, focusing on all aspects impacted by both a youth's DEB and obesity. This study will outline best practices for the treatment of DEBs in children and youth with obesity from a multidisciplinary lens.

MULTIDISCIPLINARY CARE
Psychological Care

In youth aged 13 to 18 years, the lifetime prevalence of developing an ED is 2.7%.[10] While prevalence rates for comorbid DEBs in children and adolescents with obesity are more difficult to ascertain, a Canadian sample of 3043 adolescents found that the prevalence of the range of DEBs was higher in adolescents with obesity (9.3% in male individuals and 20.2% in female individuals) when compared with their peers with healthy weight (2.1% male individuals and 8.4% female individuals).[11,12] A recent study examining the prevalence of EDs and psychiatric comorbidities in children aged 9 and 10 years found that children diagnosed with an ED were 71.4% more likely to also be diagnosed with an anxiety disorder, 47.9% more likely to be diagnosed with attention deficit/hyperactivity disorder, 45% more likely to be diagnosed with disruptive/impulse control disorders, 29.6% more likely to be diagnosed with a mood disorder, and 28.8% more likely to be diagnosed with obsessive-compulsive disorder.[13] Of note, a history of trauma, specifically sexual trauma, is often more prevalent in individuals diagnosed with an ED as well, though recent research has found that

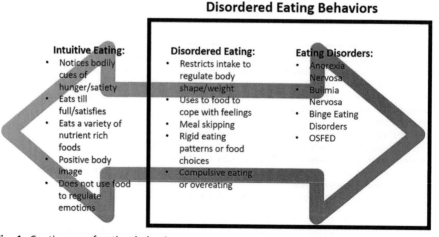

Fig. 1. Continuum of eating behaviors.

experiencing any type of traumatic event is associated with BED.[14] The high prevalence of both DEBs in children and youth with obesity continues to add credence to the importance of screening for both EDs and psychiatric conditions in pediatric weight management (PWM) in order to provide best treatment. **Table 1** provides an overview of brief validated screeners, some of which can be used in young children.

For youth that screen positive for an ED or who endorse subclinical DE that could complicate obesity treatment (ie, binge episode 1× per week with or without compensatory behaviors with marked distress afterward), it is important to treat these conditions using evidence-based treatment. Treatments of ED and DE are multidisciplinary, with psychological care provided by a psychologist, mental health provider (ie, licensed professional counselor [LPC], marriage and family therapist [MFT]), or clinical social worker (ie, licensed clinical counselor [LCSW]).

Evidence-Based Treatments of Eating Disorder

There are several evidenced-based treatments of EDs. These include enhanced cognitive-behavioral therapy (CBT-E), dialectical behavior therapy-eating disorders, and interpersonal therapy for eating disorders (IPT-ED). Several of these treatment approaches have been adapted for use with adolescents specifically, including dialectical behavior therapy for adolescents (DBT-A).

Enhanced Cognitive-Behavioral Therapy

CBT-E is a model designed to treat a range of ED behaviors that occur across multiple ED diagnoses. This model posits that all EDs share many of the same features including intense concern with weight and shape and/or difficulty coping with strong

Table 1
Screeners

Screener Name	Ages Validated	Number of Items	Screens for	Validated in
Children's Brief Binge-Eating Questionnaire[13]	7–18 y old	7 items	BED	PWM setting
Child-Binge Eating disorder Scale[16]	5–13 y old	7 items	BED	General population
Eating Disorders Screen for primary care[17]	18 y+	4 items	Anorexia, nervosa, BN, and BED	Primary care
Sick, Control, One, Fat, & Food[18]	12 y+	5 items	Anorexia, nervosa, BN, and BED	Eating disorders setting
Adolescent Binge Eating disorder Scale Questionnaire[19]	12 y+	6 items	BED	Primary care
Screen for Disordered Eating[20]	18 y+	5 items	Anorexia, nervosa, BN, and BED	Primary care
Eating disorder diagnostic scale[21]	13 y+	22 items	Anorexia, nervosa, BN, and BED	EDs setting
Eating Disorders Questionnaire-Short form[22]	14 y+	12 items	Anorexia, nervosa, BN, and BED	ED population
Eating Disorders Examination-Questionnaire[23]	7–18 y+	8 items	Anorexia, nervosa, BN, and BED	General population

emotions. CBT-E is a time-limited treatment, typically including 20 sessions over 20 weeks for individuals with BED and BN. CBT-E includes 4 treatment stages that focus on consistent eating, maintenance of ED triggers (ie, concern over body shape), and alternative coping strategies. Research has shown that for adults and adolescents diagnosed with either BN or BED, CBT-E is effective at alleviating ED features and general psychopathology.[24–28]

Dialectical Behavior Therapy for Adolescents

DBT emphasizes teaching and integration of coping skills and is a type of cognitive behavioral therapy (CBT). For adolescents with comorbid EDs and mood concerns, DBT-A is effective at treating both presenting problems concurrently.[29,30] DBT-A includes skills training sessions, individual therapy, and phone coaching for both caregivers and adolescents. Multiple studies have reported that DBT is an effective treatment of ED.[31–33]

Interpersonal Psychotherapy for Eating Disorders

IPT-ED is adapted from interpersonal psychotherapy (IPT) for the specific treatment of ED. IPT notes that interpersonal difficulties are common in individuals with EDs and often serve to maintain the DEB.[34] IPT-ED helps individuals address interpersonal difficulties, removing processes that maintain the ED and decreases ED symptoms. It typically involves 16 to 20 50 minute sessions over the course of 4 to 5 months. Research has shown IPT-ED to be efficacious in the treatment of BED and BN, but not AN.[35–37]

Treatments of Obesity and Disordered Eating Behaviors

As rates of obesity have continued to rise, there has been a growing recognition within the obesity medicine community that DEBs, often binge eating behaviors and loss of control while eating, as well as food restriction, are prevalent and impede treatment of obesity.[38] There is a need to develop treatments that combine both DEB treatment and medical weight management. Several studies have looked at interventions that address comorbid obesity and EDs, though the majority of these are adult focused. These include CBT, behavioral weight loss therapy (BWLT), and integrated treatment approaches such as a healthy approach to weight management and food in eating disorders (HAPIFED). Research has shown that while CBT often results in a remission of binge eating symptoms, BWLT often results in a greater weight loss than CBT, though this weight loss is minimal (ie, -2.1 kg/m^2).[39] Individuals who exhibit remission from binge eating have significant reductions in BMI compared to participants who did not have remission from binge eating. Combined treatments (ie, CBT + caloric restriction + sertraline + topiramate) have resulted in more significant weight loss (ie, average loss of 12 kg) and binge eating at 6 months from start of treatment.[40–42] Hay and colleagues found that HAPIFED and CBT-E show reductions in stress, improvement in mental-health related quality of life, reduction of binge eating severity, and global reduction in ED symptoms. However, adding weight management to ED treatment (in the HAPIFED approach) did not have any beneficial effects on metabolic outcomes, including blood test results for glucose, insulin, triglycerides, and cholesterol.[43]

Recommendations

- Due to the known prevalence of DEBs in children and adolescents with obesity, screening for DEBs at the start of PWM is recommended to determine best course of treatment.

- Rates of other mental health conditions are often comorbid with EDs, making screening for these conditions a recommendation as well. Treatment of comorbid mental health treatment is recommended in conjunction with PWM.
- There are several validated treatments of EDs in adolescents. Recent treatments of both DEBs and obesity have been trialed in adults, with varying results. Research combining treatments of both obesity in children and adolescents with DEBs needs to be done.

Nutrition Care

Nutrition care for patients with DEBs is important for the treatment and prevention of developing a clinically diagnosed ED.[44] Special care should be taken when working with youth with obesity as the use of unhealthy eating behaviors to lose weight and a significant history of dieting are common.[45] When a patient with obesity presents for treatment, a thorough nutrition assessment is necessary. **Fig. 2** compares the aspects of a nutrition assessment based on the Academy of Nutrition and Dietetics recommendations for patients with overweight/obesity and patients with an ED.[44,46]

Potential indicators for DEBs are listed in **Fig. 3** and indicate a need for further assessment.[44-46] Given the prevalence of DEB in youth with obesity, it is important to monitor and screen for DEBs at the onset of treatment. This should be a regular practice and will enhance treatment.[45,46]

Nutrition Intervention for Disordered Eating Behaviors and Obesity: Is There Overlap?

Appropriate nutrition interventions are determined by various factors including patients' medical history, patients' goals/desires for treatment, overall nutrition assessment, and clinical judgment. If there is a concern for DEB, the pediatric clinician should determine if a referral to a dietitian or psychologist is needed to further assess and provide treatment. Not all nutrition interventions commonly used for patients with obesity are appropriate for patients who have subclinical or clinical DEBs or EDs. Examples of inappropriate treatments may include calorie-defined plans, unbalanced macronutrients, meal replacements, and intermittent energy restriction. **Fig. 3** describes the intersection of nutrition interventions for patients with overweight and obesity compared to nutrition interventions for the treatment of ED s. It may be beneficial to

Nutrition Assessment for Overweight/ Obesity	Nutrition Assessment for Eating Disorders
• Obesity- BMI >/= 95%ile • Presence of comorbidities • Mental health status • Level of family involvement • Socioeconomic status (SES) • Pharmacotherapy • Hx of bariatric surgery (patient and family members) • Readiness and ability to follow recommended dietary changes advised • Growth pattern/trends in anthropometric measures • Biochemical data, medical tests and procedure assessment • Food and nutrient intake including composition, adequacy, meal and snack patterns, and appropriateness related to food allergies and intolerances (including current and historical efforts to use specialized and structured diets like low fat, low carbohydrate/high protein, liquids only, vegan/vegetarian, macrobiotic, food category restriction)	• Risk for malnutrition from nutrition screening documentation (diet history, physical assessment data, belief systems around eating, environmental barriers to adequate nutrition, including food security) • Development, onset, and history of eating disorder(s) and related factors (eg food issues, weight history, physical activity, sport-specific activities, previous dieting methods) • Growth pattern/trends in anthropometric measures • Mental health status • Biochemical data, medical tests and procedure assessment • Food and nutrient intake including composition, adequacy, meal and snack patterns, and appropriateness related to food allergies and intolerances • Pharmacotherapy, medication, and supplement use • Readiness for change • Level of family involvement • Socioeconomic status (SES)

Fig. 2. Nutrition assessment for overweight/obesity[44] and EDs.[46]

- Sneaking or hiding of food
- Extensive dieting history
- Emotional eating behaviors
- Feelings of loss of control around food
- Feelings of guilt or shame after eating
- Skipped meals
- Compensatory behaviors (restriction of food)
- Eating in isolation/away from others
- Reading diet books
- Increased picky eating, especially eating only "healthy foods"
- The habit of always going to the bathroom immediately after eating

Fig. 3. Indicators for further assessment.[44,47]

take an integrative approach to treatment that is weight-inclusive rather than weight-centric and with a focus on shared risk factors[45,48–50] (**Fig. 4**).

Intuitive Eating Outcomes on Health

Mindful eating interventions have shown promising results, with patients reporting an improvement in their relationship with food, increased PA, and a better sense of hunger/satiety cues.[49,52–54] It is also known that adolescents prefer interventions that focus on and target overall health improvement rather than weight alone.[49] Furthermore, research has shown the same or similar improvement in cardio-metabolic factors as well as weight loss in those participating in a mindful eating and weight neutral approach compared to those in a traditional weight management intervention.[49,53,54]

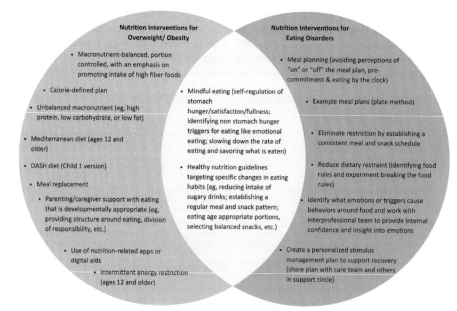

Fig. 4. Nutrition interventions for overweight/obesity,[46] EDs,[44,51] and overlapping interventions.[46,51]

Weight-focused conversations that place a high emphasis on weight or body dissatisfaction as motivation for behavior change have been shown to increase the risk for DEBs and increased the risk for the development of an ED.[45,49] Diets and calorie counting are ineffective in weight management due to lack of sustainability as well as promotion of an unhealthy relationship with food.[53,55] Furthermore, most participants will eventually experience weight regain.[55] Informing patients that dieting can be counterproductive and unsustainable long-term has shown to be more beneficial, as well as encouraging regular family meals.[45]

Nutrition Plan of Care for Disordered Eating Behaviors

The intersection of DEBs and obesity can make nutrition intervention more challenging due to other medical comorbidities that may indicate serious need for dietary and lifestyle changes (eg, metabolic dysfunction-associated steatotic liver disease [MASLD], type II diabetes mellitus [DM], hypertension, and so forth). Balancing the need for behavioral and nutritional changes in light of medical comorbidities as well as promoting a healthy and long-term relationship with food, eating, and body is vital. Given this complexity, collaboration within a multidisciplinary team and other health care professionals is an important aspect of nutrition intervention for patients with obesity and DEBs.[44,46,56]

Emphasis should be placed on interventions that overlap to prevent DE and/or progression of DEBs.[49,50] Discussing how to identify what is too much or too little food, consistency of meals and snacks, and inclusion of a variety of food groups should be incorporated into nutritional counseling with children and adolescents with obesity and DEBs.[45,46,51] Helping children and adolescents identify hunger and fullness cues, as well as the difference between physical hunger versus emotional hunger is also important. These discussions equip both patients and families with the knowledge and tools to promote a healthy relationship with food, body attunement, and overall health.[45,46,51,53]

Recommendations

- Emerging research shows promise with mindful eating interventions and weight-inclusive approaches in pediatrics. It is important to consider focusing on interventions that are shared between the 2 conditions as to not further promote DEBs unintentionally.
- Overall discussions around a healthy relationship with food, education revolving around the importance of fiber and nutrient density, consistency of meals and snacks throughout the day, recognition of hunger/fullness cues, and identification of age and gender-appropriate portion sizes should be the primary focus of conversations given the prevalence of DEBs in this population.

Physical Activity Care

Increasing PA has been identified as a pillar within comprehensive obesity treatment and prevention given the overwhelming benefits of regular PA engagement.[57–59] Regular PA engagement in childhood improves cardiometabolic health, weight status and weight-related comorbidities, cardiorespiratory and muscular fitness, cognition and academic performance, and mental health.[60–62] Evidence is also mounting to support the integration of PA into the treatment of DEBs.[63–70] PA may improve DEB through multiple pathways. PA has been shown to help decrease food cravings and food addiction[71] and may positively impact appetite control,[72] which could improve DEBs. Activity engagement also has a known positive effect on mood, stress, anxiety, and depressive symptoms that are linked to DEBs.[61,71,73] Exercise has also been shown to reduce drive for thinness and decrease body dissatisfaction.[74,75] Given the benefits of activity engagement on both obesity and DEBs, PA intervention may play an important role in the treatment of youth with obesity and comorbid DEB.

A primary goal of PA intervention for youth with obesity is to promote physical literacy development and a positive relationship with PA that will support activity engagement throughout the life span.[58,76] This can be complicated in youth with obesity secondary to a range of environmental, interpersonal, and individual barriers (Table 2).[77] O'Malley and colleagues highlight how neuromusculoskeletal impairments and pain also present as common barriers to activity engagement for youth with obesity.[78] If such barriers are identified, it would be appropriate to refer to a physical therapist to manage pain, improve function, and support the individual's activity engagement.

A key consideration when working with youth with DEB is to assess for dysfunctional exercise, which is seen in up to 80% of those with an ED and across the spectrum of DEBs.[63,79,80] Dysfunctional exercise, which can include compulsive exercise, exercise addiction, obligatory exercise, and exercise dependence, can result in physical and psychological health consequences and can exacerbate DEBs.[80] While dysfunctional exercise may include excessive quality or intensity of exercise, it also includes the emotions, cognitions, and motivations surrounding activity engagement.[63,81] Dysfunctional exercise may include exercising as a means of compensating or purging following food consumption, coping with feelings of guilt, or attempting to control body shape or size secondary to negative body image or body dissatisfaction.[8,63,81] Table 2 highlights additional signs that may indicate dysfunctional exercise. The compulsive exercise test (CET) is a screening tool that has been used in adolescents with ED and may help clinicians identify dysfunctional

Table 2
Barriers and physical activity behaviors to consider

Barriers to Physical Activity[77,78]	Signs of Dysfunctional Exercise[86–90]	Healthy Activity Behaviors[65,66,76,78,84,85]
• Pain • Injury and fear of injury • Excessive physical discomfort • Decreased balance and coordination • Decreased strength and endurance • Low self-esteem and self-efficacy with PA • Perceived inferiority in social settings and social anxiety • Weight-related teasing/bullying • Limited family PA engagement • Lack of access to PA facilities • Unsafe neighborhood and play spaces • Financial barriers to organized PA and sport	• Excessive exercise (duration, frequency, and intensity) • Rigidity with exercise routines • Guilt, shame, and distress if unable to exercise • Exercise interfering with daily life, social and family events, or sleep • Exercising despite pain, injury, or excessive fatigue • Exercise as permission to eat or as means of purging • Exercise to change body shape and control weight • Exercise to control emotions	• Activity engagement for fun and enjoyment • Positive social interactions during PA • Focus on positive physical and mental health benefits • Willingness to explore and try new PA • PA incorporated into daily life • Variability in types of activity engagement • Family PA engagement • Appropriate awareness of fatigue, injury, and pain

exercise behaviors that require further treatment.[82,83] If identified it is important that dysfunctional exercise is addressed, ideally within the context of a multidisciplinary team where exercise specialists, such as physical therapists, and psychologists can collaborate to provide psychoeducation that challenge distorted cognitions about exercise, encourage healthy activity behaviors (see **Table 2**), and provide supervised exposure to healthy PA engagement.[65,66]

To promote physical literacy development and a healthy relationship with PA, clinicians should focus on helping youth find ways to be active that are fun and enjoyable, promote positive social interactions, and encourage well-being and self-care (**Table 3**).[65,76,78] Similar to nutrition recommendations, taking a weight-neutral approach to PA that focuses on self-acceptance and health at every size versus engaging in body shape or weight-control could be particularly important for youth with obesity.[49,84] Gathering a thorough history and taking time to understand the child's past experiences, barriers, motivators, and emotions surrounding PA engagement will aide in providing tailored activity recommendations.[76,78] Clinicians should encourage exploration of PA experiences that could include various forms of free play, organized sport, supervised strength training, walking, outdoor adventures, and active video games, among many other activities. Clinicians can also connect families to community-based activity programs and other places to be active, such as recreation centers, parks, and playgrounds.[76,85] Activity recommendations should be matched to the child's physical capabilities, confidence, and interests, and should start at an appropriate frequency and intensity.[66,76,78] Youth should be encouraged to "listen to one's body" to guide activity progression and modification.[66] Lastly, it is important that clinicians closely monitor and follow up with youth regarding activity engagement. Clinicians should monitor for dysfunctional exercise behaviors and pain/injury, address barriers that arise, provide new ideas for activity engagement, and progress frequency and intensity of activity engagement as appropriate.

Recommendations

- While it may be ideal for PA intervention for youth with obesity and DEBs to be provided within the context of a multidisciplinary treatment team including physical therapists or exercise specialists, all health care professionals can take steps to support healthy PA behaviors for youth.
- Clinicians should assess for dysfunctional exercise behaviors, pain, and neuromusculoskeletal impairments in youth with obesity and DEBs and make appropriate referrals when identified.
- PA intervention should focus on enjoyment and exploration, promote positive social interactions, and encourage well-being and self-care rather than engaging in PA to control body shape or weight.

Medical Care and Considerations

Regardless of body size, the medical complications from DE can be present, serious, and deadly.[91,92] A thorough medical evaluation is necessary for patients with obesity and DE. Medical complications vary based on the ED behaviors present, so it is important to identify these behaviors, including intentional restriction, purging and/or bingeing, their intensity, frequency, and duration. Often DE symptoms present as a cycle of restriction, bingeing, and purging, utilizing one or many compensatory behaviors.

DEBs can affect all organ systems, so a complete review of medical and mental health symptoms can help guide medical assessment, increase a child's or youth's urgency for treatment, and help provide education on the physical consequences of

Table 3
Considerations for activity promotion in youth with comorbid and disordered eating behavior

Collaboration within a multidisciplinary team to support activity engagement	• *Pediatric clinician*: Medical safety and clearance for PA • *Psychologist*: Support positive behaviors and emotions, body image, and cognitions surrounding PA • *Dietician*: Ensure appropriate nutrition to support and optimize PA • *Physical therapy*: Provide positive activity experience, address pain and neuromusculoskeletal impairment, and progress activity engagement
Screen for pain and neuromusculoskeletal impairments that limit activity engagement	• Question child and family regarding pain, discomfort, and difficulty during PA • Refer to physical therapy if barriers are identified
Screen for dysfunctional exercise behaviors	• Assess activity behaviors and motivations for activity engagement (see **Table 2**) or use a screening tool such as the CET • Address within multidisciplinary team or refer to psychologist and exercise specialist
Promote a positive relationship with PA	• Focus on activity engagement for positive physical and mental health benefits (see **Table 2**). • Avoid focus on activity for shape and weight change.
Focus on fun, enjoyment, and exploration with PA	• Encourage engagement in enjoyable activities based off the child's interests. • Refer to community-based programs and local resources that support PA
Start slow and low, then gradually progress	• Start with lighter and less frequent PA and encourage "listening to one's body" • Gradually increase activity engagement based on response
Continuous monitoring and follow up	• Continuously monitor for pain, injury, or onset of dysfunctional exercise • Progress activity frequency and intensity when appropriate • Continue to provide new ideas and resources for activity engagement

their behaviors. Assessing for syncopal episodes, dizziness, palpitations, constipation, early satiety, nausea, bloating, amenorrhea, low libido, increased bleeding, increased frequency of stress fractures, and cold intolerance is important in assessing medical stability and how DE is affecting patients.

In children and youth in larger bodies, research has shown an increase in prevalence not only of EDs but also of mental health conditions, including depression, anxiety, and attention deficit hyperactivity disorder. In adolescents with obesity, being male, having a higher BMI, and being in late adolescence have all been associated with having a mental health comorbidity.[93] There is also a high prevalence of depression and anxiety in adolescents diagnosed with an ED. Individuals with an ED are twice as likely to also have depression or anxiety. One study found that close to 50% of adolescents with EDs also had high levels of anxiety and depression.[94] Due to the high prevalence of comorbid mental health conditions in adolescents with overweight and obesity as well as adolescents diagnosed with an ED, it is important to screen for mental health conditions as part of holistic medical assessment.

A physical examination with appropriate size gown, blood pressure cuff, and scale can help decrease weight stigma and accurately assess for physical symptoms associated with DEBs. Vital signs should include orthostatic heart rate, blood pressure, height, and weight (ideally postvoided and blinded). Reviewing growth chart history is important to identify if weight loss is present, and if so, at what rate and how much weight has been lost to accurately diagnose malnutrition.

Laboratory evaluation can be helpful to assess medical stability, rule out other illnesses, and help educate the child or youth on negative effects of DEBs. It is important to recognize that the lack of abnormal laboratory values does not rule out an ED or indicate no medical harm is occurring. Remarkably, children's and youth's bodies can compensate for severe behaviors over long periods to maintain medical stability. Laboratory work to consider includes but is not limited to complete blood count with differential, comprehensive metabolic panel to assess for electrolytes, and potentially dangerous hypokalemia or hypophosphatemia, or altered liver enzymes, thyroid studies, and measures of gonadotropins and sex steroids. An electrocardiogram may be necessary if there is significant malnutrition, bradycardia, syncope, or potential electrolyte abnormalities. These are the most common reasons for patients to require medical hospitalization for acute medical stabilization, at any weight. Further diagnostic tests may include a bone density study (dual energy X-ray absorptiometry [DEXA] scan) for biologic female individuals with more than 6 months of amenorrhea or any male patients with weight loss. Of note, bone loss demineralization is the one of the irreversible medical complications of food restriction in adolescents, due to the window of bone growth, which occurs within adolescence.[95]

Early adolescence is a crucial period of growth and development, and if weight loss is present, the body may slow or halt puberty to conserve energy. Regardless of body size or weight at presentation, weight suppression can have serious medical consequences. Individuals who have suppressed more than 20% of their body mass in 1 year or 10% of body mass in 6 months are at the highest risk for medical complications including bradycardia, hypotension, and refeeding hypophosphatemia and hypokalemia.[96] Studies have found atypical AN is 2 to 3 times more common than AN.[97] Of note, those at higher weight with primary restrictive behaviors are at risk of the same physical complications as those who have a BMI lower than 18.[98] In a retrospective study from the Royal Children's Hospital, patients with atypical AN had a similar rate of bradycardia, hypotension, amenorrhea, and required hospitalization at the same rate as those who were medically diagnosed as underweight. However, those with atypical AN had lost more weight (17.6 kg vs 11 kg) over a longer time (13.3 vs 10.2 months).[92] Therefore, regardless of body size, children and youth with restrictive behaviors and weight suppression need to be monitored medically to ensure stability.

For those with purging behaviors, the method and type of purging is important to elucidate. Purging by self-induced vomiting can cause significant metabolic abnormalities, including, but not limited to hypokalemia, hypophosphatemia, and potentially permanent dental erosions. An important purging behavior to be aware of is insulin omission as a form of weight control. Patients with type 1 DM have a higher estimated prevalence of EDs at approximately 7%.[99] The prevalence of insulin omission is 2% in preteens, 11% to 15% in mid-teens, and 30% to 39% for late teens/early adults.[95] Of note, patients with comorbid AN and type 1 DM have 3 times higher risk of going into diabetic ketoacidosis and 6 fold increased risk of death than those without EDs.[100]

Lastly, if a child or youth is struggling with binge episodes, it will be important to consider medical complications. Available data indicate that individuals with binge-eating disorder have a greater frequency of metabolic syndrome components (ie, dyslipidemia, hypertension, and type 2 DM) and cardiometabolic risk than those with no history of an ED or without obesity.[101] Clients with BED also have a higher prevalence of type 2 DM, especially in those with higher BMI, ranging from 1.4% to 25.6%.[102]

Recommendations

- Serious medical complications can occur in patients with DEBs no matter their body size.
- It is important to complete a thorough medical evaluation to assess for complications associated with DEBs and rule out comorbidities.
- If a patient has DM, it is important to screen for DEBs and insulin misuse as medical consequences and morbidity increases in this population.

CLINICS CARE POINTS

- There are multiple validated screeners that can be used to assess for disordered eating in children and youth with overweight and obesity prior to starting treatment.
- Multidisciplinary care is essential for the assessment and treatment of children and youth with overweight and obesity.

DISCLOSURE

All authors report no conflicts of interest and have nothing to disclose.

REFERENCES

1. Rodgers RF, Watts AW, Austin SB, et al. Disordered eating in ethnic minority adolescents with overweight. Int J Eat Disord 2017;50(6):665–71.
2. van Eeden AE, Oldehinkel AJ, van Hoeken D, et al. Risk factors in preadolescent boys and girls for the development of eating pathology in young adulthood. Int J Eat Disord 2021;54(7):1147–59.
3. Barakat S, McLean SA, Bryant E, et al. Risk factors for eating disorders: findings from a rapid review. J Eat Disord 2023;11:8.
4. Spitzer RL, Yanovski S, Wadden T, et al. Binge eating disorder: its further validation in a multisite study. Int J Eat Disord 1993;13(2):137–53.
5. Decaluwé V, Braet C. Prevalence of binge-eating disorder in obese children and adolescents seeking weight-loss treatment. Int J Obes Relat Metab Disord J Int Assoc Study Obes 2003;27(3):404–9.
6. Allison KC, Crow SJ, Reeves RR, et al. Binge eating disorder and night eating syndrome in adults with type 2 diabetes. Obes Silver Spring Md 2007;15(5): 1287–93.
7. Nagata JM, Garber AK, Tabler JL, et al. Prevalence and correlates of disordered eating behaviors among young adults with overweight or obesity. J Gen Intern Med 2018;33(8):1337–43.
8. Hayes JF, Fitzsimmons-Craft EE, Karam AM, et al. Disordered eating attitudes and behaviors in youth with overweight and obesity: implications for treatment. Curr Obes Rep 2018;7(3):235–46.

9. Zachurzok A, Springwald A, Gibała P, et al. Current therapeutic strategies in treating obesity in children and adolescents – review of the literature. Dev Period Med 2017;21(3):286–92.

10. Eating disorders - National Institute of Mental Health (NIMH). Available at: https://www.nimh.nih.gov/health/statistics/eating-disorders. [Accessed 28 February 2024].

11. Flament MF, Henderson K, Buchholz A, et al. Weight status and DSM-5 diagnoses of eating disorders in adolescents from the community. J Am Acad Child Adolesc Psychiatry 2015;54(5):403–11.e2.

12. Chaves E, Jeffrey DT, Williams DR. Disordered eating and eating disorders in pediatric obesity: assessment and next steps. Int J Environ Res Publ Health 2023;20(17):6638.

13. Convertino AD, Blashill AJ. Psychiatric comorbidity of eating disorders in children between the ages of 9 and 10. JCPP (J Child Psychol Psychiatry) 2022; 63(5):519–26.

14. Convertino AD, Morland LA, Blashill AJ. Trauma exposure and eating disorders: Results from a United States nationally representative sample. Int J Eat Disord 2022;55(8):1079–89.

15. Franklin EV, Simpson V, Berthet-Miron M, et al. A pilot study evaluating a binge-eating screener in children: Development of the Children's Brief Binge-Eating Questionnaire in a Pediatric Obesity Clinic. Clin Pediatr (Phila) 2019;58(10): 1063–71.

16. Shapiro JR, Woolson SL, Hamer RM, et al. Evaluating binge eating disorder in children: development of the children's binge eating disorder scale (C-BEDS). Int J Eat Disord 2007;40(1):82–9.

17. Cotton MA, Ball C, Robinson P. Four simple questions can help screen for eating disorders. J Gen Intern Med 2003;18(1):53–6.

18. Morgan JF, Reid F, Lacey JH. The SCOFF questionnaire. West J Med 2000; 172(3):164–5.

19. Chamay-Weber C, Combescure C, Lanza L, et al. Screening obese adolescents for binge eating disorder in primary care: the adolescent binge eating scale. J Pediatr 2017;185:68–72.e1.

20. Maguen S, Hebenstreit C, Li Y, et al. Screen for Disordered Eating: Improving the accuracy of eating disorder screening in primary care. Gen Hosp Psychiatr 2018;50:20–5.

21. Krabbenborg MAM, Danner UN, Larsen JK, et al. The eating disorder diagnostic scale: psychometric features within a clinical population and a cut-off point to differentiate clinical patients from healthy controls. Eur Eat Disord Rev J Eat Disord Assoc 2012;20(4):315–20.

22. Gideon N, Hawkes N, Mond J, et al. Development and Psychometric Validation of the EDE-QS, a 12 Item Short Form of the Eating Disorder Examination Questionnaire (EDE-Q). PLoS One 2016;11(5). e0152744.

23. Kliem S, Schmidt R, Vogel M, et al. An 8-item short form of the Eating Disorder Examination-Questionnaire adapted for children (ChEDE-Q8). Int J Eat Disord 2017;50(6):679–86.

24. Nohara N, Yamanaka Y, Matsuoka M, et al. A multi-center, randomized, parallel-group study to compare the efficacy of enhanced cognitive behavior therapy (CBT-E) with treatment as usual (TAU) for anorexia nervosa: study protocol. Biopsychosoc Med 2023;17(1):20.

25. Poulsen S, Lunn S, Daniel SIF, et al. A randomized controlled trial of psychoanalytic psychotherapy or cognitive-behavioral therapy for bulimia nervosa. Am J Psychiatr 2014;171(1):109–16.

26. Fairburn CG, Bailey-Straebler S, Basden S, et al. A transdiagnostic comparison of enhanced cognitive behaviour therapy (CBT-E) and interpersonal psychotherapy in the treatment of eating disorders. Behav Res Ther 2015;70:64–71.

27. Wonderlich SA, Peterson CB, Smith TL, et al. Integrative cognitive-affective therapy for bulimia nervosa. In: The treatment of eating disorders: a clinical handbook. The Guilford Press; 2010. p. 317–38.

28. Dalle Grave R, Calugi S, Sartirana M, et al. Transdiagnostic cognitive behaviour therapy for adolescents with an eating disorder who are not underweight. Behav Res Ther 2015;73:79–82.

29. Wisniewski L, Ben-Porath DD. Dialectical behavior therapy and eating disorders: the use of contingency management procedures to manage dialectical dilemmas. Am J Psychother 2015;69(2):129–40.

30. Fleischhaker C, Böhme R, Sixt B, et al. Dialectical Behavioral Therapy for Adolescents (DBT-A): a clinical Trial for Patients with suicidal and self-injurious Behavior and Borderline Symptoms with a one-year Follow-up. Child Adolesc Psychiatr Ment Health 2011;5(1):3.

31. Bankoff SM, Karpel MG, Forbes HE, et al. A systematic review of dialectical behavior therapy for the treatment of eating disorders. Eat Disord 2012;20(3):196–215.

32. Vogel EN, Singh S, Accurso EC. A systematic review of cognitive behavior therapy and dialectical behavior therapy for adolescent eating disorders. J Eat Disord 2021;9:131.

33. Lammers MW, Vroling MS, Crosby RD, et al. Dialectical behavior therapy adapted for binge eating compared to cognitive behavior therapy in obese adults with binge eating disorder: a controlled study. J Eat Disord 2020;8:27.

34. Karam AM, Fitzsimmons-Craft EE, Tanofsky-Kraff M, et al. Interpersonal Psychotherapy and the Treatment of Eating Disorders. Psychiatr Clin 2019;42(2):205–18.

35. Wilfley DE, Welch RR, Stein RI, et al. A randomized comparison of group cognitive-behavioral therapy and group interpersonal psychotherapy for the treatment of overweight individuals with binge-eating disorder. Arch Gen Psychiatr 2002;59(8):713–21.

36. Wilson GT, Wilfley DE, Agras WS, et al. Psychological treatments of binge eating disorder. Arch Gen Psychiatr 2010;67(1):94–101.

37. National Collaborating Centre for Mental Health (UK). Eating Disorders: Core Interventions in the Treatment and Management of Anorexia Nervosa, Bulimia Nervosa and Related Eating Disorders. British Psychological Society (UK). 2004. Available at: http://www.ncbi.nlm.nih.gov/books/NBK49304/. [Accessed 28 February 2024].

38. Jebeile H, Gow ML, Baur LA, et al. Treatment of obesity, with a dietary component, and eating disorder risk in children and adolescents: A systematic review with meta-analysis. Obes Rev Off J Int Assoc Study Obes 2019;20(9):1287–98.

39. Grilo CM, Masheb RM, Wilson GT, et al. Cognitive-behavioral therapy, behavioral weight loss, and sequential treatment for obese patients with binge-eating disorder: a randomized controlled trial. J Consult Clin Psychol 2011;79(5):675–85.

40. Brambilla F, Samek L, Company M, et al. Multivariate therapeutic approach to binge-eating disorder: combined nutritional, psychological and pharmacological treatment. Int Clin Psychopharmacol 2009;24(6):312–7.

41. da Luz FQ, Hay P, Touyz S, et al. Obesity with Comorbid Eating Disorders: Associated Health Risks and Treatment Approaches. Nutrients 2018;10(7):829.

42. Palavras MA, Hay P, Touyz S, et al. Comparing cognitive behavioural therapy for eating disorders integrated with behavioural weight loss therapy to cognitive behavioural therapy-enhanced alone in overweight or obese people with bulimia nervosa or binge eating disorder: study protocol for a randomised controlled trial. Trials 2015;16:578.

43. Hay P, Palavras MA, da Luz FQ, et al. Physical and mental health outcomes of an integrated cognitive behavioural and weight management therapy for people with an eating disorder characterized by binge eating and a high body mass index: a randomized controlled trial. BMC Psychiatr 2022;22(1):355.

44. Hackert AN, Kniskern MA, Beasley TM. Academy of nutrition and dietetics: revised 2020 standards of practice and standards of professional performance for registered dietitian nutritionists (Competent, Proficient, and Expert) in Eating Disorders. J Acad Nutr Diet 2020;120(11):1902–19.e54.

45. Taylor SA, Ditch S, Hansen S. Identifying and preventing eating disorders in adolescent patients with obesity. Pediatr Ann 2018;47(6):e232–7.

46. Kirk S, Ogata B, Wichert E, et al. Treatment of pediatric overweight and obesity: position of the academy of nutrition and dietetics based on an umbrella review of systematic reviews. J Acad Nutr Diet 2022;122(4):848–61.

47. Pediatric Nutrition Care - Nutrition Care Manual. Available at: https://www.nutritioncaremanual.org/pediatric-nutrition-care. [Accessed 28 February 2024].

48. Bacon L, Stern JS, Van Loan MD, et al. Size acceptance and intuitive eating improve health for obese, female chronic dieters. J Am Diet Assoc 2005;105(6):929–36.

49. Hoare JK, Lister NB, Garnett SP, et al. Weight-neutral interventions in young people with high body mass index: A systematic review. Nutr Diet 2023;80(1):8–20.

50. Leme ACB, Haines J, Tang L, et al. Impact of strategies for preventing obesity and risk factors for eating disorders among adolescents: a systematic review. Nutrients 2020;12(10):3134.

51. Gruenewald H. Understanding Binge Eating Behaviors: A Guide to Dietary Exposures and Behavioral Interventions. Presented at: Eating Recovery Center Pathlight Academy webinar. 2023. Available at: https://www.eatingrecoverycenter.com/professionals/education-events.

52. Beccia AL, Ruf A, Druker S, et al. Women's Experiences with a Mindful Eating Program for Binge and Emotional Eating: A Qualitative Investigation into the Process of Change. J Altern Complement Med N Y N 2020;26(10):937–44.

53. Fuentes Artiles R, Staub K, Aldakak L, et al. Mindful eating and common diet programs lower body weight similarly: Systematic review and meta-analysis. Obes Rev Off J Int Assoc Study Obes 2019;20(11):1619–27.

54. Denny KN, Loth K, Eisenberg ME, et al. Intuitive eating in young adults. Who is doing it, and how is it related to disordered eating behaviors? Appetite 2013;60(1):13–9.

55. Mann T, Tomiyama AJ, Westling E, et al. Medicare's search for effective obesity treatments: diets are not the answer. Am Psychol 2007;62(3):220–33.

56. Ozier AD, Henry BW, American Dietetic Association. Position of the American Dietetic Association: nutrition intervention in the treatment of eating disorders. J Am Diet Assoc 2011;111(8):1236–41.

57. Fitch A, Alexander L, Brown CF, et al. Comprehensive care for patients with obesity: An Obesity Medicine Association Position Statement. Obes Pillars 2023;7:100070.

58. Hampl SE, Hassink SG, Skinner AC, et al. Clinical Practice Guideline for the Evaluation and Treatment of Children and Adolescents With Obesity. Pediatrics 2023;151(2). e2022060640.

59. Wyszyńska J, Ring-Dimitriou S, Thivel D, et al. Physical Activity in the Prevention of Childhood Obesity: The Position of the European Childhood Obesity Group and the European Academy of Pediatrics. Front Pediatr 2020;8. Available at: https://www.frontiersin.org/articles/10.3389/fped.2020.535705. [Accessed 23 January 2024].

60. Piercy KL, Troiano RP. Physical Activity Guidelines for Americans From the US Department of Health and Human Services. Circ Cardiovasc Qual Outcomes 2018;11(11). e005263.

61. US Department of Health and Human Services. Physical activity guidelines for Americans. 2nd edition. Washington, DC: US Dept of Health and Human Services; 2018.

62. Murthy VH. Physical Activity: An Untapped Resource to Address Our Nation's Mental Health Crisis Among Children and Adolescents. Public Health Rep 2023;138(3):397–400.

63. Calogero RM, Pedrotty-Stump KN. Chapter 25 - Incorporating exercise into eating disorder treatment and recovery: cultivating a mindful approach. In: Maine M, McGilley BH, Bunnell DW, editors. Treatment of eating disorders. Academic Press; 2010. p. 425–41.

64. Cena H, Vandoni M, Magenes VC, et al. Benefits of Exercise in Multidisciplinary Treatment of Binge Eating Disorder in Adolescents with Obesity. Int J Environ Res Publ Health 2022;19(14):8300.

65. Ralph AF, Brennan L, Byrne S, et al. Management of eating disorders for people with higher weight: clinical practice guideline. J Eat Disord 2022;10:121.

66. Cook B, Wonderlich SA, Mitchell J, et al. Exercise in Eating Disorders Treatment: Systematic Review and Proposal of Guidelines. Med Sci Sports Exerc 2016; 48(7):1408–14.

67. Toutain M, Gauthier A, Leconte P. Exercise therapy in the treatment of anorexia nervosa: Its effects depending on the type of physical exercise—A systematic review. Front Psychiatr 2022;13. Available at: https://www.frontiersin.org/journals/psychiatry/articles/10.3389/fpsyt.2022.939856. [Accessed 26 February 2024].

68. Vancampfort D, Vanderlinden J, De Hert M, et al. A systematic review of physical therapy interventions for patients with anorexia and bulimia nervosa. Disabil Rehabil 2014;36(8):628–34.

69. Vancampfort D, Vanderlinden J, Stubbs B, et al. Physical Activity Correlates in Persons with Binge Eating Disorder: A Systematic Review. Eur Eat Disord Rev 2014;22(1):1–8.

70. Mathisen TF, Sundgot-Borgen J, Bulik CM, et al. The neurostructural and neurocognitive effects of physical activity: A potential benefit to promote eating disorder recovery. Int J Eat Disord 2021;54(10):1766–70.

71. Blanchet C, Mathieu MÈ, St-Laurent A, et al. A Systematic Review of Physical Activity Interventions in Individuals with Binge Eating Disorders. Curr Obes Rep 2018;7(1):76–88.

72. King NA, Horner K, Hills AP, et al. Exercise, appetite and weight management: understanding the compensatory responses in eating behaviour and how they contribute to variability in exercise-induced weight loss. Br J Sports Med 2012;46(5):315–22.

73. Zschucke E, Heinz A, Ströhle A. Exercise and Physical Activity in the Therapy of Substance Use Disorders. Sci World J 2012;2012. e901741.

74. Thien V, Thomas A, Markin D, et al. Pilot study of a graded exercise program for the treatment of anorexia nervosa. Int J Eat Disord 2000;28(1):101–6.

75. Cook BJ, Hausenblas HA. The role of exercise dependence for the relationship between exercise behavior and eating pathology: mediator or moderator? J Health Psychol 2008;13(4):495–502.

76. Paponetti MK, Zwolski C, Porter R, et al. Leveraging the construct of physical literacy to promote physical activity for youth with obesity – A qualitative analysis of physical therapists' perceptions. Obes Pillars 2023;5:100054.

77. Stankov I, Olds T, Cargo M. Overweight and obese adolescents: what turns them off physical activity? Int J Behav Nutr Phys Activ 2012;9:53.

78. O'Malley GC, Shultz SP, Thivel D, et al. Neuromusculoskeletal Health in Pediatric Obesity: Incorporating Evidence into Clinical Examination. Curr Obes Rep 2021; 10(4):467–77.

79. Dalle Grave R, Calugi S, Marchesini G. Compulsive exercise to control shape or weight in eating disorders: prevalence, associated features, and treatment outcome. Compr Psychiatr 2008;49(4):346–52.

80. Quesnel DA, Cooper M, Fernandez-del-Valle M, et al. Medical and physiological complications of exercise for individuals with an eating disorder: A narrative review. J Eat Disord 2023;11:3.

81. Voelker DK, Reel JJ, Greenleaf C. Weight status and body image perceptions in adolescents: current perspectives. Adolesc Health Med Therapeut 2015;6: 149–58.

82. Schlegl S, Vierl L, Kolar DR, et al. Psychometric properties of the Compulsive Exercise Test in a large sample of female adolescent and adult inpatients with anorexia nervosa and bulimia nervosa. Int J Eat Disord 2022;55(4):494–504.

83. Taranis L, Touyz S, Meyer C. Disordered eating and exercise: development and preliminary validation of the compulsive exercise test (CET). Eur Eat Disord Rev J Eat Disord Assoc 2011;19(3):256–68.

84. Bacon L, Aphramor L. Weight Science: Evaluating the Evidence for a Paradigm Shift. Nutr J 2011;10:9.

85. Lobelo F, Muth ND, Hanson S, et al. Physical activity assessment and counseling in pediatric clinical settings. Pediatrics 2020;145(3). e20193992.

86. Alcaraz-Ibáñez M, Paterna A, Sicilia Á, et al. Morbid exercise behaviour and eating disorders: A meta-analysis. J Behav Addict 2020;9(2):206–24.

87. Diagnostic and Statistical Manual of Mental Disorders. DSM Library. Available at: https://dsm.psychiatryonline.org/doi/book/10.1176/appi.books.9780890425-787. [Accessed 18 February 2024].

88. Gorrell S, Flatt RE, Bulik CM, et al. Psychosocial etiology of maladaptive exercise and its role in eating disorders: A systematic review. Int J Eat Disord 2021;54(8):1358–76.

89. Lichtenstein MB, Hinze CJ, Emborg B, et al. Compulsive exercise: links, risks and challenges faced. Psychol Res Behav Manag 2017;10:85–95.

90. Noetel M, Dawson L, Hay P, et al. The assessment and treatment of unhealthy exercise in adolescents with anorexia nervosa: A Delphi study to synthesize clinical knowledge. Int J Eat Disord 2017;50(4):378–88.

91. Peebles R, Hardy KK, Wilson JL, et al. Are diagnostic criteria for eating disorders markers of medical severity? Pediatrics 2010;125(5):e1193–201.

92. Sawyer SM, Whitelaw M, Le Grange D, et al. Physical and Psychological Morbidity in Adolescents With Atypical Anorexia Nervosa. Pediatrics 2016; 137(4). e20154080.

93. Galler A, Thönnes A, Joas J, et al. Clinical characteristics and outcomes of children, adolescents and young adults with overweight or obesity and mental health disorders. Int J Obes 2024;48(3):423–32.

94. Patton GC, Coffey C, Sawyer SM. The outcome of adolescent eating disorders: findings from the Victorian Adolescent Health Cohort Study. Eur Child Adolesc Psychiatr 2003;12(Suppl 1):I25–9.

95. Donini LM. Eating disorders: a comprehensive guide to medical care and complications (fourth edition). Eat Weight Disord - Stud Anorex Bulim Obes 2022; 27(8):2987–8.

96. Garber AK. Moving Beyond "Skinniness": Presentation Weight Is Not Sufficient to Assess Malnutrition in Patients With Restrictive Eating Disorders Across a Range of Body Weights. J Adolesc Health Off Publ Soc Adolesc Med 2018; 63(6):669–70.

97. Stice E, Marti CN, Rohde P. Prevalence, incidence, impairment, and course of the proposed DSM-5 eating disorder diagnoses in an 8-year prospective community study of young women. J Abnorm Psychol 2013;122(2):445–57.

98. Golden NH, Mehler PS. Atypical anorexia nervosa can be just as bad. Cleve Clin J Med 2020;87(3):172–4.

99. Winston AP. Eating Disorders and Diabetes. Curr Diab Rep 2020;20(8):32.

100. Gibbings NK, Kurdyak PA, Colton PA, et al. Diabetic Ketoacidosis and Mortality in People With Type 1 Diabetes and Eating Disorders. Diabetes Care 2021; 44(8):1783–7.

101. Roehrig M, Masheb RM, White MA, et al. The Metabolic Syndrome and Behavioral Correlates in Obese Patients With Binge Eating Disorder. Obes Silver Spring Md 2009;17(3):481–6.

102. Crow S, Kendall D, Praus B, et al. Binge eating and other psychopathology in patients with type II diabetes mellitus. Int J Eat Disord 2001;30(2):222–6.

The Genetics of Obesity

Juwairriyyah Siddiqui, MD[a,1], Clint E. Kinney, PhD[a,2],
Joan C. Han, MD[a,*]

KEYWORDS

- Leptin pathway • Monogenic obesity • Genetic obesity syndromes
- Polygenic obesity • Syndromic obesity

KEY POINTS

- Monogenic defects of the leptin pathway cause severe hyperphagia and early childhood-onset obesity.
- Many syndromic obesity disorders also converge on the leptin pathway.
- Common sequence and epigenetic variants of the genes implicated in rare obesity disorders contribute to population variance in body weight.

INTRODUCTION

Obesity is a complex disorder that is influenced by genetic, socioeconomic, and environmental factors.[1] The increase in obesity prevalence over the past several decades has been attributed to increased energy intake from excess consumption of highly palatable, readily available energy-dense food and reduced energy expenditure owing to sedentary behavior fostered by recent technological advancements. Genetic selection, however, evolved during millennia of food scarcity and high-energy demands for survival, leading to physiologic mechanisms that promote weight gain and protect against weight loss. The resulting mismatch in energy balance in this modern era has contributed to the current obesity epidemic.[2]

Elucidating the role of genetic variations that affect energy homeostasis can shed light on potential targets for obesity prevention and treatment. Pooled anthropometric data from greater than 50 twin studies conducted in greater than 20 countries across the world have compared the concordance in body mass index (BMI) between monozygotic and dizygotic twins, who share essentially 100% versus 50% genetic

[a] Division of Pediatric Endocrinology and Diabetes, Department of Pediatrics, Mount Sinai Hospital, Diabetes, Obesity, and Metabolism Institute, Mindich Child Health and Development Institute, Icahn School of Medicine at Mount Sinai, 1 Gustave L. Levy Place, New York, NY 10029, USA
[1] Present address: 1468 Madison Avenue, Box 1616, New York, NY 10029.
[2] Present address: 1257 Park Avenue #2S, New York, NY 10029.
* Corresponding author. Division of Pediatric Endocrinology and Diabetes, Mount Sinai Hospital, 1468 Madison Avenue, Box 1616, New York, NY 10029.
E-mail address: joan.han@mssm.edu

Pediatr Clin N Am 71 (2024) 897–917
https://doi.org/10.1016/j.pcl.2024.06.001
0031-3955/24/© 2024 Elsevier Inc. All rights reserved, including those for text and data mining, AI training, and similar technologies.
pediatric.theclinics.com

similarity, respectively. Based on these twin studies, the estimated heritability of BMI is approximately 70% to 80% during childhood and adolescence, with a progressive decline after young adulthood to 50% to 60% by the eighth decade of life owing to the increasing contribution of environmental factors.[3] Thus, the role of genetics in body weight regulation is critical to understanding obesity as a physiologic disorder, which can be modified by lifestyle changes, but fundamentally is driven by biological mechanisms.[1]

DEFINITIONS

Genetic factors driving obesity risk can be broadly divided into monogenic, syndromic, and polygenic categories.

- *Monogenic obesity* is caused by single-gene disorders, typically within or affecting the leptin signaling pathway, that cause significant loss of protein function, leading to high phenotypic penetrance, usually presenting as severe hyperphagia and obesity in early childhood.
- *Syndromic obesity* can be caused by single-gene disorders (and can, therefore, be considered a subset of monogenic obesity) or can involve multiple contiguous genes within a chromosomal region, including one or more genes that affect energy homeostasis. Syndromic obesity is typically characterized by the presence of additional pleotropic effects beyond excess weight gain, such as intellectual disability, dysmorphic facial and other phenotypic features, and multi-organ involvement.
- *Polygenic obesity*, which is much more common than monogenic and syndromic forms of obesity, results from the combined effect of numerous genetic polymorphisms that each have a small contribution to energy balance and together underlie the population variance in BMI. These genetic variants often also involve the leptin signaling pathway but cause less protein dysfunction and, hence, have lower penetrance of phenotypic effect in isolation, but when combined with other genetic variants, form the basis for the high heritability of obesity risk within families.[4]

GENETIC TESTING GUIDELINES

In the evaluation of childhood obesity, testing for monogenic and syndromic causes of obesity (**Fig. 1**) is recommended for the following conditions[1,5]:

- Severe obesity (BMI $\geq$ 120% of the 95th percentile for age and sex)
- Early-onset obesity (before age 5 years)
- Hyperphagia (insatiable hunger, severe preoccupation with food, and distress if denied food)[1]
- Clinical features of genetic obesity syndromes (developmental and physical abnormalities)
- Family history of consanguinity (increased risk of recessive conditions)
- Family history of severe obesity/bariatric surgery (suggests dominant inheritance pattern)

In tertiary referral centers for obesity, a genetic obesity disorder was identified in 7 to 13% of patients in pediatric cohorts enriched for the above criteria.[6,7] It is anticipated that this percentage may increase as genetic testing becomes more affordable and next-generation sequencing methods become more widely available. With broader genetic screening capabilities, milder deficits may also be recognized in less severe

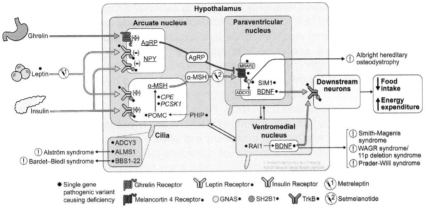

Fig. 1. LEP pathway disruption by genetic obesity disorders. Pathogenic variants of the LEP signaling pathway can be targeted with specific medications to restore energy homeostasis. Ghrelin, AgRP (MC4R antagonist), and NPY are orexigenic. LEP, insulin, and POMC are anorexigenic. POMC is cleaved by PCSK1 and CPE to form α-MSH, which is an MC4R agonist. MC4R and SIM1 are expressed in the PVH. MC4R is coupled to GNAS, which activates ADCY3. Further downstream of MC4R is the neurotransmitter BDNF, which activates TrkB/NTRK2, leading to decreased food intake and increased energy expenditure. ADCY3, adenylyl cyclase 3; AgRP, Agouti-related protein; ALMS1, Alström syndrome centrosome and basal body associated protein; BBS, Bardet-Beidl syndrome; GNAS, guanine nucleotide binding protein alpha stimulating; MRAP2, melanocortin receptor accessory protein 2; PHIP, pleckstrin homology domain-interacting protein; PVH, paraventricular hypothalamic nucleus; RAI1, retinoic-acid induced 1; SH2B1, Src-homology 2B adaptor protein 1. Green arrow = agonist; red bar = antagonist; +, activation; −, suppression; underline = neurotransmitter.

forms of obesity, bridging the spectrum between rare monogenic/syndromic disorders and common polygenic obesity (**Fig. 2**).

MONOGENIC OBESITY: SINGLE-GENE DISORDERS OF THE LEPTIN PATHWAY

Leptin (LEP) is an adipocyte-derived hormone that is secreted in proportion to fat mass and serves as a messenger of body fat status to the hypothalamus, the master regulator of energy balance.[8] Under normal physiologic conditions, loss of fat mass leads to a drop in circulating LEP concentration, which then triggers food-seeking

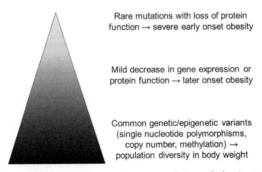

Fig. 2. Spectrum of genetic obesity. Rare and common forms of obesity comprise a spectrum of genetic disorders with the severity of the defect in gene products influencing the severity of obesity.

behavior and conservation of energy by reducing expenditure as a protective survival mechanism. Binding of LEP to the leptin receptor (LEPR) leads to activation of neurons that express proopiomelanocortin (POMC), a peptide prohormone that is cleaved by proprotein convertase subtilisin/kexin type 1 (PCSK1) and carboxypeptidase E (CPE) to produce α-melanocyte stimulating hormone (α-MSH), which activates the melanocortin-4 receptor (MC4R) and downstream signaling by brain-derived neurotrophic factor (BDNF) at its receptor, tropomyosin-related kinase B (TrkB)/neurotrophic receptor tyrosine kinase 2 (NTRK2). Pathologic disruptions in LEP secretion or its downstream mediators are misinterpreted by the hypothalamus as a state of perceived starvation, leading to a persistent and severe hunger drive. Therefore, hyperphagia is a common characteristic of disorders affecting the LEP-melanocortin pathway, with additional features distinguishing each condition (**Fig. 3**).

Leptin

Clinical presentation

Congenital LEP deficiency is an autosomal recessive and rare cause of monogenic obesity, predominantly occurring in families with parental consanguinity.[9] The estimated prevalence for homozygosity or compound heterozygosity of deleterious *LEP* gene variants is 1 in 4.4 million to 17.8 million individuals, with differences ranging by race and ethnicity.[10,11] Patients typically have a normal birth weight followed by rapid weight gain during infancy. They exhibit intense hyperphagia with impaired satiety, severe early-onset obesity, and obesity-associated metabolic disorders, including dyslipidemia, insulin resistance, and hepatic steatosis. However, blood pressure is lower than expected for the severity of obesity owing to the role of the

Key Features of Leptin Pathway Deficiencies

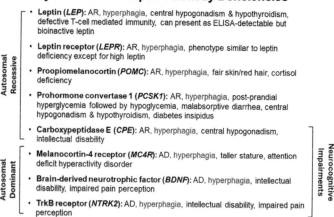

Autosomal Recessive

- **Leptin (*LEP*):** AR, hyperphagia, central hypogonadism & hypothyroidism, defective T-cell mediated immunity, can present as ELISA-detectable but bioinactive leptin
- **Leptin receptor (*LEPR*):** AR, hyperphagia, phenotype similar to leptin deficiency except for high leptin
- **Proopiomelanocortin (*POMC*):** AR, hyperphagia, fair skin/red hair, cortisol deficiency
- **Prohormone convertase 1 (*PCSK1*):** AR, hyperphagia, post-prandial hyperglycemia followed by hypoglycemia, malabsorptive diarrhea, central hypogonadism & hypothyroidism, diabetes insipidus
- **Carboxypeptidase E (*CPE*):** AR, hyperphagia, central hypogonadism, intellectual disability

Autosomal Dominant

- **Melanocortin-4 receptor (*MC4R*):** AD, hyperphagia, taller stature, attention deficit hyperactivity disorder
- **Brain-derived neurotrophic factor (*BDNF*):** AD, hyperphagia, intellectual disability, impaired pain perception
- **TrkB receptor (*NTRK2*):** AD, hyperphagia, intellectual disability, impaired pain perception

Neurocognitive Impairments

Fig. 3. Key features of monogenic LEP pathway deficiencies. Hyperphagia is a common characteristic of LEP pathway disorders. *LEP, LEPR, POMC, PCSK1,* and *CPE* disorders, which form the proximal components of the LEP pathway, exhibit an autosomal recessive (AR) pattern of inheritance, typically in the setting of consanguinity. *MC4R, BDNF,* and *NTRK2* disorders, which compromise the distal portions of the LEP pathway, present with an autosomal dominant (AD) pattern of inheritance, presenting as either de novo variants or generationally passed down in approximately half of family members. Because the downstream mediators of the LEP pathway also serve as convergence points for other signaling pathways, additional neurologic abnormalities (eg, executive function deficits, developmental delays, and impaired nociception) are observed in *CPE, MC4R, BDNF,* and *NTRK2* disorders. Distinguishing features associated with each gene defect are noted.

LEP pathway in stimulating sympathetic nervous system tone. Because of LEP's permissive role for puberty, patients with untreated LEP deficiency display hypogonadotropic hypogonadism, and although childhood height is normal, adult height is reduced owing to lack of a pubertal growth spurt. A subset of patients have central hypothyroidism, attributed to a potential role of LEP in hypothalamic thyrotropin-releasing hormone secretion. Recurrent infections occur owing to the role of LEP in T-cell lymphocyte-mediated immune function leading to higher rates of mortality from pulmonary and gastrointestinal infections.[12] There are no dysmorphic features or malformations. Overall intellectual function appears to be grossly intact in early childhood, although motor delays owing to high body weight impeding sitting, crawling, and walking are observed. Over time, learning difficulties and poor school performance have been reported, which may be attributed to multiple factors, including the effects of recurrent illnesses and psychosocial stressors related to severe obesity.[12]

Diagnosis

Because biologically inactive[13] and antagonistic variants[14] of LEP can be detected by the antibodies used in LEP immunoassays, which would quantify LEP as appropriately elevated for the degree of adiposity (and, hence, leading to a missed diagnosis of functional LEP deficiency), genetic sequencing of the *LEP* is the recommended method for screening. *LEP* and the downstream genes listed in later discussion are included on most commercially available standard gene panels for early-onset obesity.

Treatment

Treatment with metreleptin, a recombinant analogue of LEP, induces weight loss and also reverses the hormonal and immune abnormalities.[15] The development of neutralizing antibodies to metreleptin has been observed, leading to concerns about long-term efficacy of metreleptin. Furthermore, metreleptin is currently only Food and Drug Administration (FDA)-approved for the treatment of LEP deficiency owing to congenital and acquired generalized lipodystrophy. Under development are other LEPR agonists that may have lower immunogenicity, such as mibavademab, a monoclonal antibody that activates the LEPR and shows promise in recent phase 1 clinical trials.[16]

Leptin Receptor

Clinical presentation

LEPR deficiency resembles the inheritance pattern (autosomal recessive) and clinical features of LEP deficiency, including hyperphagia, early-onset obesity, hypogonadism, and immune dysfunction. Although central hypothyroidism and growth hormone deficiency have been reported in association with LEPR deficiency,[17] this has not been consistently observed.[18] The estimated prevalence of biallelic deleterious variants of the *LEPR* gene is 1 in 80,000 to 750,000 individuals, varying based on the population.[19,20]

Diagnosis

Serum LEP levels are elevated and overlap with the range found in BMI-matched controls who lack *LEPR* variants.[18] Thus, reliance on LEP concentration measurement is not definitive, and sequencing of the *LEPR* gene is the recommended method of screening.

Treatment

Treatment of obesity in LEPR deficiency relies on bypassing LEPR through activation of its downstream mediator, MC4R. Setmelanotide is an MC4R agonist that was approved by the FDA in 2020 for patients aged ≥ 6 years with obesity caused by LEPR, POMC, or PCSK1 deficiencies, which comprise the portions of the LEP-melanocortin pathway between LEP and MC4R. Common adverse effects of setmelanotide include injection site reactions, skin hyperpigmentation (owing to melanocortin-1 receptor [MC1R] activation), nausea, headache, diarrhea, abdominal pain, back pain, fatigue, vomiting, depression, upper respiratory tract infection, and spontaneous penile erection.[21] Although setmelanotide is effective for weight loss in patients with LEPR deficiency, immune dysfunction and hypogonadism persist.

Proopiomelanocortin

Clinical presentation

POMC deficiency is a rare autosomal recessive disorder, with an estimated prevalence of 1 in 500,000 individuals.[20] POMC is a precursor protein that is secreted in response to LEPR activation by LEP. POMC is cleaved by prohormone convertase enzymes into smaller peptides, including ACTH, melanocyte-stimulating hormones (α-, β-, and γ-MSH) and β-endorphin. These POMC derivatives act through various melanocortin receptors, and the loss of activation at these receptors causes the key symptoms of POMC deficiency. Lack of MC1R activation by α-MSH causes hypopigmentation of skin, hair, and iris, leading to paler complexion, lighter-colored or red hair, and blue eyes.[22,23] Lack of MC2R activation by ACTH causes adrenal glucocorticoid insufficiency, which can present in infancy as life-threatening hypoglycemia, cholestatic jaundice, and hypotension. The primary role of POMC in body weight regulation is mediated through MC4R activation by α-MSH, the lack of which causes severe hyperphagia and early-onset obesity.[24] The effect of reduced MC3R and MC5R signaling has not been fully elucidated, but these receptors appear to also play important roles in energy balance and adipocyte biology.[25,26] Some case reports describe central hypothyroidism, hypogonadism, and growth hormone deficiency, but these are not consistent features and appear to be transient in several reports.[23]

Diagnosis

Sequencing of the POMC gene is the recommended method of screening. Furthermore, when evaluating cortisol deficiency, it is important to note that POMC variants with defective cleavage sites can produce bioactive ACTH that can be detected in immunoassays as elevated. This can lead to potential misdiagnosis of primary adrenal deficiency.

Treatment

The MC4R agonist setmelanotide induces weight loss and increases pigmentation in patients with POMC deficiency. Adrenal insufficiency, however, still necessitates continued glucocorticoid replacement. Typically, mineralocorticoid (aldosterone) deficiency is not observed, but in situations of extreme stress, transient fludrocortisone therapy may be needed to treat hyponatremia owing to urinary salt wasting.[27]

Proprotein Convertase Subtilisin/Kexin Type 1

Clinical presentation

PCSK1 deficiency is a rare autosomal recessive disorder, with an estimated prevalence of 1 in 36,000 individuals.[20] PCSK1, also known as prohormone convertase 1/3, is chiefly expressed in the pituitary, hypothalamus, and pancreas. PCSK1 deficiency causes reduced processing of several other prohormone peptides besides POMC, including hypothalamic-releasing hormones (gonadotropin-releasing hormone, thyrotropin-releasing hormone, growth hormone–releasing hormone), provasopressin, proglucagon, and proinsulin, with each of these conferring additional features, including central hypogonadism, central hypothyroidism, growth hormone deficiency, diabetes insipidus, malabsorptive diarrhea (owing to altered gastrointestinal peptide secretion), and postprandial hyperglycemia followed several hours later with hypoglycemia (owing to lack of cleavage of proinsulin to insulin and persisting elevation of proinsulin, which is a weak agonist at the insulin receptor).[28,29]

Diagnosis
Sequencing of the PCSK1 gene is the recommended method of screening. Elevated fasting proinsulin, which is available in most commercial diagnostic laboratories, has been suggested as an additional biomarker for screening if genetic testing is not available.[30]

Treatment
Severe malabsorptive diarrhea may require parenteral nutrition particularly during the first 2 years of life.[31] Subsequent excess weight gain and obesity can be treated with the MC4R agonist setmelanotide.[32]

Carboxypeptidase E

Clinical presentation
CPE deficiency is a rare autosomal recessive disorder with only a few cases reported in the medical literature. CPE is a membrane-bound enzyme that aids in the conversion of precursor peptides to biologically active peptides and acts as a sorting receptor in the secretory pathway of POMC, proinsulin, and BDNF.[33] Patients present with hyperphagia and childhood obesity. In some cohorts, dysmorphic features have been noted, including full cheeks, micrognathia, and a round face. Other clinical features include hypogonadotropic hypogonadism, reduced muscle strength and coordination, learning and memory deficits, and low bone mineral density.[34]

Diagnosis
Sequencing of the CPE gene is the recommended method of screening.

Treatment
Efficacy of the MC4R agonist setmelanotide as a weight loss treatment in patients with CPE deficiency is under investigation (ClinicalTrials.gov Identifier: NCT0496323).

Melanocortin-4 Receptor

Clinical presentation
MC4R deficiency owing to loss-of-function (LoF) variants of the MC4R gene is inherited in an autosomal codominant manner and is the most common cause of monogenic obesity, with an estimated prevalence of 2% to 5% among children and 1% of adults with severe obesity.[35–37] Individuals with biallelic homozygous or compound heterozygous LoF variants typically have more severe obesity than heterozygous individuals, but variants with a dominant negative effect, mediated through receptor dimerization, can also cause extreme obesity in the heterozygous state.[38–40] Besides hyperphagia and obesity, additional characteristics of MC4R deficiency include increased linear growth, bone mineral density, and lean body mass (attributed to hyperinsulinemia)[41] and lower blood pressure than expected for degree of obesity (attributed to reduced sympathetic nervous system tone).[35,42] Global intellectual function appears to be preserved, but higher prevalence of attention-deficit/hyperactivity disorder has been described.[43–45]

Diagnosis

When interpreting *MC4R* sequencing results, understanding the functional effect of each variant is critical because MC4R coding variants are very common in the general population (estimated 7%).[46] Many variants are benign, have uncertain functional effects, or cause gain-of-function and are, therefore, protective against obesity.

Treatment

Specific treatments for MC4R deficiency are under investigation, including aminoglycoside-mediated read-through of premature stop variants, trafficking chaperones for misfolding variants, and high-affinity agonists for variants that cause reduced binding of endogenous α-MSH. All these approaches are still in preclinical phases except for some limited clinical data for setmelanotide as a potential rescue for a subset of MC4R variants, specifically C271Y, which both in vitro and in a patient with heterozygosity for this variant displayed a robust response to setmelanotide.[41,47,48]

Brain-Derived Neurotrophic Factor

Clinical presentation

BDNF deficiency is a rare autosomal dominant disorder. BDNF is abundantly expressed throughout the nervous system and has an important role in neuronal development, survival, and function. In the hypothalamus, BDNF is a downstream mediator of MC4R signaling within the LEP pathway. Binding of BDNF to its receptor TrkB/NTRK2 leads to decreased food intake and increased energy expenditure.[49] In the hippocampus, BDNF functions in learning and memory, and in the dorsal spinal column, BDNF serves as an amplifier for nociceptive sensory inputs.[49] Heterozygous LoF *BDNF* gene variants are associated with hyperphagia and severe early-onset obesity, with intellectual disability and impaired pain perception in some but not all patients.[50–54]

Diagnosis

Serum BDNF concentrations are reduced in *BDNF* haploinsufficiency, but definitive diagnosis of heterozygous variants and microdeletions is confirmed with gene sequencing and comparative genomic hybridization microarray.

Treatment

Homozygosity for complete LoF variants is embryologically lethal such that reported cases of BDNF insufficiency in the extant literature are in heterozygous persons. Therefore, augmentation of BDNF expression from the remaining functional allele of affected individuals is a strategy undergoing investigation.[32]

Tropomyosin-Related Kinase B/Neurotrophic Receptor Tyrosine Kinase 2

Deficiency of the BDNF receptor, TrkB/NTRK2, is a rare autosomal dominant monogenic obesity disorder with similar features to BDNF deficiency. In addition to hyperphagia and obesity, patients have learning difficulties, repetitive behaviors, aggression, impaired nociception, hyperactivity, and other neurodevelopmental disorders.[52,54–56]

SYNDROMIC OBESITY: MULTISYSTEM DISORDERS WITH IMPAIRED ENERGY HOMEOSTASIS

Syndromic obesity disorders are frequently recognized by their neurodevelopmental and other phenotypic characteristics (**Table 1**). Understanding the underlying genetic cause of syndromic obesity disorders is essential for developing targeted therapies and providing anticipatory guidance and appropriate screening for associated

Table 1
Genetic syndromes with obesity from leptin pathway disruption

Syndrome	Genetics/Effect on Leptin Pathway	Clinical Presentation
Prader-Willi	Imprinting disorder: absence of paternally expressed genes in the chromosome 15q11.2-q13 region Key genes: MAGEL2, NDN, SNORD116 Leptin pathway disruption: Reduced expression of LEPR, POMC, PCSK1, BDNF	Hypotonia and poor feeding in infancy, followed by weight gain and hyperphagia in early childhood. Almond-shaped eyes, thin upper lip and downturned corners of mouth, narrow bitemporal distance, small hands and feet, intellectual disability, pain insensitivity, aggressiveness, temper tantrums, rigidity, self-injury, central and obstructive sleep apnea, narcolepsy, strabismus, scoliosis, endocrine abnormalities (growth hormone deficiency, central adrenal insufficiency, central hypothyroidism, hypogonadism, and type 2 diabetes)
Bardet-Biedl	Autosomal recessive: biallelic homozygous or compound heterozygous pathogenic variants of BBS genes (BBS1-BBS22) Leptin pathway disruption: ciliopathy affecting LEPR trafficking and POMC neuronal function	Normal birth weight, hyperphagia, and obesity begins in infancy. Postaxial polydactyly, retinal cone-rod dystrophy, renal abnormalities (dysplastic cystic disease, hydronephrosis, and chronic kidney disease), hypogonadism. Narrow forehead, depressed nasal bridge, retrognathia, down-slanting palpebral fissures, macrocephaly, neurodevelopmental abnormalities include intellectual disability, speech delay, ataxia, and poor coordination. Behavioral issues include obsessive-compulsive disorder and emotional outbursts.[72] Setmelanotide is an MC4R agonist FDA-approved for treating obesity in ages $\geq$6 y
Alström	Autosomal recessive: biallelic homozygous or compound heterozygous pathogenic variants of ALMS1 Leptin pathway disruption: ciliopathy affecting LEPR trafficking and POMC neuronal function	Normal birth weight, hyperphagia, and obesity begin in infancy. Dilated cardiomyopathy in infancy, restrictive cardiomyopathy in adolescence and adulthood, retinal cone-rod dystrophy, progressive sensorineural hearing loss, renal dysfunction, hypothyroidism hypogonadism, developmental delays mainly learning and receptive language due to hearing and retinal deficits, may also have gross/fine motor delays, coordination, and balance but intellectual functioning generally in normal range[73]

(continued on next page)

Table 1
(continued)

Syndrome	Genetics/Effect on Leptin Pathway	Clinical Presentation
Carpenter	Autosomal recessive: biallelic homozygous or compound heterozygous pathogenic variants of *RAB23* (type 1) or *MEGF8* (type 2) Leptin pathway disruption: for *RAB23*, ciliopathy affecting LEPR trafficking and POMC neuronal function; mechanism under investigation for *MEGF8*	High birth weight, subsequent obesity. Central nervous system malformations, intellectual disability, multiple suture craniosynostosis, heart defects, umbilical hernia, cryptorchidism, hypoplastic testes, broad or bifid thumbs, absent or small middle phalanges, polysyndactyly, bowed femur/tibia. Facial features: flat nasal bridge, down-slanting palpebral fissures, low-set and abnormally shaped ears, underdeveloped upper and lower jaws[64]
MORM	Autosomal recessive: biallelic homozygous or compound heterozygous pathogenic variants of *INPP5E* Leptin pathway disruption: ciliopathy affecting LEPR trafficking and POMC neuronal function	Childhood-onset truncal obesity, intellectual disability, retinal dystrophy, and micropenis[64]
Chung-Jansen	Autosomal dominant: heterozygous pathogenic variants of *PHIP* Leptin pathway disruption: POMC	Pleckstrin homology domain interacting protein (PHIP) is a nuclear protein involved in insulin signaling, pancreatic beta-cell growth, and *POMC* transcription.[74] Clinical features include neonatal hypoglycemia, developmental delay, intellectual disability, hypotonia, and increasing obesity with age (gradual increase in early childhood, then steep increase after age 12 y).[75] Anxiety, depression, attention-deficit/hyperactivity disorder, constipation, visual problems, and cryptorchidism in male patients are also common features.[76] Dysmorphisms include large ears/earlobes, prominent eyebrows, anteverted nares, long philtrum, deep-set eyes, tapering fingers, syndactyly, and clinodactyly[75]
Albright Hereditary Osteodystrophy	Autosomal dominant: heterozygous pathogenic variants of *GNAS* Leptin pathway disruption: MC4R	*GNAS* encodes the alpha-subunit of the stimulatory guanine nucleotide-binding protein ($G\alpha_s$). MC4R is a G-protein–coupled receptor (GPRC) that depends on $G\alpha_s$ to facilitate signal transduction. Clinical features include obesity, developmental delay, short stature, brachydactyly of the fourth and fifth metacarpals, and facial dysmorphisms (round face, depressed nasal bridge). *GNAS* is an imprinted gene with silencing of the paternal allele in certain tissues (kidney, pituitary, thyroid, and

Gene	Inheritance / Pathway	Description
		gonads), which causes patients with maternally inherited *GNAS* pathogenic variants to also exhibit resistance to hormones that bind GPRCs in these tissues, including parathyroid hormone, growth hormone–releasing hormone, thyroid-stimulating hormone, and gonadotropins. Isolated obesity has been reported among individuals with *GNAS* pathogenic variants[77]
SIM1	Autosomal dominant: heterozygous pathogenic variants of *SIM1* Leptin pathway disruption: MC4R	SIM1 is an important regulator for the development of the paraventricular nucleus of the hypothalamus (PVH) and is co-expressed with MC4R in a subset of PVH neurons. Arcuate POMC neurons that project to the PVH release α-MSH onto these neurons, leading to decreased food intake.[78] Clinical features of SIM1 deficiency include hyperphagia and obesity, with variable degrees of neurodevelopmental abnormalities, including hypotonia, developmental delay, and intellectual disability[79,80]
MRAP2	Autosomal dominant: heterozygous pathogenic variants of *MRAP2* Leptin pathway disruption: MC4R	Melanocortin receptor accessory protein 2 (MRAP2) is highly expressed in hypothalamus and brain stem. Studies in mice have shown that *MRAP2* enhances α-MSH–stimulated MC4R signaling.[81] Heterozygous variants in the *MRAP2* gene have been identified in individuals with hyperphagia and extreme early-onset obesity.[82] Hyperglycemia and hypertension have also been described, which is in contrast with MC4R deficiency, which is typically associated with reduced sympathetic nervous system tone[83]
ADCY3	Autosomal codominant: monoallelic and biallelic pathogenic variants of *ADCY3* Leptin pathway disruption: MC4R	Adenylyl cyclase 3 (ADCY3) is an enzyme that is activated by $G\alpha_s$ and catalyzes the conversion of adenosine triphosphate to cyclic adenosine monophosphate and is an important part of intracellular signaling cascades downstream of $G\alpha_s$-coupled GPCRs, including MC4R. ADCY3 colocalizes with MC4R in the primary cilia of PVH neurons.[84] Heterozygous pathogenic variants and increased DNA methylation (which has a silencing effect) of *ADCY3* have been associated with increased obesity.[85] Individuals with biallelic homozygous or compound heterozygous pathogenic variants of *ADCY3* present with hyperphagia, severe obesity, and in some patients, anosmia and neurodevelopmental deficits[85–87]

(continued on next page)

Table 1
(continued)

Syndrome	Genetics/Effect on Leptin Pathway	Clinical Presentation
WAGR(O)/ 11p Deletion	Autosomal dominant: heterozygous deletion of contiguous genes in the chromosome 11p region containing *BDNF* Leptin pathway disruption: BDNF	WAGR/11p deletion syndrome is a rare disorder that is caused by a heterozygous deletion of contiguous genes in the chromosome 11p13 region, inclusive of 2 genes, *WT1* and *PAX6*. WAGR is an acronym for the clinical features of the disorder: Wilms tumor, aniridia, genitourinary anomalies, and a range of developmental disorders. The *BDNF* gene is located at 11p14, adjacent to the core WAGR deletion region. Individuals with deletion boundaries that encompass *BDNF* form a subset of patients who exhibit additional features, including hyperphagia, obesity, impaired nociception, and more severe intellectual disability[49,88–91]
SH2B1/16p11 Deletion	Autosomal dominant: heterozygous pathogenic variants of *SH2B1* or deletion of the chromosome 16p11.2 region containing *SH2B1* Leptin pathway disruption: LEPR, BDNF, NTRK2	Src-homology-2 B adapter protein 1 (SH2B1) is an essential adaptor protein that associates with LEPR, TrkB/NTRK2, and the insulin receptor.[92,93] SH2B1 enhances the function of BDNF-induced neuronal differentiation and also binds to the BDNF receptor TrkB.[94] Individuals with heterozygous *SH2B1* pathogenic variants or 16p11.2 deletion encompassing *SH2B1* have severe hyperphagia and early-onset obesity, with disproportionate hyperinsulinism.[95] Other features include short stature, speech and language delay, and maladaptive behaviors[92]
Smith-Magenis	Autosomal dominant: heterozygous pathogenic variants of *RAI1* (10% of cases) or deletions of the chromosome 17p11.2 region containing *RAI1* (90% of cases) Leptin pathway disruption: BDNF	Retinoic acid–induced 1 (RAI1) is a transcriptional factor involved in neurodevelopment, including *BDNF* expression.[49] Infants have poor weight gain, difficulty feeding, and hypotonia. In childhood, hyperphagia (particularly nighttime food foraging) and abdominal obesity develop. Dysmorphisms include brachycephaly, broad forehead, up-slanting palpebral fissures, short-upturned nose, downturned upper lip, and progressive coarsening of facial features with age. Neurodevelopmental abnormalities include intellectual disability, significant sleep disturbance, self-injurious behaviors, and stereotyped behaviors, particularly spasmodic upper-body self-hugging[96]

conditions. For many families, these syndromic symptoms are the primary focus of medical attention, whereas the obesity risk component may initially seem of secondary importance. However, over time, the emergence of severe hyperphagic behaviors that disrupt daily routines and social interactions can lead to significant caregiver distress.[57] Emerging evidence connects the hyperphagia of syndromic obesity disorders to LEPR, POMC, MC4R, and/or BDNF deficits, whereas neurodevelopmental abnormalities, including intellectual disability, maladaptive behaviors, and impaired pain perception, point to involvement of defective BDNF signaling in particular. Prader-Willi syndrome (PWS) and ciliopathies are the most common syndromic obesity disorders and are highlighted in later discussion, with other syndromes summarized in **Table 1**.

Prader-Willi Syndrome

Clinical presentation

PWS is a methylation disorder characterized by a lack of expression of paternally inherited genes within the chromosome 15q11.2-q13 region owing to deletion of the paternal region (65%–75%), duplication of the maternal imprinted (methylated/silenced) region owing to uniparental disomy (20%–30%), or inappropriate methylation of paternal genes owing to an imprinting defect (<5%). The prevalence of PWS is estimated to be 1 in 10,000 to 30,000. Infants with PWS have hypotonia and poor feeding, followed by weight gain and hyperphagia in early childhood, with progression to morbid obesity if food intake is not controlled. Dysmorphic features include almond-shaped eyes, thin upper lip and downturned corners of mouth, narrow bitemporal distance, and small hands and feet. Patients have motor and language delay, intellectual disability, and pain insensitivity. Behavior difficulties include aggressiveness, temper tantrums, rigidity, and self-injury. Sleep disturbances include both central and obstructive sleep apnea and narcolepsy. Strabismus and scoliosis are common. Endocrine abnormalities include growth hormone deficiency, central adrenal insufficiency, central hypothyroidism, hypogonadism with hypogenitalism, and development of type 2 diabetes in patients with obesity.[58]

Diagnosis

DNA methylation testing of the 15q11.2-q13 region identifies all 3 subtypes of PWS and, therefore, should be used as the initial testing method. Deletion detection methods, such as fluorescence in situ hybridization (FISH), should not be used as a first-line test because only two-thirds of cases are due to deletion, resulting in false negative results for one-third of cases. After confirmation of an aberrant methylation pattern, further defining the subtype can be achieved using microarray and FISH methods. The deletion subtype is associated with hypopigmentation of skin, hair, and eyes owing to haploinsufficiency of a gene in the PWS region, OCA2, which causes oculocutaneous albinism.

Involvement of the leptin pathway

Multiple genes in the 15q11.2-q13 region are involved in the regulation of energy balance. MAGEL2 and NDN are involved in LEPR trafficking and POMC neuronal response to LEP.[59] SNORD116 is involved in PCSK1 expression.[60] BDNF, as a downstream mediator of these LEP pathway components, has been shown to be reduced in PWS, and replacement using a viral vector system ameliorates the metabolic and behavioral phenotype of a mouse model of PWS.[61,62] Other treatments for PWS are under investigation in preclinical studies and clinical trials, but none are currently FDA-approved for treatment.[32]

Ciliopathies

Primary (immotile) cilia are antennae-like structures that are found as a single projection on the surface of most mammalian cells, serving as sensory receptors, and play important roles in intracellular transport and cell-cell communication. Ciliopathies are a group of disorders caused by autosomal recessive LoF variants in the genes involved in the assembly and function of cilia.[63] Bardet-Biedl, Alström, Carpenter, and MORM syndromes are clinically recognized as ciliopathies associated with early-onset obesity.[64] Intracellular trafficking of LEPR as well as the function and stability of neurons that express POMC rely on normal ciliary activities, which, when disrupted, leads to hyperphagia and obesity.[65,66] The clinical features of these syndromes are shown in **Table 1**. Treatment with the MC4R agonist setmelanotide was FDA-approved in 2022 for the treatment of obesity in patients with Bardet-Biedl syndrome aged ≥6 years. Clinical trials are ongoing for setmelanotide in other ciliopathies.[32]

POLYGENIC OBESITY

Unlike monogenic obesity, which is estimated to comprise only a small subset of the population with obesity, polygenic obesity is much more common (~95% of individuals with obesity) and is caused by the cumulative effect of inherited susceptibility variants in multiple genes. It is estimated that person-to-person genetic differences account for 40% to 70% of variation in susceptibility to obesity.[2] With advances in genetics, genome-wide association studies (GWAS) have led to the discovery of many obesity-susceptibility loci. *FTO* (fat mass and obesity associated gene) was the first identified obesity susceptibility gene and was shown to mediate its effects through altered food preference and intake. Furthermore, although *FTO* does not influence physical activity level, individuals who do engage in higher activity levels have attenuated impact of FTO on obesity risk, suggesting that behavior changes can modify genetic predisposition.[67]

In subsequent GWAS, more than a thousand genetic loci associated with BMI have been identified, many of which include genes that comprise or converge upon the LEP pathway, indicating that common variants of these genes confer a milder, but additive risk for obesity compared with the severe obesity caused by rare LoF variants of these same genes. However, the aggregate of these loci's contributions still only explains 6% of the population variance in BMI.[68] Creation of polygenic risk scores (PRS) that incorporate millions of single-nucleotide polymorphisms (SNPs) has improved prediction capability to 23%.[69] A recent functional data analysis of a small, but deeply characterized longitudinal pediatric cohort identified 24 SNPs selected based on longitudinal weight gain patterns, to calculate a PRS that explained 52% of the in-sample variability in growth curves during the first 3 years of life.[70]

In addition to genetic sequence variants, epigenetic variability of DNA methylation and histone modification factors that affect gene expression also plays an important role in the regulation of body weight and risk for obesity. For example, studies focusing on the *POMC* gene revealed that hypermethylation of variably methylated regions of *POMC* resulted in decreased gene expression and an increased risk for obesity.[71] Using a methylation risk score for ~400 CpG methylation sites, 32% of the variance in adult BMI could be predicted. However, in a pediatric study of 135 CpG sites, only 2% to 3% of the variance in BMI could be explained in children.[68] Thus, further studies are needed that combine polygenic and methylation risk scores in larger and diverse cohorts to provide more robust prediction models. As with the finding of physical activity interacting with *FTO*, identifying modifiable lifestyle behaviors or targeted medications based on individual polygenic and methylation patterns could become a precision therapy approach for treating obesity.

SUMMARY

Obesity, a multidimensional disorder influenced by both genetic and environmental factors, continues to pose significant global health challenges. Recent advancements in genomic research have significantly expanded the understanding of the genetic basis of obesity. In this context, obesity can be categorized into 3 main groups: *monogenic*, *syndromic*, and *polygenic*. Genetic testing plays a crucial role in diagnosing monogenic and syndromic obesity disorders, which are caused by single-gene or single-chromosomal region pathogenic variants. Identifying an underlying genetic cause allows for tailored medical management, early intervention, and informed genetic counseling. Polygenic obesity involves multiple genes with smaller individual effects, but when combined, accounts for a large portion of individual obesity risk. Unraveling the genetic complexities of obesity provides new opportunities for targeted treatments. Because the genes involved in rare and common obesity disorders appear on a spectrum of severity, studies of precision therapies for rare disorders can serve as a model for expansion to treatment of common disorders. As the intricate interplay between genes and environment continues to be explored, genetic testing remains pivotal in improving patient outcomes and curbing this serious worldwide epidemic.

CLINICS CARE POINTS

- Monogenic obesity:
  - Single-gene variants of the leptin-melanocortin pathway can cause severe hyperphagia and early-onset obesity.
  - Precision medicine treatments are available for leptin, leptin receptor, proopiomelanocortin, and proprotein convertase subtilisin/kexin type 1 deficiencies.

- Syndromic obesity:
  - Characteristic clinical features may appear before hyperphagia or obesity develops.
  - Early diagnosis with genetic testing permits anticipatory guidance, appropriate screening for comorbidities, and obesity prevention counseling.
  - Precision medicine treatment with setmelanotide (MC4R agonist) is available for Bardet-Biedl syndrome.

- Polygenic obesity:
  - Common genetic variants in many genes have a combined contribution to body weight.
  - Clinical testing is not widely available for polygenic obesity risk but is being studied in research contexts.
  - Lifestyle interventions, such as exercise, reduce the impact of *FTO*-associated obesity risk and potentially other common gene variants.

DISCLOSURES

J.C. Han is a clinical trial investigator for multisite research studies sponsored by Rhythm Pharmaceuticals. The remaining authors have no disclosures.

REFERENCES

1. Hampl SE, Hassink SG, Skinner AC, et al. Clinical practice guideline for the evaluation and treatment of children and adolescents with obesity. Pediatrics 2023; 151(2).
2. Heymsfield SB, Wadden TA. Mechanisms, pathophysiology, and management of obesity. N Engl J Med 2017;376(3):254–66.

3. Silventoinen K, Jelenkovic A, Yokoyama Y, et al. The CODATwins project: the current status and recent findings of collaborative project of development of anthropometrical measures in twins. Twin Res Hum Genet 2019;22(6):800–8.

4. Loos RJF, Yeo GSH. The genetics of obesity: from discovery to biology. Nat Rev Genet 2022;23(2):120–33.

5. Styne DM, Arslanian SA, Connor EL, et al. Pediatric obesity-assessment, treatment, and prevention: an endocrine society clinical practice guideline. J Clin Endocrinol Metab 2017;102(3):709–57.

6. Farooqi S, O'Rahilly S. Genetics of obesity in humans. Endocr Rev 2006;27(7):710–8.

7. Mainieri F, La Bella S, Rinaldi M, et al. Rare genetic forms of obesity in childhood and adolescence, a comprehensive review of their molecular mechanisms and diagnostic approach. Eur J Pediatr 2023;182(11):4781–93.

8. Friedman JM. Leptin and the endocrine control of energy balance. Nat Metab 2019;1(8):754–64.

9. Montague CT, Farooqi IS, Whitehead JP, et al. Congenital leptin deficiency is associated with severe early-onset obesity in humans. Nature 1997;387(6636):903–8.

10. Rajcsanyi LS, Zheng Y, Fischer-Posovszky P, et al. Prevalence estimates of putatively pathogenic leptin variants in the gnomAD database. PLoS One 2022;17(9):e0266642.

11. Nunziata A, Borck G, Funcke JB, et al. Estimated prevalence of potentially damaging variants in the leptin gene. Mol Cell Pediatr 2017;4(1):10.

12. Saeed S, Khanam R, Janjua QM, et al. High morbidity and mortality in children with untreated congenital deficiency of leptin or its receptor. Cell Rep Med 2023;4(9):101187.

13. Wabitsch M, Funcke JB, von Schnurbein J, et al. Severe early-onset obesity due to bioinactive leptin caused by a p.N103K mutation in the leptin gene. J Clin Endocrinol Metab 2015;100(9):3227–30.

14. Funcke J-B, Moepps B, Roos J, et al. Rare antagonistic leptin variants and severe, early-onset obesity. N Engl J Med 2023;388(24):2253–61.

15. Farooqi IS, Matarese G, Lord GM, et al. Beneficial effects of leptin on obesity, T cell hyporesponsiveness, and neuroendocrine/metabolic dysfunction of human congenital leptin deficiency. J Clin Invest 2002;110(8):1093–103.

16. Gewitz A, Mendell J, Wang Y, et al. Pharmacokinetics and pharmacodynamics of mibavademab (a leptin receptor agonist): Results from a first-in-human phase I study. Clin Transl Sci 2024;17(4):e13762.

17. Clement K, Vaisse C, Lahlou N, et al. A mutation in the human leptin receptor gene causes obesity and pituitary dysfunction. Nature 1998;392(6674):398–401.

18. Farooqi IS, Wangensteen T, Collins S, et al. Clinical and molecular genetic spectrum of congenital deficiency of the leptin receptor. N Engl J Med 2007;356(3):237–47.

19. Kleinendorst L, Abawi O, van der Kamp HJ, et al. Leptin receptor deficiency: a systematic literature review and prevalence estimation based on population genetics. Eur J Endocrinol 2020;182(1):47–56.

20. Ayers KL, Glicksberg BS, Garfield AS, et al. Melanocortin 4 receptor pathway dysfunction in obesity: patient stratification aimed at MC4R agonist treatment. J Clin Endocrinol Metab 2018;103(7):2601–12.

21. Kanti V, Puder L, Jahnke I, et al. A Melanocortin-4 receptor agonist induces skin and hair pigmentation in patients with monogenic mutations in the leptin-melanocortin pathway. Skin Pharmacol Physiol 2021;34(6):307–16.

22. Krude H, Biebermann H, Luck W, et al. Severe early-onset obesity, adrenal insufficiency and red hair pigmentation caused by POMC mutations in humans. Nat Genet 1998;19(2):155-7.
23. Gregoric N, Groselj U, Bratina N, et al. Two cases with an early presented proopiomelanocortin deficiency-a long-term follow-up and systematic literature review. Front Endocrinol 2021;12:689387.
24. Krude H, Grüters A. Implications of Proopiomelanocortin (POMC) Mutations in Humans: The POMC Deficiency Syndrome. Trends Endocrinol Metabol 2000; 11(1):15-22.
25. Demidowich AP, Jun JY, Yanovski JA. Polymorphisms and mutations in the melanocortin-3 receptor and their relation to human obesity. Biochim Biophys Acta, Mol Basis Dis 2017;1863(10 Pt A):2468-76.
26. Ji LQ, Hong Y, Tao YX. Melanocortin-5 receptor: pharmacology and its regulation of energy metabolism. Int J Mol Sci 2022;23(15).
27. Darcan S, Can S, Goksen D, et al. Transient salt wasting in POMC-deficiency due to infection induced stress. Exp Clin Endocrinol Diabetes 2010;118(4):281-3.
28. Frank GR, Fox J, Candela N, et al. Severe obesity and diabetes insipidus in a patient with PCSK1 deficiency. Mol Genet Metabol 2013;110(1-2):191-4.
29. O'Rahilly S, Gray H, Humphreys PJ, et al. Brief report: impaired processing of prohormones associated with abnormalities of glucose homeostasis and adrenal function. N Engl J Med 1995;333(21):1386-90.
30. Pepin L, Colin E, Tessarech M, et al. A New Case of PCSK1 pathogenic variant with congenital proprotein convertase 1/3 deficiency and literature review. J Clin Endocrinol Metab 2019;104(4):985-93.
31. Ramos-Molina B, Martin MG, Lindberg I. PCSK1 variants and human obesity. Prog Mol Biol Transl Sci 2016;140:47-74.
32. Han JC, Rasmussen MC, Forte AR, et al. Management of monogenic and syndromic obesity. Gastroenterol Clin N Am 2023;52(4):733-50.
33. Durmaz A, Aykut A, Atik T, et al. A new cause of obesity syndrome associated with a mutation in the carboxypeptidase gene detected in three siblings with obesity, intellectual disability and hypogonadotropic hypogonadism. J Clin Res Pediatr Endocrinol 2021;13(1):52-60.
34. Alsters SIM, Goldstone AP, Buxton JL, et al. Truncating homozygous mutation of carboxypeptidase E (CPE) in a morbidly obese female with type 2 diabetes mellitus, intellectual disability and hypogonadotrophic hypogonadism. PLoS One 2015;10(6):e0131417.
35. Farooqi IS, Keogh JM, Yeo GS, et al. Clinical spectrum of obesity and mutations in the melanocortin 4 receptor gene. N Engl J Med 2003;348(12):1085-95.
36. Wade KH, Lam BYH, Melvin A, et al. Loss-of-function mutations in the melanocortin 4 receptor in a UK birth cohort. Nat Med 2021;27(6):1088-96.
37. Stutzmann F, Tan K, Vatin V, et al. Prevalence of melanocortin-4 receptor deficiency in Europeans and their age-dependent penetrance in multigenerational pedigrees. Diabetes 2008;57(9):2511-8.
38. Tarnow P, Rediger A, Brumm H, et al. A heterozygous mutation in the third transmembrane domain causes a dominant-negative effect on signalling capability of the MC4R. Obes Facts 2008;1(3):155-62.
39. Alfieri A, Pasanisi F, Salzano S, et al. Functional analysis of melanocortin-4-receptor mutants identified in severely obese subjects living in Southern Italy. Gene 2010;457(1-2):35-41.
40. Biebermann H, Krude H, Elsner A, et al. Autosomal-dominant mode of inheritance of a melanocortin-4 receptor mutation in a patient with severe early-onset obesity

is due to a dominant-negative effect caused by receptor dimerization. Diabetes 2003;52(12):2984–8.

41. Collet TH, Dubern B, Mokrosinski J, et al. Evaluation of a melanocortin-4 receptor (MC4R) agonist (Setmelanotide) in MC4R deficiency. Mol Metabol 2017;6(10): 1321–9.

42. Greenfield JR, Miller JW, Keogh JM, et al. Modulation of blood pressure by central melanocortinergic pathways. N Engl J Med 2009;360(1):44–52.

43. Agranat-Meged A, Ghanadri Y, Eisenberg I, et al. Attention deficit hyperactivity disorder in obese melanocortin-4-receptor (MC4R) deficient subjects: a newly described expression of MC4R deficiency. Am J Med Genet B Neuropsychiatr Genet 2008;147B(8):1547–53.

44. Porfirio MC, Giovinazzo S, Cortese S, et al. Role of ADHD symptoms as a contributing factor to obesity in patients with MC4R mutations. Med Hypotheses 2015; 84(1):4–7.

45. Pott W, Albayrak O, Hinney A, et al. Successful treatment with atomoxetine of an adolescent boy with attention deficit/hyperactivity disorder, extreme obesity, and reduced melanocortin 4 receptor function. Obes Facts 2013;6(1):109–15.

46. Namjou B, Stanaway IB, Lingren T, et al. Evaluation of the MC4R gene across eMERGE network identifies many unreported obesity-associated variants. Int J Obes 2021;45(1):155–69.

47. Brumm H, Muhlhaus J, Bolze F, et al. Rescue of melanocortin 4 receptor (MC4R) nonsense mutations by aminoglycoside-mediated read-through. Obesity 2012; 20(5):1074–81.

48. Huang H, Wang W, Tao YX. Pharmacological chaperones for the misfolded melanocortin-4 receptor associated with human obesity. Biochim Biophys Acta, Mol Basis Dis 2017;1863(10 Pt A):2496–507.

49. Han JC. Rare syndromes and common variants of the brain-derived neurotrophic factor gene in human obesity. Prog Mol Biol Transl Sci 2016;140:75–95.

50. da Fonseca ACP, Abreu GM, Palhinha L, et al. A rare potential pathogenic variant in the BDNF gene is found in a brazilian patient with severe childhood-onset obesity. Diabetes Metab Syndr Obes 2021;14:11–22.

51. Serra-Juhe C, Martos-Moreno GA, Bou de Pieri F, et al. Heterozygous rare genetic variants in non-syndromic early-onset obesity. Int J Obes 2020;44(4): 830–41.

52. Stahel P, Sud SK, Lee SJ, et al. Phenotypic and genetic analysis of an adult cohort with extreme obesity. Int J Obes 2019;43(10):2057–65.

53. Gray J, Yeo GS, Cox JJ, et al. Hyperphagia, severe obesity, impaired cognitive function, and hyperactivity associated with functional loss of one copy of the brain-derived neurotrophic factor (BDNF) gene. Diabetes 2006;55(12):3366–71.

54. Sonoyama T, Stadler LKJ, Zhu M, et al. Human BDNF/TrkB variants impair hippocampal synaptogenesis and associate with neurobehavioural abnormalities. Sci Rep 2020;10(1):9028.

55. Farooqi IS. Monogenic human obesity syndromes. Handb Clin Neurol 2021;181: 301–10.

56. Gray J, Yeo G, Hung C, et al. Functional characterization of human NTRK2 mutations identified in patients with severe early-onset obesity. Int J Obes 2007;31(2): 359–64.

57. Heymsfield SB, Avena NM, Baier L, et al. Hyperphagia: current concepts and future directions proceedings of the 2nd international conference on hyperphagia. Obesity 2014;22(Suppl 1):S1–17.

58. Butler MG, Miller JL, Forster JL. Prader-Willi Syndrome - Clinical Genetics, Diagnosis and Treatment Approaches: An Update. Curr Pediatr Rev 2019;15(4): 207–44.

59. Wijesuriya TM, De Ceuninck L, Masschaele D, et al. The Prader-Willi syndrome proteins MAGEL2 and necdin regulate leptin receptor cell surface abundance through ubiquitination pathways. Hum Mol Genet 2017;26(21):4215–30.

60. Burnett LC, LeDuc CA, Sulsona CR, et al. Deficiency in prohormone convertase PC1 impairs prohormone processing in Prader-Willi syndrome. J Clin Invest 2017; 127(1):293–305.

61. Han JC, Muehlbauer MJ, Cui HN, et al. Lower brain-derived neurotrophic factor in patients with prader-willi syndrome compared to obese and lean control subjects. J Clin Endocrinol Metab 2010;95(7):3532–6.

62. Queen NJ, Zou X, Anderson JM, et al. Hypothalamic AAV-BDNF gene therapy improves metabolic function and behavior in the Magel2-null mouse model of Prader-Willi syndrome. Mol Ther Methods Clin Dev 2022;27:131–48.

63. Hildebrandt F, Benzing T, Katsanis N. Ciliopathies. N Engl J Med 2011;364(16): 1533–43.

64. Brewer KM, Brewer KK, Richardson NC, et al. Neuronal cilia in energy homeostasis. Front Cell Dev Biol 2022;10:1082141.

65. Seo S, Guo DF, Bugge K, et al. Requirement of Bardet-Biedl syndrome proteins for leptin receptor signaling. Hum Mol Genet 2009;18(7):1323–31.

66. Davenport JR, Watts AJ, Roper VC, et al. Disruption of intraflagellar transport in adult mice leads to obesity and slow-onset cystic kidney disease. Curr Biol 2007;17(18):1586–94.

67. Loos RJ, Yeo GS. The bigger picture of FTO: the first GWAS-identified obesity gene. Nat Rev Endocrinol 2014;10(1):51–61.

68. Keller M, Svensson SIA, Rohde-Zimmermann K, et al. Genetics and epigenetics in obesity: what do we know so far? Curr Obes Rep 2023;12(4):482–501.

69. Khera AV, Chaffin M, Wade KH, et al. Polygenic prediction of weight and obesity trajectories from birth to adulthood. Cell 2019;177(3):587–596 e589.

70. Craig SJC, Kenney AM, Lin J, et al. Constructing a polygenic risk score for childhood obesity using functional data analysis. Econom Stat 2023;25:66–86.

71. Kuehnen P, Mischko M, Wiegand S, et al. An Alu element-associated hypermethylation variant of the POMC gene is associated with childhood obesity. PLoS Genet 2012;8(3):e1002543.

72. Forsythe E, Beales PL. Bardet–Biedl syndrome. Eur J Hum Genet 2013; 21(1):8–13.

73. Marshall JD, Beck S, Maffei P, et al. Alström syndrome. Eur J Hum Genet 2007; 15(12):1193–202.

74. Marenne G, Hendricks AE, Perdikari A, et al. Exome Sequencing Identifies Genes and Gene Sets Contributing to Severe Childhood Obesity, Linking PHIP Variants to Repressed POMC Transcription. Cell Metabol 2020;31(6): 1107–19.e1112.

75. Kampmeier A, Leitao E, Parenti I, et al. PHIP-associated Chung-Jansen syndrome: Report of 23 new individuals. Front Cell Dev Biol 2022;10:1020609.

76. Sudnawa KK, Calamia S, Geltzeiler A, et al. Clinical phenotypes of individuals with Chung-Jansen syndrome across age groups. Am J Med Genet 2024; 194(3):e63471.

77. Mendes de Oliveira E, Keogh JM, Talbot F, et al. Obesity-Associated GNAS Mutations and the Melanocortin Pathway. N Engl J Med 2021;385(17): 1581–92.

78. Nyamugenda E, Griffin H, Russell S, et al. Selective Survival of Sim1/MC4R Neurons in Diet-Induced Obesity. iScience 2020;23(5):101114.

79. Ramachandrappa S, Raimondo A, Cali AM, et al. Rare variants in single-minded 1 (SIM1) are associated with severe obesity. J Clin Invest 2013; 123(7):3042–50.

80. Bonnefond A, Raimondo A, Stutzmann F, et al. Loss-of-function mutations in SIM1 contribute to obesity and Prader-Willi-like features. J Clin Invest 2013;123(7): 3037–41.

81. Schonnop L, Kleinau G, Herrfurth N, et al. Decreased melanocortin-4 receptor function conferred by an infrequent variant at the human melanocortin receptor accessory protein 2 gene. Obesity 2016;24(9):1976–82.

82. Asai M, Ramachandrappa S, Joachim M, et al. Loss of function of the melanocortin 2 receptor accessory protein 2 is associated with mammalian obesity. Science 2013;341(6143):275–8.

83. da Fonseca ACP, Abreu GM, Zembrzuski VM, et al. Study of LEP, MRAP2 and POMC genes as potential causes of severe obesity in Brazilian patients. Eating and Weight Disorders - Studies on Anorexia, Bulimia and Obesity 2021;26(5): 1399–408.

84. Siljee JE, Wang Y, Bernard AA, et al. Subcellular localization of MC4R with ADCY3 at neuronal primary cilia underlies a common pathway for genetic predisposition to obesity. Nat Genet 2018;50(2):180–5.

85. Grarup N, Moltke I, Andersen MK, et al. Loss-of-function variants in ADCY3 increase risk of obesity and type 2 diabetes. Nat Genet 2018;50(2):172–4.

86. Ozcabi B, Durmaz A, Aykut A, et al. A Rare Case of Monogenic Obesity due to a Novel Variant in the ADCY3 Gene: Challenges in Follow-up and Treatment. J Clin Res Pediatr Endocrinol 2023. https://doi.org/10.4274/jcrpe.galenos.2023.2023-7-2.

87. Saeed S, Bonnefond A, Tamanini F, et al. Loss-of-function mutations in ADCY3 cause monogenic severe obesity. Nat Genet 2018;50(2):175–9.

88. Han JC, Liu QR, Jones M, et al. Brain-derived neurotrophic factor and obesity in the WAGR syndrome. N Engl J Med 2008;359(9):918–27.

89. Han JC, Thurm A, Golden Williams C, et al. Association of brain-derived neurotrophic factor (BDNF) haploinsufficiency with lower adaptive behaviour and reduced cognitive functioning in WAGR/11p13 deletion syndrome. Cortex 2013;49(10): 2700–10.

90. Sapio MR, Iadarola MJ, LaPaglia DM, et al. Haploinsufficiency of the brain-derived neurotrophic factor gene is associated with reduced pain sensitivity. Pain 2019;160(5):1070–81.

91. Duffy KA, Trout KL, Gunckle JM, et al. Results From the WAGR Syndrome Patient Registry: Characterization of WAGR Spectrum and Recommendations for Care Management. Front Pediatr 2021;9:733018.

92. Doche ME, Bochukova EG, Su H-W, et al. Human SH2B1 mutations are associated with maladaptive behaviors and obesity. J Clin Investig 2012;122(12): 4732–6.

93. Cote JL, Vander PB, Ellis M, et al. The nucleolar δ isoform of adapter protein SH2B1 enhances morphological complexity and function of cultured neurons. J Cell Sci 2022;135(3).

94. Shih CH, Chen CJ, Chen L. New function of the adaptor protein SH2B1 in brain-derived neurotrophic factor-induced neurite outgrowth. PLoS One 2013;8(11): e79619.

95. Hanssen R, Auwerx C, Joeloo M, et al. Chromosomal deletions on 16p11.2 encompassing SH2B1 are associated with accelerated metabolic disease. Cell Rep Med 2023;4(8):101155.
96. Smith A.C.M., Boyd K.E., Brennan C., et al., Smith-Magenis syndrome. 2001, [Updated 2022 Mar 10]. In: Adam M.P., Feldman J., Mirzaa G.M., et al., editors. GeneReviews® [Internet]. University of Washington, Seattle; Seattle (WA), 1993-2024. Available at: https://www.ncbi.nlm.nih.gov/books/NBK1310/.

Overview of the Treatment of Pediatric Obesity and the 2023 Clinical Practice Guidelines

Pamela Hu, MD[a],*, Stephanie Samuels, MD[a],
Mona Sharifi, MD, MPH[a]

KEYWORDS

- Pediatric obesity • Overweight • Practice guideline • Anti-obesity agents
- Healthy lifestyle

KEY POINTS

- The 2023 AAP Clinical Practice Guidelines (CPG) for the treatment of pediatric obesity address evidence-based screening, diagnosis, evaluation, and treatment for children and adolescents with overweight and obesity.
- Obesity is now recognized as a complex chronic disease that needs to be proactively addressed by pediatric clinicians through comprehensive, patient-centered, intensive, evidence-based treatment options.
- Multi-level barriers to evaluation and treatment of pediatric obesity remain at the practice and provider level as well as at the policy, community, and population levels. The CPG provides practical resources to acknowledge and address these challenges.

OVERVIEW OF THE DEVELOPMENT OF THE NEW CLINICAL PRACTICE GUIDELINE

In 2023, the American Academy of Pediatrics (AAP) published its first clinical practice guideline (CPG) for the treatment of pediatric obesity. The CPG is organized by key action statements (KAS) and consensus recommendations that address screening,

Funding: Dr P. Hu's research is supported by the National Institute of Diabetes and Digestive and Kidney Diseases (R01DK111038, R01DK099039). Dr M. Sharifi's research is supported by the National Heart, Lung, and Blood Institute (R01HL151603), the National Institute on Minority Health and Health Disparities (R01MD014853) of the National Institutes of Health and by the American Academy of Pediatrics. Dr S. Samuels' research is supported by the American Diabetes Association (7-22-JDFN-03), the Yale Center for Clinical Investigation, and the Doris Duke Foundation. The content of this article is solely the responsibility of the authors and does not necessarily represent the official views of the National Institutes of Health or the American Academy of Pediatrics.
a Yale University School of Medicine, 333 Cedar Street, PO Box 208064, New Haven, CT 06520-8064, USA
* Corresponding author. Yale University School of Medicine, 333 Cedar Street, PO Box 208064, New Haven, CT 06520-8064.
E-mail address: pamela.hu@yale.edu

diagnosis, and evaluation of children and adolescents with obesity, assessment of comorbidities, and evidence-based treatment options. The evidence base for each KAS and recommendation is detailed alongside care recommendations. The CPG writing committee used the AAP's evidence grading matrix to develop the KAS for the CPG.[1] The strength of each KAS was determined by the quality of the evidence and determination of whether benefit or harm predominated or was balanced. The strength of each recommendation was also considered in terms of clinicians' intended obligation to follow the recommendation.

WHAT'S NEW FROM PREVIOUS RECOMMENDATIONS?

The AAP guidelines address several advancements in the medical community's understanding of obesity since the publication of prior AAP expert committee recommendations in 2007.[2] Obesity is now recognized as a complex chronic disease, and the physiologic impacts of social determinants of health on obesity are more completely understood. Substantial evidence shows that weight bias and stigma are pervasive and harmful and can be barriers to treatment. Weight stigma is associated with decreased exercise and physical activity, social isolation, poor academic outcomes, unhealthy eating behaviors, negative emotional psychologic effects, and worsening obesity.[3] The CPG acknowledges the multiple levels of risks children and families face and calls for pediatric clinicians to provide a safe space for families to engage in non-stigmatizing conversation about obesity as a chronic disease occurring in the context of a family's lived experience and environment. The goal of these conversations is to achieve a shared understanding that ongoing evaluation of obesity and co-morbidities is needed to support the child's long-term growth and development.

Obesity is often an indicator of structural inequities including unjust food systems, health inequities, variable built environment, and community factors. The guidelines cite research supporting the multifactorial etiology of obesity including genetics, obesity-promoting environments, and life experiences combined with inequities in structural barriers to healthy living. Historic and current structural racism contributes to the higher burden of obesity in historically marginalized communities. Understanding and acknowledging these barriers can inform and strengthen therapeutic relationships with families.

Despite the complex nature of the disease of obesity, multiple randomized controlled trials and comparative effectiveness studies show that obesity treatment can be successful.[4,5] Prior recommendations focused on staged treatment intensity, yet the technical reports researched in the process of writing the CPG did not identify any evidence to support this approach. To that end, the CPG recommendations are grounded in the following principles that are new from prior recommendations.

- Communication needs to be patient-centered and non-stigmatizing
- Treatment should be offered early and without delay
- Treatment of obesity and comorbid conditions should be concurrent
- Multiple evidence-based strategies can be used to deliver intensive and tailored obesity treatment
- Structured, supervised weight management interventions decrease current and future risk for eating disorder symptoms

CLINICAL PRACTICE GUIDELINE ALGORITHM

The CPG algorithm was designed to be a clinically useful tool in clinical practice. It provides a quick guide to the weight category and age associated with each key action statement, such as what ages and body mass index (BMI) categories to measure alanine aminotransferase in, for instance, and then what to do with the result. The comorbidities section also connects readers to other CPGs for guidance on comorbidity treatment. This is a helpful tool when thinking about decision points for the clinical team and health information technical supports. The complete algorithm can be accessed here: https://downloads.aap.org/AAP/PDF/Obesity/CPG-Obesity%20Algorithm%2011.17.pdf.

EVALUATION RECOMMENDATIONS

The KAS topics focus on 4 main areas of evaluation. These are discussed in more detail in the following article, but as follows is a brief overview.

- BMI measurement–KAS1: *"Pediatricians and other Pediatric Health Care Providers (PHCPs) should measure height and weight, calculate BMI, and assess BMI percentile using age- and sex-specific Centers for Disease Control and Prevention growth charts or growth charts for children with severe obesity at least annually for all children 2 to 18 y of age to screen for overweight (BMI ≥ 85th percentile to <95th percentile), obesity (BMI ≥ 95th percentile), and severe obesity (BMI ≥ 120% of the 95th percentile for age and sex)."* BMI is a clinically useful tool to measure weight trajectory over time. While BMI does have limitations, specifically potential for over- or under-detecting adiposity in certain racial and ethnic groups, it is an accessible measure that can help triage when patients and families should be referred for a higher level of care.
- Comprehensive evaluation–KAS2: *"Pediatricians and other PHCPs should evaluate children 2 to 18 y of age with overweight (BMI ≥ 85th percentile to <95th percentile) and obesity (BMI ≥ 95th percentile) for obesity-related comorbidities by using a comprehensive patient history, mental and behavioral health screening, SDoH evaluation, physical examination, and diagnostic studies."* Each patient should have a comprehensive evaluation based on age and overweight/obesity status. This includes all the elements of a well child visit (full personal and family medical and surgical history, physical examination, review of systems) with attention to social determinants of health and mental and behavioral health components as well.
- Risk assessment: An important component of a comprehensive evaluation is to assess a patient's risk factors for developing overweight/obesity. These risk factors occur at an individual, social, and contextual level.[6] While there is significant heritability of obesity, many policies and environmental risk factors are potentially modifiable through advocacy but to a lesser degree at the individual level. Early identification of individual/family-level modifiable risk factors and concerted efforts to support families in mitigating them during clinic encounters may help decrease incidence and severity of obesity for a family. The CPG has a consensus recommendation regarding risk assessment.
  - The CPG authors recommend pediatricians and other PHCP: perform initial and longitudinal assessment of individual, structural, and contextual risk factors to provide individualized and tailored treatment of the child or adolescent with overweight or obesity.
- Comorbidity evaluation–KAS3: *"In children aged 10 years and above, pediatricians and other PHCPs should evaluate for lipid abnormalities, abnormal glucose metabolism, and abnormal liver function in children and adolescents with obesity (BMI ≥ 95th percentile) and for lipid abnormalities in children and adolescents with overweight (BMI ≥ 85th percentile to <95th percentile)."* KAS specifically

address high-risk comorbidities that should be evaluated and at what ages. These include dyslipidemia (KAS5), impaired glucose metabolism (KAS6), non-alcoholic fatty liver disease (KAS7), and hypertension (KAS8). In addition to these KAS, the CPG also includes consensus recommendations for other comorbid conditions addressed in an appendix to the CPG including:

- Obstructive sleep apnea (OSA)
- Polycystic ovarian syndrome (PCOS)
- Depression
- Blount Disease
- Slipped capital femoral epiphysis
- Idiopathic intracranial hypertension

TREATMENT RECOMMENDATIONS

When it comes to treatment recommendations, one of the most important recommendations is to start treatment immediately and to deliver it intensively. There is no evidence to support a "watchful waiting" approach. What does this look like in practice?

As stated in the CPG algorithm, "providers should treat overweight/obesity and comorbidities concurrently (KAS 4) following the principles of the medical home and chronic care model, using a family-centered and non-stigmatizing approach that acknowledges obesity's biologic, social, and structural drivers (KAS 9)"

Treatment is comprised of 4 main evidence-based elements.

- Motivational interviewing (KAS 10)
- Intensive health behavior and lifestyle treatments (IHBLT) (KAS 11)
- Weight loss pharmacotherapy (KAS 12)
- Referral to metabolic and bariatric surgery programs (KAS 13)

Each of these treatment elements is reviewed in detail in other articles in this volume. In addition, evidence supports concurrent treatment of overweight/obesity and comorbidities rather than a stepwise approach. Co-morbidities such as OSA, depression, PCOS, and so forth should be addressed while directly addressing the overweight/obesity itself.

Barriers to Clinical Practice Guideline Implementation

The CPG highlights several barriers along with recommendations to overcome these barriers for CPG implementation. Three categories of barriers are described—at the Policy Level, Community and Population Level, and Practice and Provider level—and summarized in **Table 1**.

Advocacy Recommendations

Many implementation barriers require advocacy efforts outside the clinic walls and beyond the influence of the clinician-family therapeutic relationship, as many of the challenges exist at the policy and community/population levels. Advocacy is needed to push for adequate recognition of the obesity epidemic and the resources to address it. Despite evidence that childhood obesity screening and high-intensity, family-based behavioral treatment are effective, there continues to be lack of payment by insurers for childhood obesity treatment. The CPG calls for advocates to partner and demand more of insurers and our government to support obesity care. At the community/population levels, the CPG calls on different community entities (public health agencies, community organizations, health care systems and providers) to partner to increase access to evidence-based obesity treatment programs and address social

Table 1
Summary of barriers to implementation and clinical practice guideline recommendations to address these barriers

Levels	Examples of Barriers at Each Level	Implementation Consensus Recommendation (Summary)
Policy	Widespread lack of payment for intensive health and behavior lifestyle treatment (IHBLT) programs and other evidence-based treatment strategies by insurers despite 2017 USPSTF designation of a grade B classification for evidence of effectiveness childhood obesity screening and IHBLT[a] Consequences: • Direct costs to families for evaluation and therapy not covered by insurers, including high co-pays and deductibles (eg, laboratory testing, office visits, treatment programs) • Indirect costs to families (eg, time and costs associated with healthier foods and exercise) Structural racism has historically influenced federal, state, and local policies	*The subcommittee recommends that the AAP and its membership strongly promote supportive payment and public health policies that cover comprehensive obesity prevention, evaluation, and treatment... targeted policies are needed to purposefully address the structural racism in our society that drives the alarming and persistent disparities in childhood obesity and obesity-related comorbidities.*
Community/ Population	Social determinants of health can limit implementation of health behavior recommendations (eg, food insecurity, safe neighborhoods, health literacy, parenting skills, transportation access) Many communities lack access to evidence-based IHBLT in clinical or community settings Digital access disparities limit use of technology-based obesity interventions, including telehealth, for populations disparately impacted by obesity	*The subcommittee recommends that public health agencies, community organizations, health care systems, health care providers, and community members partner with each other to expand access to evidence-based pediatric obesity treatment programs and to increase community resources that address social determinants of health in promoting healthy, active lifestyles.*
Practice/ Provider	Providers may lack time, resources, knowledge, awareness, and self-efficacy (confidence) in their ability to counsel pediatric patients with overweight/obesity Limitations of electronic health record (EHR) systems may impact ability of	*The subcommittee recommends that EHR vendors, health systems, and practices implement clinical decision support (CDS) systems broadly in EHRs to provide prompts and facilitate best practices for managing children and adolescents with obesity.*

(continued on next page)

Table 1 (continued)		
Levels	Examples of Barriers at Each Level	Implementation Consensus Recommendation (Summary)
	pediatric providers and practices to implement innovations rapidly	*The subcommittee recommends that medical and other health professions schools, training programs, boards, and professional societies improve education and training opportunities related to obesity for both practicing providers and in training programs.*

[a] Grossman DC, Bibbins-Domingo K, Curry SJ, et al; US Preventive Services Task Force. Screening for obesity in children and adolescents: US Preventive Services Task Force recommendation statement. JAMA. 2017;317(23): 2417–2426.

Data summarized from Hampl SE, Hassink SG, Skinner AC, Armstrong SC, Barlow SE, Bolling CF, Avila Edwards KC, Eneli I, Hamre R, Joseph MM, Lunsford D, Mendonca E, Michalsky MP, Mirza N, Ochoa ER, Sharifi M, Staiano AE, Weedn AE, Flinn SK, Lindros J, Okechukwu K. Clinical Practice Guideline for the Evaluation and Treatment of Children and Adolescents With Obesity. Pediatrics. 2023 Feb 1;151(2):e2022060640. https://doi.org/10.1542/peds.2022-060640. Erratum in: Pediatrics. 2024 Jan 1;153(1): PMID: 36622115.

determinants of health. At the practice and provider levels, successful implementation at the practice level will also require advocacy work to integrate obesity medicine into training curriculums.

Implementation Recommendations for Clinical Practice

Acceptance of obesity as a chronic disease is an important barrier to implementation that intersects with policy, community, and provider level barriers. This includes acceptance by the patient and the family, policy makers, communities, and even providers, that obesity is a complex chronic disease that requires proactive treatment. The concept of offering pharmacotherapy and potentially bariatric surgery at younger ages than previously thought is a big change that should be recognized and addressed. The CPG seeks to provide tools to pediatric clinicians to increase their knowledge base in this area and feel comfortable with the data. Then, in the clinic, becoming adept at motivational interviewing to gauge patient acceptance and readiness will be critical. In addition, as overweight/obesity and weight-related comorbidities often affect multiple family members, understanding caregivers' experience with obesity may be warranted as well. Careful consideration of appropriate terminology for the family, patient-focused language to explain importance of evaluation and treatment of overweight/obesity and comorbidities, and shared decision-making are approaches will be important aspects of incorporating obesity care into your practice.

Applying these recommendations to daily practice will require a concerted effort from providers. The CPG asks pediatric clinicians to dedicate significant time and thoughtful care to the treatment of children with overweight/obesity. Very few pediatricians or practices will be ready to check all these boxes. That is okay. There are many tools, trainings, and clinical decision supports available to help clinicians tackle certain areas bit by bit. The AAP provides a concise and practical printable summary of how to approach obesity treatment in the primary care office: https://downloads.aap.org/AAP/PDF/Obesity/Treatment%20Flow_12.19.22.pdf. In looking at this resource, it is important to remember that we are already doing many of these tasks as pediatric providers.

It is important to set realistic expectations. We are at a critical point in the field of pediatrics where clinicians are increasingly aware and appropriately concerned about the potential for causing harm in the way in which they address obesity with patients and families. This fear of violating the "first, do no harm" principle puts us at a crossroads–we can avoid and defer care for the more than 1 in 5 children in the United States already affected by obesity, or we can root out the bias in our care delivery, strengthen our capacity for high quality, non-stigmatizing, family-centered care, and advocate for policies that facilitate both evidence-based prevention and treatment. The goal of the CPG and the many resources available through the AAP Institute for Health Childhood Weight are to facilitate the latter path.

There are many implementation resources available on the AAP website: www.aap. org/obesitycpg. Please visit the website to find practice-focused tools to support understanding the recommendations and integrating them into practice. There are many free and low-cost options to educate yourself and staff teams. Some of these resources also offer continuing medical education and skill building opportunities. At a practice level, there are materials to support clinical flow in the primary care office including quick reference cards for treatment approaches, medication considerations, laboratory interpretation, coding, and so forth. There are also patient and family resources available on the website as well. If you and your team are interested in quality improvement work, there is an entire key driver diagram and change package available as well.

Given the lack of access to IHBLT programs discussed earlier, these resources present practical strategies to intensify care in settings where access to IHBLT is limited such as:

- Increasing number of touchpoints by decreasing time between appointments or contact points
- Partnering with community or other health care entities to adopt evidence-based IHBLT programs, or connect patients with existing community resources
- Exploring group visits, telehealth, or other virtual touchpoints to actualize more frequent contact
- Integrating additional providers, for example, dieticians, physical therapists, health educators, behavioral health specialists, to provide more holistic care'

At the end of the day, with each step you and others in your practice take to become familiar with and implement the CPG for pediatric obesity, you will be making incremental progress to support the long-term health of the children and families you serve.

DISCLOSURES

The authors have no conflict of interest.

REFERENCES

1. Hampl SE, Hassink SG, Skinner AC, et al. Clinical practice guideline for the evaluation and treatment of children and adolescents with obesity. Pediatrics 2023; 151(2):e2022060640 [Erratum appears in Pediatrics 2024 Jan 1;153(1): PMID: 36622115].
2. Sarah E, Expert Committee. Barlow, and the Expert Committee; Expert Committee Recommendations Regarding the Prevention, Assessment, and Treatment of Child and Adolescent Overweight and Obesity: Summary Report. Pediatrics 2007; 120(Supplement_4):S164–92.

3. Pont SJ, Puhl R, Cook SR, et al. AAP Section on Obesity, The Obesity Society. Stigma Experienced by Children and Adolescents With Obesity. Pediatrics 2017; 140(6):e20173034.
4. Skinner AC, Staiano AE, Armstrong SC, et al. Appraisal of Clinical Care Practices for Child Obesity Treatment. Part I: Interventions. Pediatrics 2023;151(2): e2022060642.
5. O'Connor EA, Evans CV, Burda BU, et al. Screening for Obesity and Intervention for Weight Management in Children and Adolescents: Evidence Report and Systematic Review for the US Preventive Services Task Force. JAMA 2017;317(23): 2427–44.
6. Available at: https://publications.aap.org/view-large/13093742. Accessed July 9, 2024.

Motivational Interviewing for the Prevention and Treatment of Pediatric Obesity

A Primer

Susan J. Woolford, MD, MPH[a],*, Juliet Villegas, MA[a],
Kenneth Resnicow, PhD[b]

KEYWORDS

- Motivational interviewing • Childhood obesity • Behavioral intervention
- Healthy lifestyle • Readiness rulers • Motivational interviewing strategies

KEY POINTS

- Motivational interviewing (MI) is an evidence-based, patient-centered counseling approach to help patients or parents adopt and maintain healthy lifestyle habits.
- Using MI strategies (such as reflective listening), providers help guide patients or parents to see the connection between the things they value and their choices.
- MI tools such as readiness rulers may be used to encourage patients or parents to engage in change talk, which makes it more likely that they will commit to making change.

WHAT IS MOTIVATIONAL INTERVIEWING?

Motivational interviewing (MI) is defined as "a collaborative, person centered form of guiding to elicit and strengthen motivation for change."[1] It is a counseling approach that encourages patients to engage in the psychologic work of verbalizing their personal reasons for and against making a behavioral change and resolving their ambivalence to change.[2–4] To achieve this, the MI counselor helps patients explore how behaviors may align with their broader values and life goals rather than directly attempting to persuade patients to change. As patients begin seeing a connection between their behaviors and what they value, they can become motivated to change in order to bring their behaviors and values into agreement.[4–6] The interaction between

[a] Department of Pediatrics, Susan B. Meister Child Health Evaluation and Research Center, University of Michigan, NCRC Building 16, 2800 Plymouth Road Room G20, Ann Arbor, MI 48109-2800, USA; [b] Department of Health Behavior and Health Education, School of Public Health, University of Michigan, 109 Observatory Street, Room 3867 SPH I, Ann Arbor, MI 48109-2029, USA
* Corresponding author.
E-mail address: swoolfor@med.umich.edu

Pediatr Clin N Am 71 (2024) 927–941
https://doi.org/10.1016/j.pcl.2024.06.006
pediatric.theclinics.com
0031-3955/24/© 2024 Elsevier Inc. All rights are reserved, including those for text and data mining, AI training, and similar technologies.

the MI provider and the patient has been described as a "dance" rather than a "boxing match" as MI providers are encouraged not to counter-punch barriers or excuses expressed by the patients but to "roll with resistance" and show empathy for the difficulties or fears that may be impeding the behavioral change.[6] This chapter will address these strategies, including reflective listening, shared agenda setting, rolling with resistance (a form of reflection), and eliciting "change talk," or verbal expressions that indicate a desire to behave differently. It will provide resources and tools to facilitate the incorporation of MI into clinical practice. Prior research demonstrates effective use of these tools, even within the context of pediatric health care visits, is associated with improved provider satisfaction with addressing childhood obesity and improved patient or parent outcomes.[7–18]

HISTORY OF MOTIVATIONAL INTERVIEWING

Since the first publication by William Miller in 1983 describing MI, his work in collaboration with Stephen Rollnick has led to MI being successfully employed in behavior change interventions for a host of conditions (eg, smoking cessation, addiction treatment, and management of adult obesity)[19–22] and in different demographic populations (including adolescents).[4,5,7–15,23] While most studies demonstrating the impact of MI on pediatric obesity have consisted of small trails,[4,7–15] a growing number of large randomized trials support the current recommendations for the use of MI in the prevention and treatment of obesity in youth.[4,9,24–27] Initially, MI was viewed as a form of counseling mainly used in specialized settings by providers with extensive training, and that it required lengthy sessions to achieve optimal benefits. However, MI approaches have been adapted and effectively implemented by a range of professionals (including physicians, nurses, registered dietitians, exercise specialists, and community health workers), often within the confines of brief (10–20 minute) clinic visits.[9,25,27,28] Beyond the in-person clinical setting, MI principles have been incorporated into digital interventions and have formed the basis for behavior modification mobile applications and artificial intelligence (AI) tools.

UNDERLYING PRINCIPLE

Though MI was not developed from any single theoretic perspective, MI can be understood through the lens of Self-Determination Theory. This theory considers motivation on a continuum from being completely amotivated (no interest or drive to change) to engage in a behavior, all the way to having intrinsic motivation (ie, not motivated by external factors) for participating in the desired behavior.[1,29] Autonomous motivation, which has been shown to be associated with sustained behavior change,[30,31] is most likely to occur when an individual's needs for autonomy, relatedness, and competence are met. MI allows providers to address these needs and to facilitate the patient's or parent's progress along the continuum of motivation. This is accomplished through both the relational and technical components of MI, which begin with "comforting the afflicted" and then strategically "afflicting the comfortable" whereby the patient sees the discordance between what they say is important to them and what they are actually doing.[5,6]

In traditional medical encounters, providers typically tell patients what they should do and why they should do it (eg, your child's Hemoglobin A1c is elevated so you should reduce their intake of sugary drinks). Unfortunately, this often leads to reactance, which means that the patient, feeling threatened by the demand for change, begins to counter-argue with reasons why they would not be able to implement the provider's plan (eg, "Kool-aid is the cheapest option for our family;" "My children won't drink anything else;" or "I give them juice because it is good for them"). In contrast to directive encounters, MI employs a non-confrontational, non-judgmental stance that supports patients in identifying their reasons for making a behavior change. It allows them to address their ambivalence about making a change, and importantly, to establish their reasons for making the change before moving on to determining how they can actually implement the new behavior.

EVIDENCE BASE FOR MOTIVATIONAL INTERVIEWING IN PEDIATRIC OBESITY IN GENERAL AND SPECIFICALLY FOR ADOLESCENTS

There is substantial evidence regarding the efficacy of MI in behavior change in general including childhood obesity.[7-15] A systematic review published in 2020 exploring the use of MI with parents of young children for the treatment of obesity initially identified 352 studies, but only 7 studies were randomized trials.[32] This review concluded that "MI, compared to usual care, revealed positive effects for parent influence on young child anthropometric measures when applied."[32] However, an earlier meta-analysis published in 2018 examining the use of MI to treat adolescents with obesity, found from 11 studies that "MI alone does not seem effective for treating overweight and obesity in adolescents".[33] The authors identified that larger studies with longer periods of treatment are needed to fully assess the impact of MI on obesity in this age group.[33] A commentary on this review suggested that methodologic limitations may have contributed to the largely null effects observed in teen trials.[34] In addition to these gaps, a 2024 study suggested that the impact of MI in pediatric obesity may differ by race or ethnicity. In this "real world" trial, MI was associated with slightly worse weight outcomes over usual care for the full sample. However, upon stratified analysis these adverse outcomes were limited to those who identified as non-Hispanic Black and Other.[34] Despite this negative study, which was conducted in the height of the coronavirus disease 2019 pandemic, MI nonetheless shows promise of positively impacting childhood obesity.[7-15] Still, attention needs to be given to delivering a sufficient dose of high fidelity MI and potentially tailoring interventions to diverse populations. In sum, MI appears to hold promise in the treatment of overweight amongst younger children, while effects in adolescents have been more mixed. Thus, it may be beneficial to tailor how MI is implemented based on sociocultural factors, for example, race or ethnicity, age, as well as behavioral and motivational factors.

THE AMERICAN ACADEMY OF PEDIATRICS 2023 GUIDELINES ON THE EVALUATION AND MANAGEMENT OF OBESITY

Based on the preponderance of the evidences, the American Academy of Pediatrics (AAP) 2023 guidelines support the use of MI in the evaluation and management of obesity.[35] A Key Action Step states that "Pediatricians and other Pediatric Health Care Providers should use Motivational Interviewing to engage patients and families in treating overweight and obesity."[35] The authors give this recommendation a Grade B indicating that there are consistent findings from multiple observational studies to support it, but trials or diagnostic studies have minor limitations.

The authors emphasize that MI can be particularly helpful in assessing readiness to change and determining when behavioral actions should be taken.[35] They acknowledge that families may face numerous competing priorities, and addressing their child's weight may compete with other needs and resources.[35] Furthermore, as obesity management is generally an undulating course with recurrent relapses, MI can be used to help those who have suffered setbacks to regain their momentum.

Due to the nature of pediatrics, there is the added nuance of intervening with young children through their parents, who must enact the change plan. While most studies to date have focused on parents as the target of MI counseling for childhood obesity, the guidelines acknowledge the importance of addressing interventions to the person with greatest control over the relevant behaviors.[35] Thus, they indicate that the focus of MI should be on the parent when patients are preadolescents and younger. However, as the locus of control changes between ages 8 and 12 years, once patients become adolescents, the target moves to the patient along with the parent.

KEY STRATEGIES

MI encounters may be viewed as having 3 or 4 phases.[1,36] The main goal of the first phase, described as Exploring by Resnicow and McMaster (or "Engaging and Focusing" in the 4-phase model of Miller and Rollick[36]) is to establish rapport and trust. As part of this process, the provider and parent or patient collaborate to set a shared agenda for their time together. It is important in this phase that patient autonomy is supported. This can involve not only shared-agenda setting but also allowing the patient to control how much information is provided, as well as the behavioral domains they may be open to addressing. By the provider embodying the spirit of MI, which is patient-centered and results in the pediatric provider (PP) speaking for less than 50% of the encounter (particularly in this initial stage where the vast majority of the speaking should be by the patient/parent). In the second phase described as Guiding (or Evoking), the provider helps the patient to engage in change talk as they home in on the reasons why they want to change and come to the point of ultimately committing to change. This leads to the final stage of Choosing (Planning) during which the patient tackles the details of how to change with the aid of the provider. This may include setting SMART goals and structuring incentives for the child to engage in the process. The PP may utilize a number of strategies to facilitate the MI encounter designed to lead to behavior change. Key strategies include:

Open-Ended Questions

The use of open-ended questions avoids "yes/no" responses and encourages patients to elaborate on their answers. While open-ended questions are generally preferred, it should be noted that some such questions might lead patients to feel judged and to become defensive if it seems that the question implies an expectation of change. For example, to explore the consumption of fast food, rather than replacing the closed-ended question "Does your child eat too much fast food?" with the open-ended question "How often does your child eat fast food?" or one might ask "How often, if ever, does your child eat fast food?" The inclusion of phrases such as "if ever", "if at all", "if anyone", or "if any", communicate to the patient that 0 or never are within the range of "normal" responses, thereby reducing possible embarrassment or shame that could occur if the question implies that 0 is out of the normal range.

Affirmations

Affirmations help build rapport, which is crucial to the success of MI encounters. By highlighting something positive that the patient has expressed or strength they have demonstrated, the patient feels understood and appreciated rather than being pathologized. Affirmations are not limited to moments when patients have successfully achieved a goal but can be used to acknowledge patient effort and even partial success. As with open-ended questions, care must be taken to avoid potential negative consequences. In this case, first-person affirmations (eg, "I am so proud of the choice you made" or "I am so happy to hear that") should be avoided as these can be perceived as paternalistic and such direct praise is not typical of the MI approach. Instead, affirmations are better if used in the second or third person. For example, "Despite being in the midst of the busy season at work, you were still able to spend time outdoors with your child twice this week." As this example illustrates, affirmations can be used to address the barriers patients' face, while still facilitating change talk. To achieve this, they frequently take the form of reflections which are described below. Affirmations can entail recognizing that the patient is taking even tiny steps toward change, such as researching gyms in the area, buying a new set of sneakers, or finding recipes online. Recognizing these "micro" steps can help the patient feel that they are progressing along the change track.

Reflective Listening

One of the hallmarks of MI is the use of reflective listening. This allows the PP to offer a hypothesis regarding the patient's perspective and to test whether they have understood them correctly. In its simplest form, it is readily implemented into provider-patient communication, though some types of complex reflections (**Table 1**) require more practice to master.

For those who are less experienced with MI and who would like to allow for the possibility that they might not have captured the patient's thoughts accurately, tentative openings may be used, such as, "If I heard you correctly..." "Correct me if I'm off here," or "It sounds like...." As confidence with MI grows, providers may drop the opening clause and merely state, "You are struggling because...." There is of course the possibility of being wrong, but this is unlikely to break rapport, and most patients will appreciate the effort to understand them and will simply provide more information to help clarify their perspective. This "foul tip" (equivalent to swinging a baseball bat and missing) as it has been called, can elicit additional information that helps achieve the ultimate goal of patient-centered behavior change. Descriptions of the 5 most common types of reflections can be found in **Table 1**.

Eliciting change talk

Eliciting Change Talk is the process of encouraging patients or parents to engage in the exploration of the benefits of change; the fantasy of life without this problem (for example, tell me what it would be like if your family began to eat a greater number of healthy meals and to be more active?) This is a central aspect of MI as the more patients hear themselves presenting the arguments supporting a particular course of action; the more likely they are to move from thinking about it, to actually taking action.[37] It can also build confidence in their own ability to make change. There are 3 main strategies for eliciting change talk.

1. *Reflect Patient's Change Talk* – One approach is to identify change talk in the patient's statements and reflect these back to encourage patients to elaborate on their reasons for change, and ultimately move toward a commitment to change. Sometimes the change talk is buried beneath barriers and sustain talk, which can be reflected first (rolling with resistance) before reflecting the change talk (**Fig. 1**). By reflecting a patient's change talk, you encourage continued exploration of the benefits of change and how the patient may go about achieving the change. The provider is encouraged to use moderate intensity or tentative words when they reflect change talk to avoid overstating patient readiness, which could in turn produce reactance. If, however, change talk is strong, more intensive change talk language can be used. Examples of tentative change talk reflection language are provided in **Box 1**.

Table 1
Five most common types of reflections

Type of Reflection	Description	Helpful Tips	Sample Reflections
Content Reflections	Typically entail the provider paraphrasing the patient's statement without making any inferences or going beyond the surface content of what was said. When done correctly, content reflections are useful in collecting background information and ensuring that the provider understands the basics of the patient's story.	Even in content reflections, the counselor is encouraged to change the words of the patient to show they are being understood. If the client's statement is repeated verbatim, which is sometimes called parroting, this can reduce rapport as it fails to show the provider has fully understood the patient.	An example of a content reflection could be, "So, you have tried many weight loss programs already, and they have not been successful."
Feeling Reflections	Generally, address how the patient feels and why they feel that way. These feeling reflections present a higher degree of skill because the provider must often guess the patient's feelings behind what has been said.	While there may be a natural tendency to understate a feeling (going with 'concerned' rather than 'frustrated') in general this is discouraged, as the patient may feel their emotions are being minimized, which can begin to break rapport. It can imply that the patient is overreacting or that they do not have the right to have a particular feeling. Instead, the PP should often intensify the feeling word used by the patient to test the ceiling of emotion. If the PP overshoots, the patient will usually downgrade the intensity. This can aid rapport if the patient feels their recalibration is understood by the provider.	For example, a provider might state "You are feeling angry about not losing weight, because you have worked so hard at it in several programs." To which the patient may recalibrate with; "well maybe not angry, but certainly frustrated."

Rolling with Resistance	Entails the provider accepting barriers or fears expressed by the client as valid. The rolling with resistance reflection communicates that the person's perspective is inherently valid and the provider is not going to try to counter-argue against the barrier. This supports the MI goal of a "dance" rather than a "boxing match".	Rolling with resistance allows patients to share their concerns without being judged or being pushed into change. This is often described as the provider "comforting the afflicted" by, in effect, appearing to agree with the patient without regard to the veracity of the patient's viewpoint. This entails pulling along side the patient and generally reflecting with whatever barrier or concern they raise. This creates a safe space for the patient to express their fears and concerns.	Some examples may include, *"You are exhausted by the thought of trying again because it is always a battle to get your family onboard."* Or *"Cooking healthier meals can be hard as it takes more time than eating fast food and your kids may refuse to eat what you make."* Or *"These changes seem daunting to you."*
Amplified Negative Reflections	Are an exceptionally useful means of helping patients when they have become mired in sustain talk, when they are stuck in a negative vortex. If rolling with resistance "comforts the afflicted" then amplified negative reflections "afflict the comfortable." This is achieved by not only reflecting to the patient their reasons for not doing something but actually exaggerating their negativity. The PP exhausts the negative side of the discussion leaving the patient with no room to be more negative.	This paradoxic approach of using an argument against change to encourage patients to form their own rationale for change is powerful but must be used judiciously to avoid appearing sarcastic. In addition, resorting to these reflections too often could diminish their impact. The language often entails statements such as "You see absolutely no benefit whatsoever of changing XX."	For example, a provider might say, *"So, from your viewpoint, there are really no benefits AT ALL of getting more sleep."* This will typically lead to a patient reversing direction and countering the extreme negativity with a response such as *"Well there are some benefits…"* followed by sharing reasons that argue for actually making the change.
Double-sided Reflections	Acknowledge ambivalence about change and the complexity of the patient's perspectives. They include compelling reasons supporting both the pros and cons of change. This allows the PP to drain the swamp of negativity while also acknowledging there is some movement toward change.	These reflections allow the provider to demonstrate an understanding of both sides of the issue, while not pressuring the client to change. It maintains rapport and reassures the patient that they are in control of whether and when to make any behavioral changes and they get to set the pace.	A typical double-sided reflection might be, *"On the one hand you would like to buy more vegetables for the family, but on the other hand you are worried about the expense and the likelihood that a lot will go to waste."*

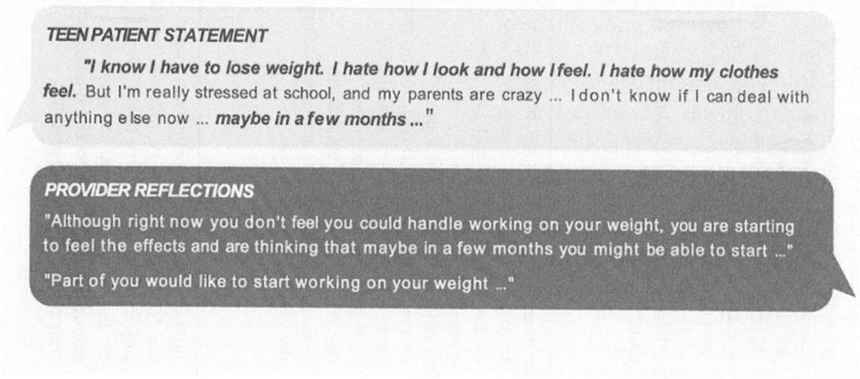

TEEN PATIENT STATEMENT

"I know I have to lose weight. I hate how I look and how I feel. I hate how my clothes feel. But I'm really stressed at school, and my parents are crazy ... I don't know if I can deal with anything else now ... *maybe in a few months ..."*

PROVIDER REFLECTIONS

"Although right now you don't feel you could handle working on your weight, you are starting to feel the effects and are thinking that maybe in a few months you might be able to start ..."

"Part of you would like to start working on your weight ..."

Fig. 1. Reflections to elicit change talk.

2. ***Change Rulers*** - Another popular approach is the use of Readiness Rulers. In this technique the provider asks the patient about 2 related aspects of their motivation: 1) the *importance* of the target behavior and 2) their *confidence* in achieving the behavior.[38] For example, "On a scale of 0 to 10 with 0 being 'not at all' and 10 being 'a lot,' how *important* is it to you to achieve your exercise goal." This should be followed by the companion question "On a scale of 0 to 10 with 0 being 'not at all' and 10 being 'a lot' how *confident* are you that you can achieve your exercise goal." Each of these questions is typically followed by a probe that is designed to encourage the patient to engage in positive change talk. For example, if the patient indicates that they are a 4 out of 10 in regard to the importance of achieving their

---

Box 1
Tentative change talk reflection language

You are starting to feel you might want a change xx

You are thinking that you may no longer want XX in your life.

You are starting to think it might be time to change...

You are starting to feel xx has gotten a little out of control

You are beginning to see the benefits of...

You are moving toward...

You are starting to worry a bit more about...

Things are fine as they are, but you are starting to feel you can't go on like this forever

You are beginning to move toward change or considering change...

You are starting to wonder what it might be like with/without XX,

You are starting to feel a little dependent on XX (for addictive behaviors)...

XX does not feel as sustainable as it once did...

XX is starting to catch up with you...

Something about XX is starting to feel not right for you...

XX is starting to bother you a bit more...

exercise goal. The provider can then ask why they did not choose a lower number. If the provider asks about a lower number, that is, "You said you are a 4, why didn't you choose, say, a 2 out of 10." This will usually elicit the desired positive change talk as the patient will list the strengths and reasons for making the change. The patient might say "I'm a 4 and not a 2 because I know if I exercise, I will feel better and I have always wanted to be fit enough to keep up with my friends." Whereas, if the provider makes the comparison with a higher number, then the patient will be most likely to give a list of barriers and reasons that argue against change. For example, if the provider gives the following probe "So you are a 4 for the importance of achieving your exercise goal, why did you choose a 4 and not something higher like an 8?" the patient will give a list of the cons and barriers of behavior change and why it is not more important to them. A possible response might be, "I'm not an 8 because I have so many other health concerns that I need to address first." For most encounters, it is best to avoid leading the patient to focus on barriers in this way. However, higher numbers can be used to elicit change talk by asking what it would take to move the patient from a 4 for behavior change to a 7 or 8 (**Fig. 2**). This type of probe is likely to help the patient or parent to focus on problem-solving the barriers that currently exist.

3. **Values/Goals Tables** – If patients or parents provide a low score on the importance ruler, a particularly helpful next step for building importance is to guide patients or parents to explore discrepancies between their current behaviors and the things they value or the goals they have, allowing what they value in life to energize their change. This can be accomplished by asking them to select the values or goals that are important to them from a list (**Fig. 3**A: Adult and 3B: Adolescent). If, for example, a parent indicates that being hardworking is a value that is important to them, the PP could help them consider how choices that lead to better health would be in keeping with this value whereas things that are detrimental to their health would impede their ability to work hard.

Self-affirmation/strength Activity – When patients or parents provide a low score on the confidence ruler, the PP may use the self-affirmations or strength activity to help increase their confidence. For this activity, the PP presents them with a list of strengths, skills, or accomplishments (**Fig. 4**) and asks them to select the ones that they think apply to them or to share one that might not be on the list. For a parent who shares that one of their strengths is being creative, the PP could state "How could your creative skills help you find the confidence to become more active along with your child?" Or "…to find new foods or recipes they may enjoy?"

Summaries are important to ensure there is a shared agreement about what was said and what the plan may be for moving forward. They can be used when key

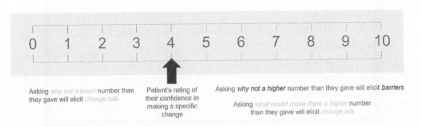

Fig. 2. Example of a readiness ruler.

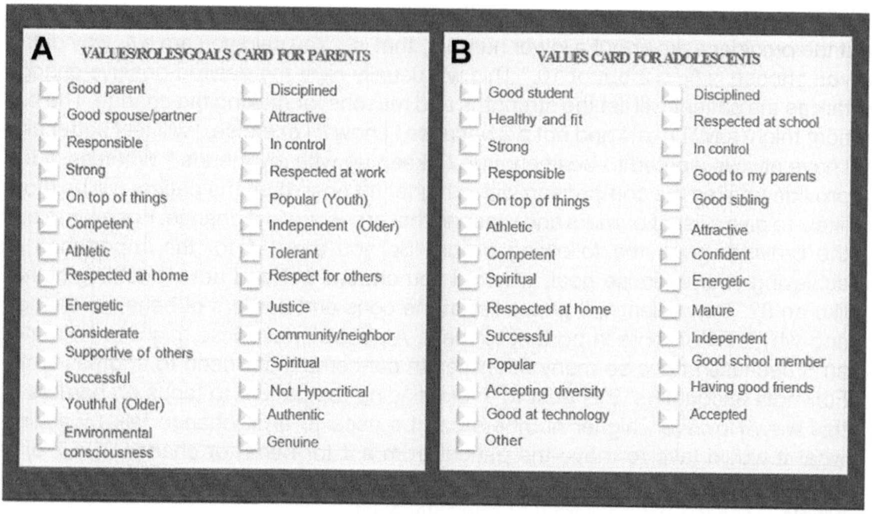

A

VALUES/ROLES/GOALS CARD FOR PARENTS

Good parent
Good spouse/partner
Responsible
Strong
On top of things
Competent
Athletic
Respected at home
Energetic
Considerate
Supportive of others
Successful
Youthful (Older)
Environmental consciousness
Disciplined
Attractive
In control
Respected at work
Popular (Youth)
Independent (Older)
Tolerant
Respect for others
Justice
Community/neighbor
Spiritual
Not Hypocritical
Authentic
Genuine

B

VALUES CARD FOR ADOLESCENTS

Good student
Healthy and fit
Strong
Responsible
On top of things
Athletic
Competent
Spiritual
Respected at home
Successful
Popular
Accepting diversity
Good at technology
Other
Disciplined
Respected at school
In control
Good to my parents
Good sibling
Attractive
Confident
Energetic
Mature
Independent
Good school member
Having good friends
Accepted

Fig. 3. Examples of values cards (*A* – Values Cards for Adults, *B* Values Cards for Adolescents).

information is discussed, or during a longer encounter they can be used periodically to convey that the PP has an accurate grasp of the patient's or parent's perspective, and at the end of a session they can be used to underscore the main points of the visit and plan next steps. They can also be used to assess where patients are regarding their decision about behavior change. After summarizing the pros and the cons provided by the patient or parent, the PP might ask "...so, I wonder, considering all these points, where are you currently in regard to eating more meals together as a family?"

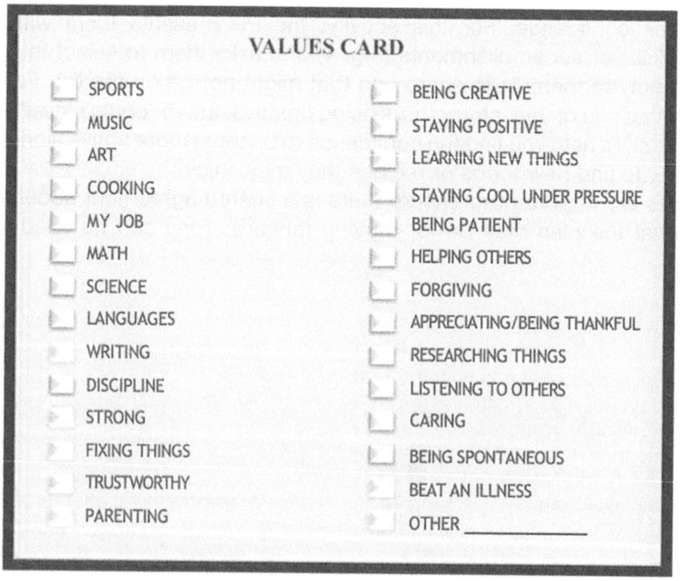

VALUES CARD

SPORTS
MUSIC
ART
COOKING
MY JOB
MATH
SCIENCE
LANGUAGES
WRITING
DISCIPLINE
STRONG
FIXING THINGS
TRUSTWORTHY
PARENTING
BEING CREATIVE
STAYING POSITIVE
LEARNING NEW THINGS
STAYING COOL UNDER PRESSURE
BEING PATIENT
HELPING OTHERS
FORGIVING
APPRECIATING/BEING THANKFUL
RESEARCHING THINGS
LISTENING TO OTHERS
CARING
BEING SPONTANEOUS
BEAT AN ILLNESS
OTHER ____________

Fig. 4. Sample list of strengths, skills, and accomplishments.

Elicit, Provide, Elicit is a framework[1] used in MI encounters to ensure that information and advice are provided in an autonomy-supportive manner, tailored to the patient or parent. The first step is to find out from the patient or parent their knowledge about the topic, what information they would like to gain about the topic, and how they would like to get that information. Once that has been elicited, the PP may move into the "provide" phase where they deliver the desired information. Information is given in small "bite-size" nuggets, usually 2 to 3 sentences in length. For the final "elicit" the PP gleans feedback from the patient or parent and explores whether they would like to receive more information. This cycle may be repeated until the patient or parent has no further requests for information.

Motivational Interviewing and GLP1 Agonists

The 2023 AAP guidelines recommend the use of medications, and specifically GLP1 receptor agonists, in the treatment of pediatric obesity.[35] These medications offer the promise of significantly increasing weight loss and improving health outcomes for many struggling with the impact of obesity. However, it should be noted that the studies demonstrating the positive effects of GLP1 receptor agonists included intensive health behavior and lifestyle therapy (IHBLT) for the intervention groups.[39,40] Thus, the AAP guidelines state that IHBLT should be offered along with medications.[35] This includes the incorporation of MI to help patients achieve healthy lifestyle habits, as well as to ensure optimal adherence to their medication regimen.

Motivational Interviewing and Generative Artificial Intelligence

AI offers the potential to improve and extend the ability for health care providers to deliver MI interventions. The AAP over a decade ago created the "Change Talk" application designed to help health care providers enhance their ability to use MI in the treatment of childhood obesity.[41] More recently, AI has been incorporated into tools to assess MI skills. One such tool is the Real-time Assessment of Dialogue in

---

Box 2
Brief MI session framework

What is the target behavior?
  Where are you?
  Where do you want to be?
  Where have you been?
  What have you done/tried/liked?

0 to 10 Importance/Confidence
  Why not lower?
  Why not higher?

What are your values?
  How are they connected to the behavior?

What strengths?
  How are they connected to the behavior?

Looking Forward/Magic Wand (eg, what would life look like with a healthy weight)

Summarize

Where does that leave you?

Find a plan

Identify Small Steps

Motivational Interviewing application, which uses natural language processing to give immediate feedback to providers about their use of MI. Beyond training, AI has been used to extend the ability to deliver MI interventions to a larger number of patients.[42] For example, the Technology Assisted Motivational Interviewing Coach uses machine learning models to deliver a tobacco cessation MI intervention. While most such programs using chatbots have been developed for use with adults to achieve their goals (ie, increase motivation, stop smoking, and lose weight),[43–46] this technology is increasingly being incorporated into interventions for adolescents.[47]

Future Directions

Future MI interventions will almost certainly include generative AI to either assist the provider in delivering care or it may directly interact with the patient. Several researchers are training AI agents to incorporate MI into the information they feed their Large Language Model agents.[48–50] As use of GLP-1 medications becomes more widespread in children and adolescents, MI interventions may begin to focus more on adherence to these medications, as well as preparing for life without the medications. Finally, MI may need to be adapted to new dietary models such as reducing ultra-processed foods and low glycemic models of eating.

CLINICS CARE POINTS

While a full MI session takes 10 to 15 minutes, studies have shown that even adding a small degree of MI, such as including 1 reflection, is associated with increased weight loss for adults and teens.[51,52] A summary of the main components of MI to incorporate in clinical encounters for pediatric weight management is provided as follows and a framework for brief MI encounters is presented in **Box 2**.

- *Ask Permission* – When addressing obesity with families, the first step is to ask permission to discuss the topic. Patients may be reluctant to discuss this sensitive issue. In some cases, they may feel that other concerns are not considered fully by health care professionals who focus on weight at times when the patient has other priorities. They may also feel they are being blamed for their child's weight. Thus, an important part of building rapport is to request permission from the patient or parent to embark upon a discussion about weight. *This allows the parent to feel in control of the encounter.*

- *Begin with Shared Agenda Setting* – This allows the patient or parent to have control over the aspects of weight management and of their behaviors they wish to address. To do this a PP might say "A number of choices can impact weight including, what we eat, physical activity, screen time, sleep, even stress. Which, if any, would you like us to focus on first today?"

- *Choose open-ended questions or reflections* – This approach creates room for patients or parents to do most of the talking and to guide the discussion to areas that are most salient to them. It also helps providers gain more insights into the issues that impact the patient's weight. For example, rather than asking a closed ended question such as "Does your child drink soda?" an open-ended option such as "Tell me about the beverages your child drinks most days" will elicit more information.

- *Don't give unsolicited advice* – A notable difference between traditional provider-patient communication and MI is the limited use of advice, which is only provided at the request of the patient or parent. When requested, the advice given is more likely to be embraced and has a greater likelihood of leading to behavior change than provider-initiated recommendations.

- *Elicit change talk* – Help patients or parents engage in change talk. This often requires listening carefully for possible opportunities to encourage the patient or parent to elaborate on the positive aspects of change.

- *Foster rapport by using a non-judgmental approach* – The connection between providers and patients or parents is a key component of MI. Showing an understanding of patient or parent perspectives, not judging, and letting patients or parents choose whether and when to change, builds trust.
- *Guide patients or parents to make a decision* – MI sessions should arrive at a conclusion that includes a decision about a change patients or parents want to undertake and their plan for follow-up. It is possible that they decide not to make a change, in which case, they may be open to scheduling an appointment to revisit the discussion in the future.

DISCLOSURE

The authors have nothing to disclose.

REFERENCES

1. Resnicow K, McMaster F. Motivational interviewing: Moving from why to how with autonomy support. Int J Behav Nutr Phys Activ 2012;9(1):19.
2. Hettema J, Steele J, Miller WR. Motivational interviewing. Annu Rev Clin Psychol 2005;1:91–111.
3. Bischof G, Bischof A, Rumpf HJ. Motivational interviewing: an evidence-based approach for use in medical practice. Dtsch Arztebl Int 2021;118(7):109–15.
4. Resnicow K, McMaster F, Woolford S, et al. Study design and baseline description of the BMI2 trial: reducing paediatric obesity in primary care practices. Pediatric obesity 2012;7(1):3–15.
5. Resnicow K, McMaster F. Motivational Interviewing: moving from why to how with autonomy support. Int J Behav Nutr Phys Activ 2012;9:19.
6. Resnicow K, McMaster F, Rollnick S. Action reflections: a client-centered technique to bridge the why-how transition in motivational interviewing. Behav Cognit Psychother 2012;1–7.
7. Spear BA, Barlow SE, Ervin C, et al. Recommendations for treatment of child and adolescent overweight and obesity. Pediatrics 2007;120(Suppl 4):S254–88.
8. Davis MM, Gance-Cleveland B, Hassink S, et al. Recommendations for prevention of childhood obesity. Pediatrics 2007;120(Supplement_4):S229–53.
9. Taveras EM, Gortmaker SL, Hohman KH, et al. Randomized controlled trial to improve primary care to prevent and manage childhood obesity: the high five for kids study. Arch Pediatr Adolesc Med 2011;165(8):714–22.
10. Resnicow K, Davis R, Rollnick S. Motivational interviewing for pediatric obesity: conceptual issues and evidence review. J Am Diet Assoc 2006;106(12):2024–33.
11. Flattum C, Friend S, Neumark-Sztainer D, et al. Motivational interviewing as a component of a school-based obesity prevention program for adolescent girls. J Am Diet Assoc 2009;109(1):91–4.
12. Brennan L, Walkley J, Fraser SF, et al. Motivational interviewing and cognitive behaviour therapy in the treatment of adolescent overweight and obesity: study design and methodology. Contemp Clin Trials 2008;29(3):359–75.
13. Carels RA, Darby L, Cacciapaglia HM, et al. Using motivational interviewing as a supplement to obesity treatment: a stepped-care approach. Health Psychol 2007;26(3):369–74.
14. Irby M, Kaplan S, Garner-Edwards D, et al. Motivational interviewing in a family-based pediatric obesity program: a case study. Fam Syst Health 2010;28(3):236–46.

15. Pakpour AH, Gellert P, Dombrowski SU, et al. Motivational interviewing with parents for obesity: an RCT. Pediatrics 2015;135(3):e644–52.

16. Winchester B, Cragun D, Redlinger-Grosse K, et al. Application of motivational interviewing strategies with the extended parallel process model to improve risk communication for parents of children with familial hypercholesterolemia. J Genet Counsel 2022;31(4):847–59.

17. Rollnick S, Butler C, Cambridge J, et al. Consultations about behaviour change. BMJ 2005;331(7522):961–3.

18. Rollnick S, Miller W, Butler C. Motivational interviewing in health care: helping patients change behavior. New York, NY: Guilford Publications; 2007.

19. Miller W. Motivational interviewing with problem drinkers. Behav Psychother 1983; 11(2):147–72.

20. Rollnick S, Heather N, Gold R, et al. Development of a short "readiness to change" questionnaire for use in brief, opportunistic interventions among excessive drinkers. Br J Addict 1992;87(5):743–54.

21. Velasquez M, Hecht J, Quinn V, et al. Application of motivational interviewing to prenatal smoking cessation: training and implementation issues. Tobac Control 2000;9(Supp III):36–40.

22. Zomahoun HTV, Guénette L, Grégoire JP, et al. Effectiveness of motivational interviewing interventions on medication adherence in adults with chronic diseases: a systematic review and meta-analysis. Int J Epidemiol 2017;46(2):589–602.

23. Hettema JE, Hendricks PS. Motivational interviewing for smoking cessation: a meta-analytic review. J Consult Clin Psychol 2010;78(6):868–84.

24. Broccoli S, Davoli AM, Bonvicini L, et al. Motivational interviewing to treat overweight children: 24-month follow-up of a randomized controlled trial. Pediatrics 2016;137(1).

25. Resnicow K, McMaster F, Bocian A, et al. Motivational interviewing and dietary counseling for obesity in primary care: an RCT. Pediatrics 2015;135(4):649–57.

26. van Grieken A, Veldhuis L, Renders CM, et al. Population-based childhood overweight prevention: Outcomes of the 'be active, eat right' study. PLoS One 2013;8(5).

27. Taylor Rachael W, Cox Adell, Knight Lee, et al. A Tailored Family-Based Obesity Intervention: A Randomized Trial. Pediatrics 2015;136(2):281–9.

28. Döring Nora, Ghaderi Ata, Benjamin Bohman, et al. Motivational interviewing to prevent childhood obesity: a cluster RCT. Pediatrics 2016;137(5):e20153104.

29. Vansteenkiste M, Williams GC, Resnicow K. Toward systematic integration between self-determination theory and motivational interviewing as examples of top-down and bottom-up intervention development: autonomy or volition as a fundamental theoretical principle. Int J Behav Nutr Phys Activ 2012;9:23.

30. Deci E, Ryan R. Intrinsic motivation and self-determination in human behavior. New York: Plenum; 1985.

31. Ryan RM, Deci EL. Self-determination theory and the facilitation of intrinsic motivation, social development, and well-being. Am Psychol 2000;55(1):68–78.

32. Suire KB, Kavookjian J, Wadsworth DD. Motivational interviewing for overweight children: a systematic review. Pediatrics 2020;146(5):e20200193.

33. Vallabhan MK, Jimenez EY, Nash JL, et al. Motivational interviewing to treat adolescents with obesity: a meta-analysis. Pediatrics 2018;142(5):e20180733.

34. Resnicow Ken, Delacroix Emerson, Sonneville Kendrin R, et al. Outcome of BMI2+: Motivational Interviewing to Reduce BMI Through Primary Care AAP PROS Practices. Pediatrics 2024;153(2). e2023062462.

35. Hampl SE, Hassink SG, Skinner AC, et al. Clinical practice guideline for the evaluation and treatment of children and adolescents with obesity. Pediatrics 2023; 151(2). e2022060640.

36. Miller WR, Rollnick S. Motivational interviewing: helping people change. 3rd ed. New York: Guilford Press; 2013.

37. Resnicow K, Gobat N, Naar S. Intensifying and igniting change talk in Motivational Interviewing: A theoretical and practical framework. European Health Psychologist 2015;17(3):102–10.

38. Hesse M. The Readiness Ruler as a measure of readiness to change poly-drug use in drug abusers. Harm Reduct J 2006;3:3. Published 2006 Jan 25.

39. Mundil D, Cameron-Vendrig A, Husain M. GLP-1 receptor agonists: A clinical perspective on cardiovascular effects. Diabetes Vasc Dis Res 2012;9(2):95–108.

40. Sandsdal RM, Juhl CR, Jensen SBK, et al. Combination of exercise and GLP-1 receptor agonist treatment reduces severity of metabolic syndrome, abdominal obesity, and inflammation: a randomized controlled trial. Cardiovasc Diabetol 2023;22:41.

41. Change Talk. Childhood obesity; motivational interviewing skill building simulation for pediatricians, nurses, family physicians, and nutritionists. Change Talk 2014. Available at: https://health.mo.gov/living/healthcondiseases/chronic/wisewoman/pdf/MIChangeTalk.pdf.

42. Hershberger PJ, Pei Y, Bricker DA, et al. Advancing motivational interviewing training with artificial intelligence: ReadMI. Adv Med Educ Pract 2021;12:613–8.

43. Saiyed A, Layton J, Borsari B, et al. Technology-assisted motivational interviewing: Developing a scalable framework for promoting engagement with tobacco cessation using NLP and machine learning. Procedia Computer Science 2022;206:121–31.

44. Chew HS. The use of Artificial Intelligence–based conversational agents (chatbots) for weight loss: Scoping review and practical recommendations. JMIR Medical Informatics 2022;10(4).

45. Galvão Gomes da Silva J, Kavanagh DJ, Belpaeme T, et al. Experiences of a motivational interview delivered by a robot: qualitative study. J Med Internet Res 2018;20(5):e116.

46. Brown A, Kumar AT, Melamed O, et al. A motivational interviewing chatbot with generative reflections for increasing readiness to quit smoking: iterative development study. JMIR Ment Health 2023;10:e49132.

47. Motivational interviewing technology helps youth experiencing homelessness. The Annie E. Casey Foundation. 2021. Available at: https://www.aecf.org/blog/motivational-interviewing-technology-helps-youth-experiencing-homelessness.

48. Pérez-Rosas V, Mihalcea R, Resnicow K, Singh S, An L. Building a motivational interviewing dataset. Proceedings of the Third Workshop on Computational Linguistics and Clinical Psychology. Published online 2016. doi:10.18653/v1/w16-0305.

49. Pérez-Rosas V, Mihalcea R, Resnicow K, et al. Understanding and predicting empathic behavior in counseling therapy. Vancouver, Canada: Published online; 2017. https://doi.org/10.18653/v1/p17-1131.

50. Pérez-Rosas V, Mihalcea R, Resnicow K, et al. Predicting counselor behaviors in motivational interviewing encounters. Vancouver, Canada: Published online; 2017. https://doi.org/10.18653/v1/e17-1106.

51. Pollak KI, Alexander SC, Coffman CJ, et al. Physician communication techniques and weight loss in adults: Project CHAT. Am J Prev Med 2010;39(4):321–8.

52. Pollak KI, Alexander SC, Østbye T, et al. Primary care physicians' discussions of weight-related topics with overweight and obese adolescents: results from the Teen CHAT Pilot study. J Adolesc Health 2009;45(2):205–7.

Lifestyle Interventions in Pediatric Primary Care

Jennifer O. Lambert, MD, MHS[a], Amy Beck, MD, MPH[b],
Nakiya N. Showell, MD, MHS, MPH[c],*

KEYWORDS

- Lifestyle interventions • Pediatric obesity • Nutrition • Physical activity • Screen time
- Sleep • Primary care

KEY POINTS

- Pediatric clinicians should ask permission to discuss obesity-related health concerns, build rapport with families, and recommend a whole family approach to lifestyle interventions.
- Pediatric clinicians should counsel on age-appropriate recommendations for nutrition, physical activity, screen time, and sleep, and help families to set goals for behavioral change using principles of shared decision-making.
- The highest priority topics for goal setting are reducing sugar-sweetened beverage intake, increasing physical activity, and reducing screen time.
- Intensive health behavior and lifestyle treatment programs are effective in addressing pediatric obesity but are not widely accessible. When unavailable or not feasible for families, pediatric clinicians should refer to other available resources including dietitians, community based physical activity programs, relevant sub-specialty clinics, and resources to address food insecurity.

INTRODUCTION

Case 1

Jackson is a 5-year-old boy presenting with his parents for well-child care. His parents express concerns about seasonal allergies but have no concerns about his growth. Jackson has a family history of type 2 diabetes in his maternal grandmother. At his well visit, Jackson's body mass index (BMI) has increased from the 80th to the 95th percentile.

[a] Johns Hopkins University School of Medicine, 200 North Wolfe Street, Room 2088, Baltimore, MD 21287, USA; [b] University of California San Francisco, 550 16th Street, San Francisco, CA 94158, USA; [c] Johns Hopkins University School of Medicine, 200 North Wolfe Street, Room 2023, Baltimore, MD 21287, USA
* Corresponding author.
E-mail address: nshowel1@jh.edu

Pediatr Clin N Am 71 (2024) 943–955
https://doi.org/10.1016/j.pcl.2024.07.004
pediatric.theclinics.com

Case 2

Mariah is a 12-year-old girl presenting with her mother after a failed vision screen at school. Her mother is concerned Mariah may need glasses but has no concerns about her growth. Mariah has a family history of type 2 diabetes in her father and both paternal grandparents and hypertension in her mother. At her primary care visit, Mariah's BMI is 98th percentile, her blood pressure is elevated, and she is found to have acanthosis nigricans.

Lifestyle interventions represent the first-line treatment for pediatric obesity at the individual and family level. Pediatric clinicians should dedicate time during clinical encounters to discuss health behavior recommendations, particularly for families of children and adolescents with obesity. In this article, we review key health behavior recommendations for nutrition, physical activity, screen time, and sleep, and provide an approach to pediatric obesity management in primary care. We utilize 2 patient cases, as outlined earlier, to explore these topics.

In both cases, the family is not presenting due to a growth concern. This is typical as obesity is often not a primary concern expressed by families in pediatric primary care. However, pediatric primary care represents the only longitudinal setting in which children are routinely screened for overweight and obesity.[1] Studies have found that caregivers expect weight status to be discussed at pediatric primary care visits,[2,3] and better understand their child's weight status when it is specifically discussed by a pediatric provider.[4] Additionally, caregivers find the doctor's office to be the most appropriate place for managing overweight and obesity.[5] Therefore, obesity is a critical topic to address in pediatric primary care.

Contrary to the belief that children are likely to "grow out of" obesity, a meta-analysis found that 55% of children with obesity will continue to have obesity in adolescence.[6] Among adolescents with obesity, approximately 80% will have obesity in adulthood.[6] Early onset of obesity is particularly worrisome. In a large cohort study in Germany, 90% of children with obesity at age 3 experienced overweight or obesity in adolescence.[7] This study also found that among adolescents with obesity, the most rapid weight gain occurred between 2 and 6 years of age.[7] As pediatric obesity is unlikely to resolve without intervention, it is important for pediatric clinicians to address this serious health risk.

HEALTH BEHAVIOR RECOMMENDATIONS

Lifestyle interventions to address pediatric obesity include promoting healthy nutritional intake, increasing physical activity, limiting screen time, and ensuring adequate sleep. Key, age-specific recommendations from the American Academy of Pediatrics (AAP),[1,8–11] United States Department of Agriculture,[12] US Department of Health and Human Services,[13] American Heart Association (AHA),[14,15] American Academy for Sleep Medicine (AASM),[16] and World Health Organization[17] are summarized in **Table 1**.

The impact of these health behavior recommendations is not limited to promoting a healthy weight status. Many of the recommended health behaviors are strongly linked to cardiometabolic health and can prevent or help treat type 2 diabetes, prediabetes, dyslipidemia, hypertension, and metabolic dysfunction-associated steatotic liver disease (MASLD). There are also mental and emotional health benefits associated with optimizing nutrition, physical activity, screen time, and sleep habits. While some of these health behavior recommendations have not been studied individually, they often comprise parts of evidence-based, comprehensive lifestyle interventions.

Table 1
Key pediatric health behavior recommendations by age

	Nutrition	Physical Activity	Screen Time	Sleep
Infants	Breastfeeding recommended No juice or SSB No added sugar	≥30 mins/d prone position "tummy time" until mobile	None except video calls with friends and family	12–16 h/d (4–12 mo)
Toddlers/Preschoolers	Limit 100% juice to 4oz/day (1–3 y) No SSB No added sugar <24 mo	≥60 mins/d and up to several h/d unstructured activity (1–3 y) ≥180 mins/d activities of varying activities throughout the day (3–5 y)	Limited high-quality programming with a caregiver (≥18 mo) No devices during meals or ≤ 1 h before bedtime	11–14 h/d (1–2 y) 10–13 h/d (3–5 y) No devices in bedroom
School-age children	Limit SSB to ≤8oz/week Limit 100% juice to 4-6oz/d (ages 4–6) or 8oz/d (ages ≥7) Limit added sugar to ≤25 g/d (less is better)	≥60 mins/d moderate or vigorous activity ≥3 d/w: vigorous activity Include muscle- and bone-strengthening activities	≤1 h high-quality programming, ideally with a caregiver (ages 2–5) Create a family media use plan No devices during meals or ≤1 h before bedtime	9–12 h/d No devices in bedroom
Adolescents	Limit SSB to ≤8oz/w Limit 100% juice to ≤8oz/d Limit added sugar to ≤25 g/d (less is better)	≥60 mins/d moderate or vigorous activity ≥3 d/w: vigorous activity Include muscle- and bone-strengthening activities	Create a family media use plan No devices during meals or ≤1 h before bedtime	8–10 h/d No devices in bedroom

Abbreviation: SSB, sugar sweetened beverages.

Highest-Priority Health Behaviors

In a busy clinical practice, it is not feasible to make all the detailed recommendations in **Table 1** at every visit. Generally, the highest priority recommendations for children and adolescents with, and at risk for, obesity, include reducing sugar-sweetened beverage (SSB) intake, increasing physical activity, and reducing screen time. Toward the end of this article, we will return to our cases to explore recommendations for Jackson and Mariah.

Nutrition

SSB intake is one of the most important health behaviors to focus on for both the prevention and treatment of childhood obesity. We define SSB as beverages with added sugar. SSB intake contributes to increasing BMI trajectory and is also associated with type 2 diabetes,[18] MASLD,[19] hypertension,[18,20] cancer,[21] and cardiovascular disease,[18] even after controlling for BMI. Intervention trials in which SSB have been removed from the diet have led to improvements in weight status,[22] insulin resistance,[23] hepatic fat fraction,[24] fasting triglycerides,[23] and diastolic blood pressure.[23] Given the wide-ranging impacts of SSB on health, the AHA advises that children aged 2 and older limit SSB intake to one 8-ounce serving per week.[14]

Beyond reduction in SSB intake, nutritional approaches to treat obesity should focus on limiting added sugar intake and reducing high calorie, low nutrient processed foods while increasing consumption of vegetables and fruits.[25] Ideally fruits and vegetables should be offered in their whole form and not as juices, as 100% fruit juice intake has been shown to be a risk factor for excess weight gain.[26] Screening for intake of foods with added sugar, processed foods, and deep fried foods can help to guide goal setting. Providers can assist families to make specific goals to reduce, but not eliminate, these foods and to identify healthier replacements. For many children, it can be practical to focus on healthy snacking and replacement of items such as chips or cookies with a fruit or vegetable served alone or in combination with a protein source to promote satiety.[27] Key age-specific nutrition recommendations are shown in **Table 1**.

It is also important to recognize that food insecurity may be a major factor in the foods that parents purchase and prepare. Thus, it is critical to refer families to governmental nutrition programs, as well as locally available food resources[28] and to make realistic recommendations regarding meal and snack planning that consider budget constraints, family preferences, and cultural norms. If available and desired, providers should refer to a dietitian or an Intensive Health Behavior and Lifestyle Treatment (IHBLT) program that can provide detailed nutritional guidance.

Physical Activity

Physical activity is a key health behavior target for lifestyle interventions addressing pediatric obesity and cardiometabolic health. Among children and adolescents with obesity, several studies have demonstrated that exercise training reduces body fat mass, insulin resistance, blood pressure, and glucose levels.[29,30] Furthermore, moderate to vigorous physical activity has been strongly linked to improvements in bone health and cardiovascular fitness.[13] In addition to its positive effects on physical health, increased physical activity has been linked to reduced depressive symptoms and higher cognitive performance.[31,32]

Given the wide-ranging benefits of physical activity, the 2018 Physical Activity Guidelines for Americans recommend that children aged 6 to 17 years have at least 60 minutes of moderate-to-vigorous physical activity daily, including vigorous-intensity activity and muscle and bone-strengthening activities at least 3 days per week.[13] Younger children aged 3 to 5 years should engage in at least 3 hours of daily varied-intensity physical activity and infants and toddlers should engage in interactive floor-based play and tummy time.[10,13,17] Age-specific physical activity recommendations are shown in **Table 1**.

Screen Time

Excess screen time is strongly linked to obesity in children and adolescents.[33] The mechanisms by which screen time impacts adiposity may include reduced physical activity time, increased exposure to food advertising, and increased caloric intake from eating while viewing.[33] Even after adjusting for physical activity, children and adolescents have higher odds of overweight or obesity if they engage in more than 2 hours of screen time daily.[34] Among adolescents with obesity, media use for over 5 hours per day is associated with insulin resistance, elevated liver enzymes, and elevated triglycerides.[35]

Therefore, the AAP recommends families avoid screen time for children under 18 month old, optionally engage in limited high-quality screen time with their children 18 to 24 month old, and limit screen time to no more than 1 hour daily of high-quality programming for children 2 to 5 years old.[8] The AAP previously recommended no more than 2 hours of screen time for older children and adolescents, but their most recent guidelines emphasize that even this limit may be too high to promote cardiometabolic health.[9] Instead the AAP now recommends creating an individualized family media use plan.[11] For all ages, media use is discouraged during meals or in bedrooms.[8,9] Age-specific pediatric screen time recommendations from the AAP are shown in **Table 1**.

Sleep

Short sleep duration has been associated with obesity, hypertension, insulin resistance, and type 2 diabetes in children and adolescents.[16,36] Age-specific pediatric sleep duration recommendations from the AASM are shown in **Table 1**, and include a recommended 9 to 12 hours of sleep per night for school-aged children and 8 to 10 hours of sleep per night for adolescents.[16] To achieve the recommended quantity of sleep and ensure good sleep quality, families should implement consistent bedtimes and bedtime routines for their children. Additionally, the AAP recommends no screen time within an hour of bedtime and that those bedrooms are kept device-free.[11]

EVIDENCE FOR LIFESTYLE INTERVENTIONS

Data on lifestyle interventions demonstrate that more hours of support for families of children and adolescents with obesity result in better outcomes. A US Preventive Services Task Force systematic review of randomized interventions to address pediatric obesity found them more effective than control groups only when there were at least 26 contact hours over 6 to 12 months.[37] A general dose-response pattern was found, where higher contact hours were associated with greater effects. A more recent appraisal of clinical care practices for pediatric obesity yielded similar results.[38]

IHBLT interventions are recommended by the AAP to treat children aged 6 and older with overweight or obesity and may also be recommended for children 2 to 5 years.[1] However, the accessibility of IHBLT programs is lacking.[39] Therefore, families of children and adolescents with obesity should be connected with the highest level of intervention available to and desired by the family. In some cases, this may be continued engagement in primary care alone or in combination with other referrals.

LIFESTYLE INTERVENTIONS TO ADDRESS PEDIATRIC OBESITY IN PRIMARY CARE

A 5-step approach to guide pediatric clinicians in addressing obesity in primary care is shown in **Fig. 1**. The order of these steps can be adjusted to accommodate the clinician and family.

Broaching the Topic

Broaching the topic of weight status with a child's family can be challenging due to the stigma associated with obesity. Thus, it is critical to first prioritize building a positive relationship with families. An important goal of the clinician and family interaction is that families will want to return to share their successes and challenges. This starts with the physical environment of the clinic, which should include appropriately sized blood pressure cuffs and gowns for children and adolescents with obesity, as well as inclusive visuals that portray individuals with a range of body sizes in a positive light. Optimally, discussions about a child's weight status would be initiated in the context of a longitudinal relationship. However, this is not always possible.

Whether or not the pediatric clinician has an established relationship with the patient and family, they should take the time to build rapport prior to addressing any aspect of weight status. This is an important part of any visit, but especially important in this setting as evidence shows physicians build less rapport with adult patients with obesity.[40] Pediatric clinicians should be mindful of the language they use when opening the discussion. One appropriate way to begin the discussion with the family is to ask, "Do you have any concerns regarding how your child is growing, with either their height or weight?" This opening question provides an opportunity to assess the family's existing understanding of their child's weight status.

History and Physical

Key history and review of systems components for children and adolescents with obesity are shown in **Box 1**. They include nutrition, physical activity, screen time, and sleep behaviors, as well as family history[41] and social history. The social history should

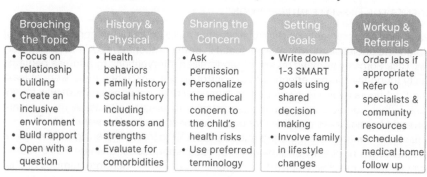

Addressing Pediatric Obesity in Primary Care

Broaching the Topic	History & Physical	Sharing the Concern	Setting Goals	Workup & Referrals
• Focus on relationship building • Create an inclusive environment • Build rapport • Open with a question	• Health behaviors • Family history • Social history including stressors and strengths • Evaluate for comorbidities	• Ask permission • Personalize the medical concern to the child's health risks • Use preferred terminology	• Write down 1-3 SMART goals using shared decision making • Involve family in lifestyle changes	• Order labs if appropriate • Refer to specialists & community resources • Schedule medical home follow up

Fig. 1. Approach to addressing pediatric obesity in primary care.

Box 1
Key history and review of systems components for pediatric obesity

Nutrition history
- Typical meals (foods, portions, where eaten, and whether shared with family)
- Typical snacks
- Typical beverages
- Meals eaten outside the home (restaurants, fast food, schools, etc.)
- Disordered eating behaviors (restricted or compulsive eating)

Physical activity history
- Typical physical activity and how vigorous it is
- Access to safe and inviting places to play
- Opportunity to engage in organized sports or activities

Sleep history
- Typical bedtime and wakeup time (weekdays vs weekends)
- Presence of screens (television, smartphone, and tablet) in the bedroom
- Use of screens within 1 hour of bedtime
- Difficulties with sleep onset or early awakening

Screen time history
- Hours per day watched
- Types of media consumed
- Whether accompanied by meals or snacks

Family history
- First- or second-degree relatives with type 2 diabetes, prediabetes, MASLD, hypertension, coronary artery disease, or dyslipidemia

Social history
- Child's primary caregiver(s)
- Where the child spends their time (including childcare or school)
- Who purchases food
- Who prepares the child's meals and snacks
- Strengths including resources that support a healthy lifestyle
- Acute stressors (eg, death of a family member)
- Chronic stressors (eg, neighborhood violence)
- Food insecurity

Review of systems
- Abdominal pain, headaches, daytime sleepiness, snoring, apnea, musculoskeletal pain, disordered sleep, polyuria, oligomenorrhea, skin or hair changes, and mental or behavioral health concerns

---

include assessing for strengths, as well as stressors such as food insecurity, which can be assessed using the "Hunger Vital Sign."[42] Given the amount of information, it is most feasible to gather these components over multiple visits. After obtaining the history, an obesity-focused physical examination should be performed as detailed in another article in this volume.

Sharing the Concern

When sharing a concern about obesity and associated comorbidities, the pediatric clinician should first ask permission from the patient and family to discuss the topic. If permission is granted, the clinician should personalize the concerns to the individual child or adolescent. This personalization can involve highlighting relevant family history or comorbidities identified during the physical examination or diagnostic workup. It is essential to employ person-first language with families, and the term "obese" should not be used. In many cases, using the word "obesity" may not be preferred in the clinical encounter. Research indicates that children, parents, and health care professionals prefer use of the term "above a healthy weight."[43]

Inquiring about the patient's or family's perspective on contributing factors to the health concern may help identify potential targets for goal setting and/or resource needs. It may also be helpful to create space for families to share difficulties in addressing the issue. In response, the pediatric clinician should express empathy, offer personalized support when possible, and acknowledge the influence of structural, environmental, and genetic factors on child weight status. It is important to convey that childhood obesity is multifactorial, and families are not at fault.

Setting Individualized Goals

The pediatric clinician should use shared decision-making[44] to set individualized goals around nutrition, physical activity, screen time, and sleep for the child or adolescent and their family. Clinicians should recommend whole family adoption of lifestyle interventions because it is most feasible for a child to make changes if all family members participate. The child or adolescent should take an active role in determining what goals to set. Ideally goals should be specific, measurable, achievable, realistic, and time-bound (SMART).[45] A good first step is to identify 1 to 3 SMART goals and write them down with the family, as families prefer written plans for lifestyle interventions.[46] Motivational interviewing may also be used and is described in depth in Susan J. Woolford and colleagues' article, "Motivational Interviewing for the Prevention and Treatment of Pediatric Obesity: A Primer," in this issue.

Workup and Referrals

As part of the workup for pediatric obesity, pediatric clinicians should routinely screen for comorbid physical and mental health conditions. This may include additional laboratory testing, ancillary studies, and specialty referrals as detailed in other articles in this volume. Referrals may also include connection to IHBLT programs, when available and preferred by the family. In the absence of an accessible program, pediatric clinicians should refer to dietitians, case managers, or social workers as appropriate. Clinicians should also refer eligible families to programs to assist with enrollment in governmental nutrition programs including the Special Supplemental Nutrition Program for Women, Infants, and Children and the Supplemental Nutrition Assistance Program (SNAP), as well as community-based organizations that provide food resources.[28] Pediatric clinicians should also refer to community-based programs that support healthy lifestyles, such as community-based physical activity programs.[47]

In addition to facilitating connection to other clinics and resources, the pediatric clinician should arrange for the patient and their family to follow-up in the medical home. Offering a mix of in person and telemedicine visits may optimize contact time with the clinician while maximizing feasibility and accessibility for families.[48]

Beyond the Clinic

In addition to the limited availability and expense of comprehensive pediatric obesity treatment programs, attempting to address the complex medical and social condition of pediatric obesity without addressing systemic inequities is often not successful. Pediatric clinicians also have a duty to serve as advocates for healthy policies in their communities to help address the systemic factors affecting children's health. These include food insecurity, poverty, structural racism, unsafe neighborhoods, lack of greenspace, toxic stress, and predatory food marketing. Please refer to other articles in this volume on obesity as a health equity issue, the built environment, and the toxic food environment for further discussion of these systemic challenges and avenues for pediatric clinicians to combat them.

CASES REVISITED
Case 1

We will revisit our case of Jackson, the 5-year-old presenting for a well visit with a recent increase in BMI percentile from 80th to 95th percentile. You first build rapport and address the family's primary concern regarding seasonal allergies. Upon further history-taking, you learn that Jackson is drinking 12 ounces of 100% apple juice daily but does not drink any SSB. After asking permission to discuss the topic, it would be appropriate to share your concern that he is now above a healthy weight and that this puts him at risk for future health problems.

After sharing your concern, you ask his parents what they think may have contributed to his recent accelerated weight gain. His parents report they have been giving him extra juice since they have limited access to affordable fruits and vegetables. He gets exercise for about 30 minutes 5 days per week and sleeps 12 hours per day. He watches television for an hour per day in addition to using a tablet during mealtimes. It is important to first praise Jackson's family for many of his healthy behaviors including avoiding SSB and ensuring an age-appropriate quantity of sleep. Recommended lifestyle interventions include limiting juice, increasing physical activity to 60 minutes per day, and avoiding screens during mealtimes. Given the presented concern for food insecurity, you should also refer to governmental nutrition programs, including SNAP, if not already enrolled, as well as locally available food resources. Using shared decision-making, you may decide to set goals to limit juice to 4 to 6 ounces per week and eliminate mealtime screen time in addition to referring the family to social work or another resource to assist with addressing food insecurity. You could also offer the family a referral to a dietitian for an in-depth nutritional assessment and guidance, and plan to have him return to your clinic in 1 to 3 months to follow-up on his progress and set new goals. Inviting the family back in 1 to 3 months' time shares with them that you see this as an important issue and that you are wanting to partner with them.

Case 2

Next, we revisit our case of Mariah, the 12-year-old presenting after a failed vision screen with BMI of 98th percentile, elevated blood pressure, and acanthosis nigricans. After building rapport and addressing their concern about the failed vision screen, you learn that Mariah is drinking 16 ounces of sweet tea daily, exercising for about 30 minutes 3 days per week, and sleeping 9 hours per night. She uses her phone for about 3 hours per day but does not use it during mealtimes or within an hour of bedtime. It would be appropriate, after asking permission to discuss the topic, to share your concern that the acanthosis suggests an increased risk of developing diabetes and elevated blood pressure poses an increased risk of developing heart disease in the future. Given her comorbidities and family history of diabetes in her father and hypertension in her mother, you should recommend lifestyle changes to reduce her risk of developing these health problems in the future.

It is valuable to praise Mariah and her family for healthy behaviors including avoiding screens in the bedroom and in the hour before bedtime and ensuring an age-appropriate quantity of sleep. Some recommended lifestyle interventions would include limiting SSB and increasing physical activity. Using shared decision-making, you may set goals to limit SSB intake to 8 ounces per week and increase physical activity to 60 minutes most days. It is important to explore potential avenues for increasing physical activity including any school or community-based programs that she could participate in, opportunities for physical activity together with peers, and whether parents or siblings can join her for activity on certain days of the week.

At the same time, you can pursue a laboratory workup including lipids, hemoglobin A1c, and alanine transaminase and plan to follow-up her blood pressure when she returns to clinic. With Mariah's family, you may decide to schedule a telemedicine visit in 1 month and an in-person visit in 3 months.

CLINICS CARE POINTS

- Broach the topic of pediatric obesity with care by creating an inclusive environment, building rapport, focusing on relationship building, and opening with a question.
- Collect a detailed history over multiple visits, including a health behavior history, family history, and social history that includes strengths and stressors, such as food insecurity.
- Ask permission to discuss obesity-related health concerns, use preferred language, and recommend a whole family approach to lifestyle interventions focused on improving health.
- In partnership with patients and families, create and write down 1 to 3 individualized SMART goals, prioritizing reducing SSB intake, increasing physical activity, and reducing screen time.
- Connect families to specialists and community resources to support healthy lifestyle changes, including IHBLT programs when accessible and feasible for the family.

FUTURE DIRECTIONS

Further research is needed to assess the effectiveness of additional approaches in pediatric obesity treatment, such as programs that promote mindfulness and resilience to stress.[49] Furthermore, there is a need for deeper investigation into enhanced models of care including integrated behavioral health and enhanced care management utilizing case managers, community health workers, or health educators. Last, thorough evaluation is necessary to understand the role of technology, including the use of mobile apps, wearables, and artificial intelligence, in addressing pediatric obesity.

SUMMARY

Pediatric clinicians play a vital role in the care of children and adolescents with obesity by providing guidance on healthy lifestyle behaviors including nutrition, physical activity, screen time, and sleep. In addition to performing an appropriate history and physical examination, pediatric primary care clinicians should thoughtfully broach the topic of unhealthy weight gain and share their concern in a way that promotes relationship building with families. Together, pediatric clinicians and families should set individualized SMART goals, with a particular focus on reducing SSB intake, increasing physical activity, and decreasing screen time. Evidence shows that lifestyle intervention programs for pediatric obesity with greater contact hours are more effective. However, intensive programs are not accessible for many families. Pediatric clinicians should refer families to the highest level of care that is accessible, based on family preferences and availability, and should continue to provide longitudinal care for these families in the medical home, which leads to effective partnership.

DISCLOSURES

The authors have nothing to disclose.

REFERENCES

1. Hampl SE, Hassink SG, Skinner AC, et al. Clinical Practice Guideline for the Evaluation and Treatment of Children and Adolescents With Obesity. Pediatrics 2023; 151(2). https://doi.org/10.1542/peds.2022-060640.
2. Bossick AS, Barone C, Alexander GL, et al. Teen, Parent, and Clinician Expectations About Obesity and Related Conditions During the Annual Well-Child Visit. J Patient Cent Res Rev 2017;4(3):114–24.
3. Uy MJA, Pereira MA, Berge JM, et al. How Should We Approach and Discuss Children's Weight With Parents? A Qualitative Analysis of Recommendations From Parents of Preschool-Aged Children to Physicians. Clin Pediatr (Phila) 2019;58(2):226–37.
4. Hernandez RG, Cheng TL, Serwint JR. Parents' Healthy Weight Perceptions and Preferences Regarding Obesity Counseling in Preschoolers: Pediatricians Matter. Clin Pediatr (Phila) 2010;49(8):790–8.
5. Eneli IU, Kalogiros ID, McDonald KA, et al. Parental preferences on addressing weight-related issues in children. Clin Pediatr (Phila) 2007;46(7):612–8.
6. Simmonds M, Llewellyn A, Owen CG, et al. Predicting adult obesity from childhood obesity: a systematic review and meta-analysis. Obes Rev 2016;17(2):95–107.
7. Geserick M, Vogel M, Gausche R, et al. Acceleration of BMI in Early Childhood and Risk of Sustained Obesity. N Engl J Med 2018;379(14):1303–12.
8. Hill D, Ameenuddin N, Reid Chassiakos YL, et al. Media and Young Minds. Pediatrics 2016;138(5). https://doi.org/10.1542/peds.2016-2591.
9. Reid Chassiakos YL, Radesky J, Christakis D, et al. Children and Adolescents and Digital Media. Pediatrics 2016;138(5). https://doi.org/10.1542/peds.2016-2593.
10. American Academy of Pediatrics. In: Hagan JF Jr, Shaw JS, Duncan PM, editors. Bright futures: guidelines for health supervision of infants, children, and adolescents. 4th edition. Itasca, IL: American Academy of Pediatrics; 2017.
11. American Academy of Pediatrics Council on Communications and Media. Media Use in School-Aged Children and Adolescents. Pediatrics 2016;138(5). https://doi.org/10.1542/peds.2016-2592.
12. US Department of Agriculture, US Department of Health and Human Services. Dietary guidelines for Americans, 2020–2025. 9th edition. Washington, DC: US Government Publishing Office; 2020.
13. US Department of Health and Human Services. Physical activity guidelines for Americans. 2nd edition. Washington, DC: US Government Publication; 2018.
14. Vos MB, Kaar JL, Welsh JA, et al. Added Sugars and Cardiovascular Disease Risk in Children: A Scientific Statement From the American Heart Association. Circulation 2017;135(19). https://doi.org/10.1161/CIR.0000000000000439.
15. Barnett TA, Kelly AS, Young DR, et al. Sedentary Behaviors in Today's Youth: Approaches to the Prevention and Management of Childhood Obesity: A Scientific Statement From the American Heart Association. Circulation 2018;138(11). https://doi.org/10.1161/CIR.0000000000000591.
16. Paruthi S, Brooks LJ, D'Ambrosio C, et al. Recommended Amount of Sleep for Pediatric Populations: A Consensus Statement of the American Academy of Sleep Medicine. J Clin Sleep Med 2016;12(06):785–6.

17. Bull FC, Al-Ansari SS, Biddle S, et al. World Health Organization 2020 guidelines on physical activity and sedentary behaviour. Br J Sports Med 2020;54(24):1451–62.

18. Li B, Yan N, Jiang H, et al. Consumption of sugar sweetened beverages, artificially sweetened beverages and fruit juices and risk of type 2 diabetes, hypertension, cardiovascular disease, and mortality: A meta-analysis. Front Nutr 2023;10. https://doi.org/10.3389/fnut.2023.1019534.

19. Chen H, Wang J, Li Z, et al. Consumption of Sugar-Sweetened Beverages Has a Dose-Dependent Effect on the Risk of Non-Alcoholic Fatty Liver Disease: An Updated Systematic Review and Dose-Response Meta-Analysis. Int J Environ Res Public Health 2019;16(12):2192.

20. Farhangi MA, Nikniaz L, Khodarahmi M. Sugar-sweetened beverages increases the risk of hypertension among children and adolescence: a systematic review and dose–response meta-analysis. J Transl Med 2020;18(1):344.

21. Arroyo-Quiroz C, Brunauer R, Alavez S. Sugar-Sweetened Beverages and Cancer Risk: A Narrative Review. Nutr Cancer 2022;74(9):3077–95.

22. de Ruyter JC, Olthof MR, Seidell JC, et al. A Trial of Sugar-free or Sugar-Sweetened Beverages and Body Weight in Children. N Engl J Med 2012;367(15):1397–406.

23. Lustig RH, Mulligan K, Noworolski SM, et al. Isocaloric fructose restriction and metabolic improvement in obese children and metabolic syndrome. Obesity 2016;24(2):453–60.

24. Schwarz JM, Noworolski SM, Erkin-Cakmak A, et al. Effects of Dietary Fructose Restriction on Liver Fat, De Novo Lipogenesis, and Insulin Kinetics in obese children. Gastroenterology 2017;153(3):743–52.

25. Liberali R, Kupek E, de Assis MAA. Dietary Patterns and Childhood Obesity Risk: A Systematic Review. Child Obes 2020;16(2):70–85.

26. Sanigorski AM, Bell AC, Swinburn BA. Association of key foods and beverages with obesity in Australian schoolchildren. Public Health Nutr 2007;10(2):152–7.

27. Magkos F. The role of dietary protein in obesity. Rev Endocr Metab Disord 2020;21(3):329–40.

28. Gitterman BA, Chilton LA, Cotton WH, et al. Promoting Food Security for All Children. Pediatrics 2015;136(5):e1431–8.

29. Sigal RJ, Alberga AS, Goldfield GS, et al. Effects of Aerobic Training, Resistance Training, or Both on Percentage Body Fat and Cardiometabolic Risk Markers in Obese Adolescents. JAMA Pediatr 2014;168(11):1006.

30. Kazeminasab F, Sharafifard F, Miraghajani M, et al. The effects of exercise training on insulin resistance in children and overweight adolescents or obesity: a systematic review and meta-analysis. Front Endocrinol 2023;14. https://doi.org/10.3389/fendo.2023.1178376.

31. Korczak DJ, Madigan S, Colasanto M. Children's Physical Activity and Depression: A Meta-analysis. Pediatrics 2017;139(4). https://doi.org/10.1542/peds.2016-2266.

32. Ardoy DN, Fernández-Rodríguez JM, Jiménez-Pavón D, et al. A Physical Education trial improves adolescents' cognitive performance and academic achievement: the <scp>EDUFIT</scp> study. Scand J Med Sci Sports 2014;24(1). https://doi.org/10.1111/sms.12093.

33. Robinson TN, Banda JA, Hale L, et al. Screen Media Exposure and Obesity in Children and Adolescents. Pediatrics 2017;140(Supplement_2):S97–101.

34. Bai Y, Chen S, Laurson KR, et al. The Associations of Youth Physical Activity and Screen Time with Fatness and Fitness: The 2012 NHANES National Youth Fitness Survey. PLoS One 2016;11(1):e0148038.

35. Sayin FK, Buyukinan M. Sleep Duration and Media Time Have a Major Impact on Insulin Resistance and Metabolic Risk Factors in Obese Children and Adolescents. Child Obes 2016;12(4):272–8.
36. Matthews KA, Dahl RE, Owens JF, et al. Sleep Duration and Insulin Resistance in Healthy Black and White Adolescents. Sleep 2012;35(10):1353–8.
37. O'Connor EA, Evans CV, Burda BU, et al. Screening for Obesity and Intervention for Weight Management in Children and Adolescents. JAMA 2017;317(23):2427.
38. Skinner AC, Staiano AE, Armstrong SC, et al. Appraisal of Clinical Care Practices for Child Obesity Treatment. Part I: Interventions. Pediatrics 2023;151(2). https://doi.org/10.1542/peds.2022-060642.
39. Thornton RLJ, Hernandez RG, Cheng TL. Putting the US Preventive Services Task Force Recommendation for Childhood Obesity Screening in Context. JAMA 2017;317(23):2378.
40. Gudzune KA, Beach MC, Roter DL, et al. Physicians build less rapport with obese patients. Obesity 2013;21(10):2146–52.
41. Corica D, Aversa T, Valenzise M, et al. Does Family History of Obesity, Cardiovascular, and Metabolic Diseases Influence Onset and Severity of Childhood Obesity? Front Endocrinol 2018;9. https://doi.org/10.3389/fendo.2018.00187.
42. Hager ER, Quigg AM, Black MM, et al. Development and Validity of a 2-Item Screen to Identify Families at Risk for Food Insecurity. Pediatrics 2010;126(1):e26–32.
43. van Maarschalkerweerd PEA, Camfferman R, Seidell JC, et al. Children's, Parents' and Healthcare Professionals' Preferences for Weight-Based Terminology in Health Care. Health Commun 2021;36(13):1805–9.
44. Charles C, Gafni A, Whelan T. Decision-making in the physician–patient encounter: revisiting the shared treatment decision-making model. Soc Sci Med 1999;49(5):651–61.
45. Deslippe AL, Bains A, Loiselle S, et al. SMART goals of children of 6–12 years enrolled in a family-centred lifestyle intervention for childhood obesity: Secondary analysis of a randomized controlled trial. Pediatr Obes 2023;18(1). https://doi.org/10.1111/ijpo.12973.
46. Cheng ER, Moore C, Parks L, et al. Human-centered designed communication tools for obesity prevention in early life. Prev Med Rep 2023;35:102333.
47. Armstrong SC, Windom M, Bihlmeyer NA, et al. Rationale and design of "Hearts & Parks": study protocol for a pragmatic randomized clinical trial of an integrated clinic-community intervention to treat pediatric obesity. BMC Pediatr 2020;20(1):308.
48. Bala N, Price SN, Horan CM, et al. Use of Telehealth to Enhance Care in a Family-Centered Childhood Obesity Intervention. Clin Pediatr (Phila) 2019;58(7):789–97.
49. Shomaker LB, Berman Z, Burke M, et al. Mindfulness-based group intervention in adolescents at-risk for excess weight gain: A randomized controlled pilot study. Appetite 2019;140:213–22.

Clinician's Guide for Pediatric Anti-obesity Medications

Wesley P. Dutton, MD[a,1], Nina Paddu, DO[b,2],
Amy Braddock, MD, MsPH[c,3], Brooke Sweeney, MD, DABOM[d,*]

KEYWORDS

- Pediatric obesity • Treatment • Pharmacotherapy • Anti-obesity medications

KEY POINTS

- Previous medication treatment gap between family based intensive health behavior and lifestyle treatment (IHBLT) and metabolic and bariatric surgery has now been filled with 4 Food and Drug Administration (FDA)-approved anti-obesity medications (AOM) commonly used in children: phentermine, phentermine/topiramate (Qsymia), liraglutide (Saxenda), and semaglutide (Wegovy).
- Orlistat and setmelanotide are also FDA-approved for pediatric use, but their application is limited. Metformin and topiramate are used off-label as well to facilitate weight loss.
- Pediatric clinicians should offer treatment for obesity that is individualized and available early in the treatment rather than offering a staged approach. Medications should be offered at 12 and older, and considered in younger children as more evidence emerges.
- AOM, in combination with IHLBT, ranges from 4% to 16% body mass index change when effective, depending on the specific treatment and response.
- Although structured weight loss in a medical setting is not associated with increased risk of eating disorders, assessment of eating disorder symptomatology or disordered eating prior to, and throughout treatment is important.

[a] Harvard Medical School, Massachusetts General Hospital, Weight Center at Massachusetts General Hospital, Boston, MA, USA; [b] Vanderbilt University Medical Center, Nashville, TN, USA; [c] Family and Community Medicine, University of Missouri, Columbia, MO, USA; [d] University of Missouri Kansas City, Children's Mercy Kansas City, Center for Children's Healthy Lifestyles & Nutrition, Kansas City, MO, USA
[1] Present address: MGH Weight Center, 50 Staniford Street Suite 430, Boston, MA 02114.
[2] Present address: 16 Serein Court, Syosset, NY 11791.
[3] Present address: 3510 Danvers Drive, Columbia, MO 65203.
* Corresponding author. 610 East 22nd Street, Kansas City, MO 64108.
E-mail address: brsweeney@cmh.edu

Pediatr Clin N Am 71 (2024) 957–980
https://doi.org/10.1016/j.pcl.2024.07.006
0031-3955/24/© 2024 Elsevier Inc. All rights reserved, including those for text and data mining, AI training, and similar technologies.

pediatric.theclinics.com

BACKGROUND

Pediatric obesity is a complex and multifactorial disease. Knowledge of the underlying pathophysiology of obesity has evolved substantially over the last 10 years with promising options for anti-obesity medications (AOMs) in adults and now children as well. The weight set point, a defended level of body-fat mass, is regulated by the brain via complex, overlapping biologic and environmental mechanisms.[1] The neurologic control over this set point results in difficulty for some to lose weight, despite significant efforts to change lifestyle, as recommended by clinicians.[2] However, the recent advent of highly effective AOMs provide pediatric clinicians a powerful tool to treat obesity.

Pediatric obesity treatment guidelines have been released and updated over time in 1998,[3] 2007,[4,5] 2017,[6] and most recently in January of 2023,[7] respectively, all reflecting continued improvements in understanding of the pathophysiology and treatment of obesity. The most recent guidelines state "pediatricians and other pediatric health care providers should offer adolescents 12 years and older with obesity (body mass index [BMI] >95th percentile) weight loss pharmacotherapy, according to medication indications, risks, and benefits, as an adjunct to health behavior and lifestyle treatment".[7] The previous treatment gap between family-based intensive health behavior and lifestyle treatment (IHBLT) and metabolic and bariatric surgery has now been filled with 6 Food and Drug Administration (FDA)-approved medications for use in pediatrics, as well as an increasing literature base for other agents used in adults that can be used in the pediatric population.

The motivations, goals, and preferences of our patients, known as 'the patient voice', should be considered as clinicians communicate about obesity. Including the patient in the conversation is especially important to empower their role in shared-decision making and to increase treatment efficacy.

ASSESSMENT PRIOR TO STARTING ANTI-OBESITY MEDICATIONS

For many pediatric patients, especially those with severe obesity (Class 2 BMI 35 or BMI percentile 120% of the 95th percentile and Class 3 BMI 40 or BMI 140% of the 95th percentile), weight set point reduction is often necessary to allow successful sustained weight reduction and improvement in cardiometabolic risk.[8,9] Because IHBLT alone is unlikely to result in clinically meaningful weight reduction, frustration among patients, their family, and clinicians is a common experience in the clinical setting. AOMs can be especially effective in patients with obesity (BMI 30 or BMI percentile 95th percentile and above) for whom behavior modification has proven suboptimal for improving the control of obesity and targeting the treatment of obesity-associated comorbidities.[7,10] Reviewing expected weight loss outcomes from each AOM and other treatments can be helpful in shared-decision making with the patient and their family. Intensive lifestyle as monotherapy typically stabilizes weight or decreases by an average 1.8% BMI change from baseline with wide variability in response.[11] AOM in combination with IHLBT results in a variable BMI change when effective (ie, 4% for liraglutide – 16% for semaglutide with others agents between), depending on the specific treatment and response and surgery brings an average 33.8% percent BMI change. Layering multiple modalities may have additive effects. Each treatment also has a bell curve of response with some high responders, most moderate responders, and some non-responders.[11] Response to AOMs can usually be determined within the first 12 weeks, after titration to a clinically effective dose. A different medication or approach should be offered to non-responders.

Key historic components to review prior to selection of AOMs may include (1) assessment of phenotypic symptomatology, (2) current eating behaviors including screening for any disordered eating, and (3) assessment of any potential undertreated or undiagnosed comorbidities or endocrinopathies or medications that contribute to significant weight gain or are contraindications to starting AOM.

Phenotypic Symptomatology

Phenotypic symptomatology is a relatively new obesity medicine construct that includes patient experience of hunger, satiety, and satiation. Phenotype for AOM selection has the preliminary data in adult studies.[12] In pediatric practice, identified symptomatology may guide initial treatment selection.[13]

Eating Disorder Symptomatology

Eating disorder symptomatology is common in pediatric patients seeking weight management services. Although structured medical weight loss is not associated with an increased risk of eating disorders,[14] assessment of eating disorder symptomatology or disordered eating, prior to and throughout AOM therapy, is essential and can guide nutrition counseling and treatment. Appropriate treatment with AOMs can assist in normalizing hunger and fullness signaling, allowing remission or sometimes resolution of previous disordered eating symptoms.

Screening for Medical Conditions and Weight Gain Promoting Medications

It is important to screen for weight-related conditions (eg, hypertension [HTN], metabolic liver diseases, prediabetes/diabetes, hyperlipidemia [HLD], and obstructive sleep apnea) and endocrinopathies associated with obesity (eg, hypothyroidism and polycystic ovarian syndrome).[6,7] It is critical to check potential drug-drug interactions or for any concomitant weight-promoting medications. Often substitutions can be made that are weight neutral or facilitate weight loss.[15]

INITIATING PEDIATRIC ANTI-OBESITY MEDICATIONS

Initiating AOM with IHLRT is an iterative process with regular clinic visits for efficacy and safety. Current evidence supports treatment for obesity that is individualized and initiated early in the disease course versus a staged approach as previously recommended.[7] Close monitoring of BMI percentile and growth curves is important during initiation of AOMs. The goal should be gradual and sustained weight loss and adjustments of medication selection or dosage may be necessary if weight loss is too rapid or unhealthy eating patterns develop due to medication-induced anorexia. It is also beneficial to prepare families for the expected weight gain with the reduction or discontinuation of medications.

If patients ask if they will need to be on medications lifelong, discuss the chronic nature of obesity as a disease, similar to high blood pressure or diabetes. Likely the medications and dosages will change over time, but most patients, including adults and children, will need lifelong treatment for this chronic disease. All medications are intended to support improved healthy lifestyle implementation in addition to weight loss and will need adjustments based on treatment response.

AOM may not be appropriate if the clinician has identified significant body dysmorphia, poor self-esteem, or disordered eating that need treatment prior to initiation. Children with obesity have an increased prevalence and stable incidence of mental health needs, including pre- and post-surgery, supporting the need for assessment and treatment of mental health concerns throughout obesity care.[16]

ANTI-OBESITY MEDICATION SELECTION

Selection of AOM is based on medical history, clinical presentation, disease severity, insurance coverage, and availability of specific medications. An AOM algorithm can assist in selection (**Fig. 1**).

There are currently 4 FDA-approved AOM commonly used in children: phentermine, phentermine/topiramate (Qsymia), liraglutide (Saxenda), and semaglutide (Wegovy). Orlistat and setmelanotide are also FDA-approved for use in pediatrics, but their use is limited. Orlistat is not recommended per adult guidelines due to its side effect profile and poor efficacy.[17] Setmelanotide is currently indicated only for patients with specific genetic obesity syndromes.[7] Metformin and topiramate are used off-label as well to facilitate weight loss through different mechanisms (see **Table 1**).

Glucagon-like Peptide-1 receptor agonists reduce weight by delaying gastric emptying, resulting in increased satiety, and decreasing appetite and hunger. The most common side effects are nausea, vomiting, and diarrhea, and generally occur in the first few weeks and resolve over time.[17] For this reason, they are started at a low dose and titrated up to a therapeutic level over weeks to months. Personal or family history of medullary thyroid cancer or multiple endocrine neoplasia type 2 is black box contraindications for this class due to thyroid C-cell tumors seen in rodents, but not yet seen in humans.[18]

Semaglutide (see **Table 1**) is a once weekly subcutaneous injection that has demonstrated the highest average weight loss response in pediatric obesity, and it is generally well-tolerated.[19,20] At a weekly dose of 2.4 mg with lifestyle intervention, semaglutide results in an average of 16.1% BMI reduction after 68 weeks[19] with a number needed to treat (NNT) of 2 to produce a BMI reduction of 5%.[19] Semaglutide is the first of the FDA-approved AOM for pediatrics to demonstrate improvement in weight-related quality of life.[19] Liraglutide is a once daily subcutaneous injection that is associated with a lower average response: 4.6% BMI reduction with an NNT of 4 to achieve a 5% BMI reduction.[21]

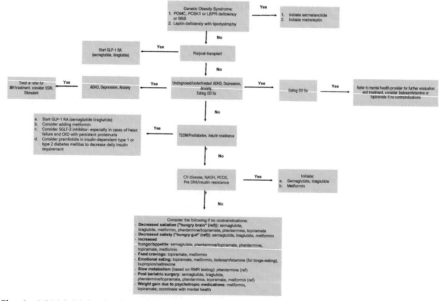

Fig. 1. AOM initial selection algorithm.

Table 1
Food and Drug Administration-approved anti-obesity medications in pediatrics

		FDA-Approved AOMs in Pediatrics		
Medication/FDA-Approval Age/ Mechanism of Action	Efficacy	Side Effects/Contraindications	Prescribing Information/ Management Tips	Ref
Semaglutide (Wegovy®) ≥ 12 year old GLP-1 receptor agonist	Mean change in BMI baseline to wk 68: −16.1% wth semaglutide and 0.6% with placebo (95% CI, −20.3 to −13.2). Change in BMI ≥l 5% reduction: 76% ≥l 10% reduction: 63% ≥l 15% reduction: 57% ≥l 20% reduction: 40%	Primary side effects: Nausea, vomiting, diarrhea, constipation, gastroesophageal reflux, eructation, abdominal pain, dizziness, fatigue Additional side effects: • Thyroid C-cell tumor (Black Box Warning) • GLP-1 RA class effects: acute pancreatitis, gallbladder disease, hypoglycemia with concurrent glucose lowering medications, acute kidney injury, diabetic retinopathy complications, HR increase, suicidal behavior/ideation Contraindications: • Personal or family history of medullary thyroid cancer (MTC) or multiple endocrine neoplasia type 2 (MEN2)	Dosing: Wks. 1–4: 0.25 mg SQ weekly Wks. 5–8: 0.5 mg SQ weekly Wks. 9–12: 1.0 mg SQ weekly Wks. 13–16: 1.7 mg SQ weekly Wks. 17+: 2.4 mg SQ weekly Management Tips: • *Primary side effects peak at initiation and dose increases, often improve with continued use at stable dose.* • *Risk of side effects may decrease with a prolonged titration strategy (>4 w per dose level).* • *Titrate to the lowest effective dose to minimize side effects.* • *Regularly spaced small meals and adequate hydration can mitigate gastrointestinal side effects.* Patient selection to maximize benefits: • *History of prediabetes or diabetes, dyslipidemia, NAFLD, PCOS* • *History of pre-existing cardiovascular disease or heart failure with preserved ejection fraction* • *Abnormal satiety/"Hungry gut"*	19,43

(continued on next page)

Table 1
(continued)

FDA-Approved AOMs in Pediatrics				
Medication/FDA-Approval Age/ Mechanism of Action	Efficacy	Side Effects/Contraindications	Prescribing Information/ Management Tips	Ref
Liraglutide (Saxenda®) ≥ 12 y old GLP-1 Receptor Agonist	Mean change in BMI baseline to w 56: −4.29% with liraglutide and 0.35% with placebo (95% CI, −7.14 to −2.14). Change in BMI ≥ 5% reduction: 43.3% ≥ 10% reduction: 26.1%	As described earlier for semaglutide	Dosing: Wk. 1: 0.6 mg SQ daily Wk. 2: 1.2 mg SQ daily Wk. 3: 1.8 mg SQ daily Wk. 4: 2.4 mg SQ daily Wk. 5+: 3.0 mg SQ daily Management Tips: • *As described earlier for semaglutide* • *The variable dose pen design allows for a broader range of possible doses that may be considered for more gradual dose escalation to further limit GI side effects* Patient selection to maximize benefits: • *As described earlier for semaglutide*	21,44
Phentermine/topiramate-ER (Qsymia®) ≥ 12 year old Phentermine - sympathomimetic amine Topiramate – increases GABA activity, antagonizes glutamate receptors, inhibits carbonic anhydrase,	Mean change in BMI baseline to wk 56: −7.11% with top-dose PHEN/ TPM (placebo subtracted −10.44%) (95% CI, −13.89 to −6.99) −4.78% with mid-dose PHEN/ TPM (placebo subtracted	Primary side effects: Dizziness, pyrexia, paresthesia, dysgeusia, depression, anxiety, insomnia Additional side effects: Embryo-fetal toxicity, HR increase, mood disorders, sleep disorders, cognitive impairment (disturbances in	Dosing: Wks. 1–2: 3.75 mg/23 mg PO daily in AM Wks. 3–14: 7.5 mg/46 mg PO daily in AM • If <3% TBWL, then discontinue or increase Wks. 15–16: 11.25 mg/69 mg daily in AM	22,45

modulates neuronal voltage gated sodium channels	−8.11%) (95% CI, −11.92 to −4.31) Change in BMI with top-dose ≥ 5% reduction: 46.9% ≥ 10% reduction: 42.5% ≥ 15% reduction: 28.3% Change in BMI with mid-dose ≥ 5% reduction: 38.9% ≥ 10% reduction: 31.5% ≥ 15% reduction: 13.0%	attention, memory, or speech/language), suicidal behavior/ideation, risk of acute myopia and secondary angle closure glaucoma, slowing of linear growth, metabolic acidosis and decrease in renal function Contraindications: • History of glaucoma or hyperthyroidism • Monoamine oxidase inhibitor (MAOI) therapy within 14 d	Wks. 17–29: 15 mg/92 mg daily in the AM • If <5% TBWL, then discontinue Management Tips: • Pregnancy test prior to initiation and prn; recommend effective contraception • Consider dose reduction or discontinuation if abnormalities arise: BP, HR, neuropsychiatric conditions, electrolytes and creatinine • *Prescribing separately off-label may help reduce the cost compared to the combination capsule* Patient selection to maximize benefits: • *Abnormal satiety/"hungry gut"* [23,46]
Phentermine ≥ 16 year old Sympathomimetic amine	Change in BMI baseline to 6 mo of phentermine 15 mg compared to standard of care was −4.1% (95% CI, −7.1 to −1.0). ≥ 5% reduction in BMI: 63.6%	Primary side effects: Dry mouth, palpitations, tachycardia, elevated BP, overstimulation, restlessness, dizziness, insomnia, euphoria, dysphoria, tremor, headache, psychosis, changes in libido Additional side effects: Primary pulmonary HTN (rare case reports), valvular heart disease (rare case reports), development of tolerance	Dosing: • Capsules: 15 mg, 30 mg, and 37.5 mg (equivalent to 30 mg base) • Tablets: 8 mg, 37.5 mg (equivalent to 30 mg base) • *Typically start at 15 mg or 18.75 mg (1/2 tablet of 37.5 mg) PO daily for 1 mo. If no improvement in obesity or weight plateaued after 1 mo, then consider increasing to phentermine 30 mg or 37.5 mg daily*

(continued on next page)

Table 1
(continued)

	FDA-Approved AOMs in Pediatrics		
Medication/FDA-Approval Age/ Mechanism of Action	Efficacy	Side Effects/Contraindications	Prescribing Information/ Management Tips	Ref
		Contraindications: • History of CV disease (eg, coronary artery disease, stroke, arrhythmias, congestive heart failure, uncontrolled HTN) • MAOI therapy within 14 d • Others: hyperthyroidism, glaucoma, agitated states, history of drug abuse	Management Tips: • Use lowest effective dose to limit side effects • Monitor BP, HR, and neuropsychiatric symptoms prior to initiation and periodically during use; consider dose reduction or discontinuation for clinically significant dysfunction • Development of tolerance to the anorexiant effect commonly develops; do not exceed recommended dose to overcome tolerance • *Long-term, off-label use of phentermine is common, but state law and state medical board guidance takes precedence* Patient selection to maximize benefits: • *Low predicted energy expenditure/"slow burn"*	

				Ref
Orlistat ≥ 12 year old Inhibits gastrointestinal lipases	The change in BMI from baseline to trail completion ranged from −1.44 to −1.3 at 6 mo and −0.55 at 12 mo. The between group differences ranged from −0.94 (95% CI, −1.58 to −3.0) to −0.50 (95% CI, −7.62-6.62) at 6 mo and −0.86 a 12 mo.	Primary side effects: Steatorrhea and oily discharge, soft stool, increased frequency/urgency of bowel movements, flatulence, fecal incontinence. Additional side effects: Decreased absorption of fat-soluble vitamins, increased urinary oxalate (calcium oxalate nephrolithiasis), cholelithiasis, liver injury. Drug interactions (cyclosporine, levothyroxine, amiodarone, warfarin, anticonvulsants, antiretrovirals, etc). Contraindications: • Chronic malabsorption • Cholestasis	Dosing: • 120 mg TID with each meal containing fat (during meal or 1 h after meal) • *Orlistat 60 mg (Alli®) is available without prescription, but it is not approved for pediatrics.* Management Tips: • Gastrointestinal symptoms are more common with a high fat diet • All patients should take a daily multivitamin that includes vitamin A, D, E, K and beta carotene • Monitor levels of other drug therapy more frequently. Patient selection to maximize benefits: • Chronic constipation • Last resort	24,47
Setmelanotide ≥ 6 year old with monogenic or syndromic obesity due to: POMC deficiency, PCSK1 deficiency, or LEPR deficiency confirmed on FDA-Approved genetic test resulting in biallelic variants interpreted as pathogenic, likely pathogenic, or undetermined significance; Bardet-Biedl Syndrome MCR-4 receptor agonist	POMC or PCSK1 • Mean % change in body weight baseline to wk 52 −25.6% (90% CI, −28.8 to −22.0) • ≥ 10% reduction in total body weight: 80% LEPR • Mean % change in body weight baseline to wk 52 −12.5% (90% CI, −16.1 to −8.8) • ≥ 10% reduction in total body weight: 45%	Primary side effects: Skin hyperpigmentation, headache, fatigue, dizziness, nausea, vomiting, diarrhea, abdominal pain, back pain, depression, and spontaneous penile erection. Additional side effects: Disturbance in sexual arousal (males and females), depression and suicidal ideation, hypersensitivity reactions, skin hyperpigmentation and	Dosing: • ≥12 year old start dose: 2 mg SQ daily • ≥6 to < 12 year old start dose: 1 mg SQ daily • Target dose: 3 mg SQ daily • Dose titration: If the starting dose is not tolerated, then reduce the dose by half. If the reduced dose is tolerated for at least 1 wk, then repeat a trial of the starting dose. If the starting dose is tolerated for 2 wk, then	25,48

(continued on next page)

Table 1
(continued)

	FDA-Approved AOMs in Pediatrics		
Medication/FDA-Approval Age/Mechanism of Action	Efficacy	Side Effects/Contraindications	Prescribing Information/Management Tips	Ref
	BBS • Mean % change in body weight baseline to wk 52 −5.2% (SD 7.9) • ≥ 10% reduction in total body weight: 32.3%	darkening of pre-existing nevi, risk of benzyl alcohol reaction in neonates Contraindications: Hypersensitivity reaction to setmelanotide or its components	increase to 3.0 mg subcutaneously once daily Management Tips: • Perform a full body skin exam prior to initiation and periodically • Seek emergency care if erection longer than 4 h • Train patients on SQ injection, and how to withdraw from the vial • Assess efficacy for weight loss at 12–16 wk in patients with POMC, PCSK1, or LEPR deficiency or 1 y in patients with BBS	

	Non-FDA-Approved Mediations Commonly Used Off-Label for Obesity		
Medication/FDA-Approved Indication/Mechanism of Action	Efficacy	Side Effects/Contraindications	Prescribing Information/Management Tips	Ref
Tirzepatide (Zepbound®) GLP-1 receptor and GIP receptor co-agonist Overweight/obesity in adults with BMI ≥27 with obesity related comorbidity or a BMI ≥30; Type 2 diabetes in adults	There is no pediatric data available at this time but in clinical trials for adolescents. Double-blinded, randomized, controlled trial in adults (n = 2539) overweight/obesity (mean BMI 38) mean % change in total body weight baseline to 72 wk: −15.0%, −19.5%, and −20.9% with tirzepatide 5.0 mg,	Primary side effects: Nausea, vomiting, diarrhea, constipation, eructation, gastroesophageal reflux, abdominal pain, hair loss, fatigue Other side effects: • Thyroid C-cell Tumor (Black Box Warning) • Other GPL-1 RA class effects (see semaglutide)	Dosing: Wks. 1–4: 2.5 mg SQ weekly *Only do subsequent dose escalation if needed for further improvement in obesity is needed.* Wks. 5–8: 5 mg SQ weekly Wks. 9–12: 7.5 mg SQ weekly Wks. 13–16: 10 mg SQ weekly Wks. 17+: 15 mg SQ weekly	49,50

			51,52,59
	10.0 mg, and 15.0 mg compared to −3.1% with placebo.	Contraindications: • Personal or family history of MTC or MEN2	Management Tips: • *As described above for semaglutide* • Recommend female patients switch to a non-oral contraceptive therapy or add a barrier method of contraception for 4 wk after initiation and subsequent dose escalations Patient selection to maximize benefits: • *As described above for semaglutide*
Dulaglutide GLP-1 receptor agonist Type 2 diabetes mellitus in patients ≥10 year old; adverse cardiovascular disease reduction in adults with type 2 diabetes and established cardiovascular disease or multiple cardiovascular disease risk factors	In a double-blinded, placebo-controlled trial of dulaglutide 0.75 mg or 1.5 mg in pediatric (n = 154) who were 10–17 y (mean 14.5) with type 2 diabetes (mean HgbA1c 8.1%) there was no significant difference in body weight end-points from baseline to 52 wk. In a randomized control trial of adult patients with type 2 diabetes inadequately controlled with metformin, dulaglutide 4.5 mg was superior to 1.5 mg and there appeared to dose response relationship with body weight reduction. The mean weight loss from baseline to wk 52 was −3.5 kg, −4.3 kg, and −5.0 with dulaglutide 1.5 mg, 3.0 mg, and 4.5 mg respectively from a baseline weight of 95.5 kg, 96.3 kg, and 95.4 kg.	As described earlier for semaglutide	Dosing: Wks. 1–4: 0.75 mg SQ weekly *Only do subsequent dose escalation if needed for further improvement in obesity. Wks. Wks. 5+: 1.5 mg SQ weekly • Only the 0.75 mg and 1.5 mg doses are approved for pediatric type 2 diabetes • 3.0 mg and 4.5 mg have not been studied in pediatrics Management Tips: As described earlier for semaglutide Patient selection to maximize benefits: • *As described above for semaglutide*

(continued on next page)

Table 1
(continued)

	Non-FDA-Approved Mediations Commonly Used Off-Label for Obesity		
Medication/FDA-Approved Indication/Mechanism of Action	**Efficacy**	**Side Effects/Contraindications**	**Prescribing Information/ Management Tips**	**Ref**
Metformin Biguanide – decreases hepatic gluconeogenesis, decreases intestinal glucose absorption, increases peripheral insulin sensitivity Type 2 diabetes mellitus in patients ≥10 year old	Systematic review and meta-analysis (8 studies, n = 616 patients 6–19 y with obesity (weighted mean BMI 36.0)) • Metformin (typical dose 1–2 g/day) with IHLBT • Change BMI z: − 0.10 (95% CI, −0.17 to −0.03) • Reduction in BMI was −0.86 (95% CI, −1.44 to −0.29).	Primary side effects: Diarrhea, flatulence, abdominal cramping, abdominal cramping, nausea/vomiting, headache Other side effects: Lactic acidosis (Black Box Warning), vitamin B12 deficiency, hypoglycemia with concurrent use of glucose lowering medications Contraindications: Acute or chronic metabolic acidosis	Dosing: Typically start at 500 mg once daily with a meal. Gradually increase by 500 mg in 1–2 divided doses every 1–2 wk. Typical top dose for obesity management is 1000 mg to 2000 mg in 1–2 divided doses depending on formulation. Management Tips: • Taking with a meal may reduce the risk of gastrointestinal side effects. • Slow dose escalation may improve tolerability Patient selection to maximize benefits: • Patients with type 2 diabetes mellitus, prediabetes, or polycystic ovarian syndrome • Patients who have experienced weight gain due to psychotropic medications	53,54

55,56

Topiramate
Increases GABA activity, antagonizes glutamate receptors, inhibits carbonic anhydrase, modulates neuronal voltage gated sodium channels
Epilepsy in patients ≥2 year old
Migraine prophylaxis in patients ≥12 year old

Retrospective study 28 patients (mean 15.2 y, SD 2.5) with obesity (mean baseline BMI 46.2, SD 10.3)
- Topiramate (most prescribed as 75 mg daily) with IHLBT
- Mean % change in BMI at 6 mo: −4.9 (95% CI, −7. to −2.8).
  ≥5% reduction in BMI: 50%
  ≥10% reduction in BMI: 13.6%

Primary side effects:
Paresthesia, hypoesthesia, changes in taste, fatigue, somnolence, dizziness, changes in mood
Additional side effects:
Acute myopia and secondary angle closure glaucoma, oligohidrosis, and hyperthermia, metabolic acidosis, nephrolithiasis, teratogenic, may decrease efficacy of oral contraceptive therapy, suicidal behavior/ideation, cognitive and psychiatric disturbances (psychomotor slowing, difficulty with memory, speech disorders, nervousness)
Contraindications:
Hypersensitivity reaction to topiramate or its components

Dosing:
Typically start at 25 mg PO daily in the evening for 2 wk then increase to 50 mg total daily dose in 1–2 divided doses.
If not experiencing improvement in obesity or improvement has plateaued, then consider increasing by 25 mg (generally, 100 mg is the maximum daily dose for obesity in most patients).
Management Tips:
- Check a basic metabolic panel at baseline and periodically to assess for metabolic acidosis
- Assess for mood disorders and changes in mood at baseline and periodically during treatment
- *Review potential to decrease efficacy of oral contraceptive therapy and recommend barrier contraception to prevent unintended pregnancy*
- *Consider evening dosing if experiencing daytime fatigue/somnolence*
Patient selection to maximize benefits:
- *Patients with migraines or idiopathic intracranial hypertension not on other carbonic anhydrase inhibiting therapy*

(continued on next page)

Table 1
(continued)

	Non-FDA-Approved Mediations Commonly Used Off-Label for Obesity		
Medication/FDA-Approved Indication/Mechanism of Action	**Efficacy**	**Side Effects/Contraindications**	**Prescribing Information/ Management Tips**	**Ref**
			• *Used in combination with concurrent sympathomimetic therapy* • *Patients with impulsive eating, emotional/stress eating, binge type eating, or night eating syndrome*	57,58
Naltrexone/bupropion ER tablets Naltrexone – opioid receptor antagonist Bupropion – inhibits reuptake of dopamine and norepinephrine Overweight/obesity in adults with BMI ≥27 with obesity related comorbidity or a BMI ≥30	There are no pediatric data available for naltrexone/ bupropion. There are no pediatric data available assessing the efficacy of naltrexone monotherapy or bupropion monotherapy on obesity. - BMI changes in adolescents (n = 296, mean age 16.3 year old) in a clinical trial evaluating bupropion for smoking cessation: decrease in BMI z-score (−0.16 (95% CI, −0.29 to −0.04)) from baseline to 6 wk in the 300 mg/day group, but this was not significant at 26 wk.	Primary Side effects: Headache, dizziness, fatigue, anxiety, irritability, insomnia, dry mouth, tremor, elevated blood pressure, palpitations, nausea, vomiting, diarrhea or constipation Other side effects: Suicidal Behavior and Ideation (Black Box Warning), neuropsychiatric symptoms have been reported in the setting of smoking cessation (Black Box Warning), increased blood pressure and heart rate, decreased seizure threshold, hepatotoxicity associated with naltrexone, angle closure glaucoma, hypoglycemia with concurrent glucose lowering medications	Dosing: • Tablet: 8 mg naltrexone/90 mg bupropion • Titration: 1 tablet once daily for 1 wk, then 1 tablet twice daily for 1 wk, next 2 tablets every morning and 1 tablet every evening for 1 wk, and lastly 2 tablets twice daily. Management Tips: • Assess for depression and suicidal ideation at baseline and periodically throughout treatment • Assess blood pressure (BP) and heart rate (HR) at baseline and periodically throughout treatment • *Prescribing separately off-label may help reduce the cost compared to the combination capsule*	

26,27

- *If prescribing separately, then may start together or sequentially.*

Patient selection to maximize benefits:
- Abnormal hedonic eating/ "Emotional hunger"

Contraindications:
- Uncontrolled hypertension
- Seizure disorders
- Anorexia nervosa or bulimia
- Abrupt discontinuation of alcohol, barbiturates, benzodiazepines, and anti-epileptic drugs
- Concurrent opiate therapies
- MAOI therapy within 14 d

Metreleptin
Leptin analogue
Leptin deficiency in patients with congenital or acquired generalized lipodystrophy

In a study of 3 pediatric patients with obesity and congenital leptin deficiency treated with recombinant human leptin, there were improvements in obesity as demonstrated by decreased BMI, decreased fat mass, and increased lean mass. There were also beneficial changes in feeding behaviors and endocrine function. The percentage BMI change from baseline to 6 mo was −13.9%, −18.1%, and −12.5% for patient A, B, and C respectively and −31.5% and −40.18% from baseline to 36 mo for patient A and B respectively.

Metreleptin has a Risk Evaluation and Mitigation Strategy (REMS) program for prescribers and pharmacies.

Primary side effects:
Headache, hypoglycemia with concurrent glucose lowering medications, decreased weight, abdominal pain, nausea, dizziness, fatigue, arthralgia

Additional side effects:
- Development of neutralizing antibodies (Black Box Warning)
- Risk of T-cell lymphoma (Black Box Warning)
- Progression of other autoimmune disorders
- Benzyl alcohol toxicity

Dosing:
- ≤ 40 kg: starting dose is 0.6 mg/ kg/day, increase or decrease by 0.02 mg/kg to a max daily dose of 0.13 mg/kg.
- > 40 kg:
  ○ Males: starting dose is 2.5 mg/ kg/day, increase or decrease by 1.25–2.5 mg/day to maximum dose of 10 mg/day
  ○ Females: starting dose is 5 mg/ kg/day, increase or decrease by 1.25–2.5 mg/day to maximum dose of 10 mg/day

Management tips:
- Test for neutralizing antibodies in patients with severe infection or loss of efficacy to therapy
- Consider benefits and risk of treatment in patients with hematologic abnormalities or acquired general lipodystrophy
- Consider dose reduction of glucose lowering medications

(continued on next page)

Table 1
(continued)

		Non-FDA-Approved Mediations Commonly Used Off-Label for Obesity		
Medication/FDA-Approved Indication/Mechanism of Action	Efficacy	Side Effects/Contraindications	Prescribing Information/ Management Tips	Ref
		Contrindications: • General obesity not associated with congenital leptin deficiency	• Use preservative-free sterile preparation in neonates and infants to avoid benzyl alcohol	

The combination oral medication phentermine/topiramate is FDA-approved for children 12 years and older with obesity. Phentermine is a monoamine sympathomimetic, which is believed to increase norepinephrine in the central nervous system (CNS) and decreased appetite. The weight loss mechanism of action of topiramate is thought to occur through modulation of gamma-aminobutyric acid receptors in the CNS.[17] Phentermine/topiramate extended release results in a 10.44% BMI reduction with an NNT of 3 to achieve a 5% BMI reduction.[22] Although uncontrolled HTN is a contraindication with phentermine, improved blood pressure was seen with phentermine/topiramate treatment. Topiramate is FDA-approved for seizures 2+ years old and migraine prophylaxis 12+ years old.[17] Female patients of child-bearing potential should be counseled of the teratogenic risks of topiramate and the importance of reliable contraception.[17] If insurance does not cover combination phentermine and topiramate, the provider can consider prescribing them separately, although results and side effects may vary with extended- versus immediate-release medications.

Tips for prescribing phentermine and topiramate separately:

- Start both together or start a single medication (phentermine or topiramate) and monitor for weight loss and tolerability for 1 month, then start the other medication if not meeting weight loss or lifestyle/comorbidity improvement goals.
- Phentermine
  - If not experiencing control of symptoms or lack of improvement in weight status after 1 month, consider increasing to phentermine 15 mg, 30 mg, or 37.5 mg daily in the morning.
- Topiramate
  - Typically start with 25 mg per os daily in the evening for 1 to 2 weeks then increase to 50 mg total daily dose in 1 or 2 daily doses.
  - If not experiencing improvement in symptoms, or weight status, consider increasing by 25 to 50 mg (generally 75–100 mg daily dose offers maximal effect for obesity; higher doses can be used if seeking migraine control).

In adolescents and children, monotherapy phentermine results in a 4.1% BMI reduction at 6 months with an NNT of 4 to achieve a 5% BMI reduction.[23] Durations of how long phentermine can be prescribed varies by state.

Orlistat is the least effective FDA-approved AOM and has the largest side effect burden. It works by inhibiting gastrointestinal tract lipase. It is generally taken 3 times a day with meals. In adolescents, orlistat has an NNT of 10 to achieve a 5% BMI reduction.[24]

Setmelanotide is a melanocortin-4-receptor agonist, which restores function in the melanocortin pathway for appetite regulation in patients with disruptions upstream of the MC4 receptor. Clinical studies are limited due to the rarity of the condition, but 80% of patients with POMC or PCSK1 deficiency and 45% of patients with LEPR deficiency achieved a 10% BMI reduction after 1 year.[25] Metreleptin is a leptin analogue used for leptin deficiency in patients with congenital or acquired generalized lipodystrophy.[26,27] In 3 pediatric patients with obesity and congenital leptin deficiency treated with recombinant human leptin, there were improvements in obesity as demonstrated by decreased percent BMI 12.3% to 18.1% at 6 months and 31.5% to 40.18% at 36 months.[26,27] Strongly consider screening children with hyperphagia and severe obesity for these genetic disorders.[7,25] Note that Bardet-Biedl Syndrome is considered a clinical diagnosis and does not require a confirmatory genetic test, as there are genes responsible that remain unknown (**Box 1**).[28]

As discussed in **Table 1**, some medications are often used off-label for weight management.[29] This means they are not FDA-approved for obesity, but show clear benefit

---

Box 1
Bardet Biedl syndrome

- Diagnosis *4 primary criteria* or *3 primary and 2+ secondary*
  - ○ Primary
    - ▪ Visual impairment (retinal abnormalities)
    - ▪ Obesity (usually by age 1)
    - ▪ Hypogonadism
    - ▪ Renal anomalies (malformation or function)
    - ▪ Learning disabilities
  - ○ Secondary
    - ▪ Developmental delays/neurologic problems
    - ▪ Olafactory dysfunction
    - ▪ Oral/dental abnormalities
    - ▪ Cardiovascular and other thoaco-abdominal abnormalities
    - ▪ GI abnormalities
    - ▪ Metabolic Abnoramlities:T2DM, metabolic syndrome, subclinical hypothyroid, PCOS
    - ▪ Strabismus, astigmatism, cataracts
    - ▪ Brachydactlyly/syndactyly

Clinical Diagnosis.[28]*Genetics not required, but may support diagnosis.

---

for weight loss. Off-label prescribing is a common and accepted practice in medicine, especially in pediatrics where pharmaceutic studies are conducted less often.[7,30] If prescribing medications off-label, be sure to discuss that the safety and side effect profiles of these medications, which are often are well-established even in pediatric patients for different indications (eg, topiramate) and document the discussion.[30]

MONITORING DURING MANAGEMENT WITH ANTI-OBESITY MEDICATIONS

hen determining effectiveness of AOM in pediatric patients, typical reference goal is 5% BMI reduction from baseline at 12 weeks.[17] In the pediatric population, weight stabilization and decreased rate of BMI% increase is also beneficial. Recommended follow-up visit after initiation of AOM is 2 to 4 weeks, depending on clinical availability. This can be facilitated by clinical nursing for "goal checks" as well. Remember to consider the "patient voice" and not use "weight check" as the reason for visit, as it can minimize the patient's efforts and overly focus on weight as a marker of improvement, rather than an improvement in quality of life, comorbidities, and lifestyle. At follow-up visits, continue to monitor any pubertal changes, anthropometrics including growth curves, side effects, and eating behaviors. Effective AOM typically leads to normalization of hunger and satiety, improved eating patterns, decreased snacking and portions, and improvement in weight.

AOMs can have central acting effects in the brain, which can disrupt the neuropsychiatric axis. Therefore, regular assessment of cognition, self-esteem, body image, and mood is essential. The clinician can consider using standardized tools such as Generalized Anxiety Disorder[31] or Beck Depression Inventory for adolescents and baseline and follow-up visits.[32,33]

Ongoing nutrition counseling after initiation of successful AOM to support healthy eating patterns, food choices, and water intake is important due to decrease in hunger and thirst cues. Some patients have AOM-induced anorexia with dramatic reduction in hunger drive with minimal consumption and/or rapid weight loss and will therefore need a reduction in dose or change to an alternate therapy to assure sufficient consumption of food throughout the day.

When initiating treatment with a GLP1 RA, the recommendation is to start with a low dose, monitoring closely for any side effects including nausea, vomiting, or other GI side effects such as diarrhea, constipation, or bloating. Antiemetics, such as ondansetron, can be used in the short term to assist. However, ongoing nausea and vomiting is an indication for dose adjustment or discontinuation.

Monitoring body composition and physical activity is also essential throughout treatment.[34] Measurement of body composition using a bioelectrical impedance scale[35] or dual energy X-ray absorptiometry would be ideal but is not available in most settings. In the absence of direct measurement availability, screening for increased fatigue, feeling unwell, weakness, or decreased exercise performance can be signs of muscle loss. Ensuring adequate protein intake and physical activity can support preservation of muscle mass. Laboratory management is also important. Based on experience in post-bariatric patients, consider checking laboratories every 6 to 12 months during weight loss, including Vitamin D, iron, B1, and B12 levels. Also consider a daily multivitamin or bariatric vitamin and 1000 to 1200 mg of calcium daily, especially if there is a concern for poor nutritional intake.[36]

Finally, we recommend treating obesity like any other chronic disease and encourage the same prescribing practices. Due to weight bias, clinicians may try to dissuade families from using indicated AOMs and place requirements prior to treatment. These can include an increased frequency of pregnancy tests or specific lifestyle changes, requiring a family to "earn" AOMs. For other chronic diseases like diabetes, for example, the patient would not have to show they can adopt a healthy lifestyle prior to an anti-diabetic prescription.

The goal of treatment in obesity medicine is to help prevent and treat weight-related comorbidities, not simply achieve a "normal" BMI. Many conditions such as HTN, metabolic liver disease, type 2 diabetes mellitus, HLD, and sleep apnea can be significantly improved with weight loss of 10% to 20% from baseline weight.[37] Because this level of weight loss is now achievable with novel medications, such as GLP-1 RA medications and setmelanotide, which target underlying physiologic abnormalities, withholding these treatments is a disservice to our patients.

SPECIAL POPULATIONS AND ANTI-OBESITY MEDICATIONS
Pre- and Post- Bariatric Surgery

It is common to use AOM pre- and post-bariatric surgery as part of an intensive multidisciplinary program. In the immediate post-operative period, medications are generally held until 3 to 6 months post-surgery. Monitoring for weight regain or failure to achieve weight loss goals can be indications for AOM support, either starting or restarting AOM from prior to surgery.[36,38] Setting expectations before surgery that AOM may still be required can be helpful.

Patients with Special Needs/Genetic Disorders of Obesity

Children with secondary diagnoses and genetic disorders of obesity often have intellectual disability and behavioral dysregulation, requiring additional psychoactive medications. These medications are necessary, especially to control symptoms of aggression, irritability, impulsivity, depression, and anxiety. AOM may be needed to counteract weight gain associated with the child's diagnosis and other medications, commonly metformin, topiramate, and attention deficit hyperactivity disorder stimulants[39,40]

INPATIENT PEDIATRIC OBESITY MANAGEMENT

Inpatient treatment provides a controlled environment to practice lifestyle modifications, close monitoring of AOM response, and the opportunity to overcome barriers to care, such as a lack of insurance coverage.[41] If obesity is considered a life-threatening risk factor, insurance coverage for potent AOMs (ie, semaglutide) can be secured through an appeal for medical-necessity prior to discharge. A timely outpatient follow-up visit should be scheduled to ensure continuity of care.

ROLE OF THE PRIMARY CARE CLINICIAN

Due to shortage of obesity specialists, the majority of obesity care will be offered by primary care providers (PCPs). However, many PCPs site significant barriers to using AOMs, including the lack of training, specialty support, time or availability, and obesity bias.[42] With additional training and support, there are advantages to PCPs managing treatment of obesity. PCPs have the benefit of managing chronic weight-related diseases in addition to obesity, which often improve with AOM therapy. The strong therapeutic relationship with the patient and their family and understanding of the patient's health goals can lead to increased efficacy of obesity treatment. Since PCPs have long-term relationships, they have many opportunities to counsel, encourage and congratulate patients on these changes.

ACCESS TO ANTI-OBESITY MEDICATIONS

Current access to AOM is, unfortunately, limited for many patients. Insurance coverage is improving but has also been limited and requires a time-consuming prior authorization process. When approved, current AOM shortages cause inconsistent treatment with patients having to stop and restart AOM. If there is a treatment gap for less than 6 weeks, it is recommended to restart at a lower dose, but not the starting dose if the patient had minimal side effects after initiation.

To facilitate starting AOM therapy, empower caregivers or patients to contact their insurance companies to inquire about coverage and, if covered, contact several pharmacies regarding supply. Consider waiting to start until they have 2 months of medication in hand. It can also be helpful to have a team to help complete prior authorizations and to follow-up with patients, as these are often required for AOM. If one AOM is denied by insurance or not available, consider using alternative oral medications, which are much less expensive (see **Table 1**). Limited insurance coverage and supply have commonly led to decreased access for those who are uninsured, underinsured, and economically disadvantaged.

SUMMARY

There is increasing evidence that obesity is a chronic disease with well-documented risks. The hesitancy of PCPs to use AOM is understandable, but also questioned, as the need for weight management is critical. PCPs are encouraged to embrace this evolving landscape, fortify their expertise, and actively engage in treating patients struggling with this chronic condition.

CLINICS CARE POINTS

- Assess patients for iatrogenic weight gain and other causes of obesity, eating disorder symptoms, and comorbidities; consider medication changes to prevent iatrogenic weight gain and treat comorbidities when uncovered.
- Discuss advanced options for weight management treatment and enter into shared decision making with the family.
- Select AOM based on patient needs, including starting BMI and symptomatology.

- Monitor for response and follow up frequently in the titration phases of AOM. Once in remission and stable at new setpoint, continue to monitor at least every 6 months as you do for other stable chronic diseases.

DISCLOSURES

Dr B. Sweeney consults without compensation for Nestle, Eli Lilly, Novo Nordisk, and Rhythm. She is an unpaid speaker for Rhythm. She is a paid investigator for Rhythm on 2 research studies. Dr W.P. Dutton, Dr N. Paddu, and Dr A. Braddock have no financial disclosures or conflicts of interest to report.

REFERENCES

1. Ganipisetti VM, Pratyusha B. Obesity and set-point theory. Available at: https://www.ncbi.nlm.nih.gov/books/NBK592402/. [Accessed 12 April 2024].
2. Schwartz MW, Seeley RJ, Zeltser LM, et al. Obesity pathogenesis: An endocrine society scientific statement. Endocr Rev 2017;38(4):267–96.
3. Barlow SE, Dietz WH. Obesity evaluation and treatment: Expert committee recommendations. The maternal and child health bureau, health resources and services administration and the department of health and human services. Pediatrics 1998;102(3):E29.
4. Barlow SE, Expert Committee. Expert committee recommendations regarding the prevention, assessment, and treatment of child and adolescent overweight and obesity: Summary report. Pediatrics 2007;120(Suppl 4):S164–92.
5. Spear BA, Barlow SE, Ervin C, et al. Recommendations for treatment of child and adolescent overweight and obesity. Pediatrics 2007;120(Suppl 4):S254–88.
6. Styne DM, Arslanian SA, Connor EL, et al. Pediatric obesity-assessment, treatment, and prevention: An endocrine society clinical practice guideline. J Clin Endocrinol Metab 2017;102(3):709–57.
7. Hampl SE, Hassink SG, Skinner AC, et al. Clinical practice guideline for the evaluation and treatment of children and adolescents with obesity. Pediatrics 2023;(2):151. https://doi.org/10.1542/peds.2022-060640.
8. Hampl SE, Hassink SG, Skinner AC, et al. Clinical practice guideline for the evaluation and treatment of children and adolescents with obesity. Pediatrics 2023.
9. Skinner AC, Perrin EM, Moss LA, et al. Cardiometabolic risks and severity of obesity in children and young adults. N Engl J Med 2015;373(14):1307–17.
10. Jebeile H, Kelly AS, O'Malley G, et al. Obesity in children and adolescents: Epidemiology, causes, assessment, and management. Lancet Diabetes Endocrinol 2022;10(5):351–65.
11. Ryder JR, Kaizer AM, Jenkins TM, et al. Heterogeneity in response to treatment of adolescents with severe obesity: The need for precision obesity medicine. Obesity (Silver Spring) 2019;27(2):288–94.
12. Acosta A, Camilleri M, Abu Dayyeh B, et al. Selection of antiobesity medications based on phenotypes enhances weight loss: A pragmatic trial in an obesity clinic. Obesity (Silver Spring) 2021;29(4):662–71.
13. Fox CK, Molitor SJ, Vock DM, et al. Appetitive and psychological phenotypes of pediatric patients with obesity. Pediatr Obes 2024;19(4):e13101.
14. Golden NH, Schneider M, Wood C, et al. Preventing obesity and eating disorders in adolescents. Pediatrics 2016;138(3). https://doi.org/10.1542/peds.2016-1649.
15. Saunders KH, Igel LI, Shukla AP, et al. Drug-induced weight gain: Rethinking our choices. J Fam Pract 2016;65(11):780–8.

16. Hunsaker SL, Garland BH, Rofey D, et al. A multisite 2-year follow up of psycho-pathology prevalence, predictors, and correlates among adolescents who did or did not undergo weight loss surgery. Journal of Adolescent Health 2018;63(2): 142–50.

17. Srivastava G, Fox CK, Kelly AS, et al. Clinical considerations regarding the use of obesity pharmacotherapy in adolescents with obesity. Obesity (Silver Spring) 2019;27(2):190–204.

18. Nordisk N. Wegovy. Available at: https://www.novo-pi.com/wegovy.pdf.

19. Weghuber D, Barrett T, Barrientos-Pérez M, et al, STEP TEENS Investigators. Once-weekly semaglutide in adolescents with obesity. N Engl J Med 2022; 387(24):2245–57.

20. Vajravelu ME, Tas E, Arslanian S. Pediatric obesity: Complications and current day management. Life (Basel) 2023;13(7). https://doi.org/10.3390/life13071591.

21. Kelly AS, Auerbach P, Barrientos-Perez M, et al, NN8022-4180 Trial Investigators. A randomized, controlled trial of liraglutide for adolescents with obesity. N Engl J Med 2020;382(22):2117–28.

22. Kelly AS, Bensignor MO, Hsia DS, et al. Phentermine/topiramate for the treatment of adolescent obesity. NEJM Evid 2022;1(6). https://doi.org/10.1056/evidoa2200014.

23. Ryder JR, Kaizer A, Rudser KD, et al. Effect of phentermine on weight reduction in a pediatric weight management clinic. Int J Obes (Lond) 2017;41(1):90–3.

24. Chanoine JP, Hampl S, Jensen C, et al. Effect of orlistat on weight and body composition in obese adolescents: A randomized controlled trial. JAMA 2005; 293(23):2873–83.

25. Trapp CM, Censani M. Setmelanotide: A promising advancement for pediatric patients with rare forms of genetic obesity. Curr Opin Endocrinol Diabetes Obes 2023;30(2):136–40.

26. Pharma A. Myalept [package insert]. 2022.

27. Farooqi IS, Matarese G, Lord GM, et al. Beneficial effects of leptin on obesity, t cell hyporesponsiveness, and neuroendocrine/metabolic dysfunction of human congenital leptin deficiency. J Clin Invest 2002;110(8):1093–103.

28. Foundation BBS. What is bbs?. Beales PL, Elcioglu N, Woolf AS, Parker D, Flinter FA. New criteria for improved diagnosis of Bardet-Biedl syndrome: results of a population survey. J Med Genet 1999; 36: 437–46.

29. San Giovanni CB, Sweeney B, Skelton JA, et al. Aversion to off-label prescribing in clinical pediatric weight management: The quintessential double standard. J Clin Endocrinol Metab 2021;106(7):2103–13.

30. Frattarelli DA, Galinkin JL, Green TP, et al, American Academy of Pediatrics Committee on Drugs. Off-label use of drugs in children. Pediatrics 2014;133(3):563–7.

31. Mossman SA, Luft MJ, Schroeder HK, et al. The generalized anxiety disorder 7-item scale in adolescents with generalized anxiety disorder: Signal detection and validation. Ann Clin Psychiatry 2017;29(4):227–234a.

32. Osman A, Kopper BA, Barrios F, et al. Reliability and validity of the beck depression inventory–ii with adolescent psychiatric inpatients. Psychol Assess 2004; 16(2):120–32.

33. Osman A, Barrios FX, Gutierrez PM, et al. Psychometric properties of the beck depression inventory-ii in nonclinical adolescent samples. J Clin Psychol 2008; 64(1):83–102.

34. Quadri M, Ariza AJ, Selvaraj K, et al. Percent body fat measurement in the medical management of children with obesity. Pediatr Ann 2018;47(12):e487–93.

35. Khalil SF, Mohktar MS, Ibrahim F. The theory and fundamentals of bioimpedance analysis in clinical status monitoring and diagnosis of diseases. Sensors (Basel) 2014;14(6):10895–928.
36. Moore JM, Haemer MA, Fox CK. Lifestyle and pharmacologic management before and after bariatric surgery. Semin Pediatr Surg 2020;29(1):150889.
37. Garvey WT. New horizons. A new paradigm for treating to target with second-generation obesity medications. J Clin Endocrinol Metab 2022;107(4):e1339–47.
38. Doyle WN, Reinhart N, Reddy NC, et al. Anti-obesity medication use for adolescent metabolic and bariatric surgery patients: A systematic literature review. Cureus 2023;15(12):e50905.
39. Sweeney B, Kelly AS, San Giovanni CB, et al. Clinical approaches to minimize iatrogenic weight gain in children and adolescents. Clin Obes 2021;11(1):e12417.
40. Dreyer Gillette ML, Killian HJ, Fernandez C, et al. Treating obesity in children and adolescents with special healthcare needs. Curr Obes Rep 2022;11(4):227–35.
41. Goldman VE, Espinoza JC, Vidmar AP. Inpatient medical management of severe pediatric obesity: Literature review and case reports. Front Pediatr 2023;11: 1095144.
42. Forman-Hoffman V, Little A, Wahls T. Barriers to obesity management: A pilot study of primary care clinicians. BMC Fam Pract 2006;7:35.
43. Nordisk N. Wegovy [package insert]. Food and Drug Administration. Available at: https://www.novo-pi.com/wegovy.pdf. [Accessed 12 February 2024].
44. Nordisk N. Saxenda [package insert]. Food and Drug Administration. Available at: https://www.novo-pi.com/saxenda.pdf. [Accessed 12 February 2024].
45. Vivus. Qsymia [package insert]. Available at: https://qsymia.com/patient/include/media/pdf/prescribing-information.pdf?v=0422. [Accessed 13 February 2024].
46. Teva Pharmaceuticals USA I. Adipex-p (phentermine hydrochloride) [package insert]. Available at: https://www.accessdata.fda.gov/drugsatfda_docs/label/2012/085128s065lbl.pdf. [Accessed 12 February 2024].
47. CHEPLAPHARM. Xenical [package insert]. 02/12/2004. Available at: https://www.accessdata.fda.gov/drugsatfda_docs/label/2022/020766s038lbl.pdf.
48. Haqq AM, Chung WK, Dollfus H, et al. Efficacy and safety of setmelanotide, a melanocortin-4 receptor agonist, in patients with bardet-biedl syndrome and alström syndrome: A multicentre, randomised, double-blind, placebo-controlled, phase 3 trial with an open-label period. Lancet Diabetes Endocrinol 2022; 10(12):859–68.
49. Jastreboff AM, Aronne LJ, Ahmad NN, et al, SURMOUNT-1 Investigators. Tirzepatide once weekly for the treatment of obesity. N Engl J Med 2022;387(3): 205–16.
50. Lilly E. Zepbound [package insert]. Available at: https://www.accessdata.fda.gov/drugsatfda_docs/label/2023/217806s000lbl.pdf. [Accessed 12 February 2024].
51. Lilly E. Trulicity [package insert]. Available at: https://www.accessdata.fda.gov/drugsatfda_docs/label/2020/125469s036lbl.pdf. [Accessed 12 February 2024].
52. Arslanian SA, Hannon T, Zeitler P, et al, AWARD-PEDS Investigators. Once-weekly dulaglutide for the treatment of youths with type 2 diabetes. N Engl J Med 2022;387(5):433–43.
53. Squibb B-M. Glucophage [package insert]. 2017.
54. O'Connor EA, Evans CV, Burda BU, et al. Screening for obesity and intervention for weight management in children and adolescents: Evidence report and systematic review for the us preventive services task force. JAMA 2017;317(23): 2427–44.

55. Fox CK, Marlatt KL, Rudser KD, et al. Topiramate for weight reduction in adolescents with severe obesity. Clin Pediatr (Phila) 2015;54(1):19–24.
56. Janssen. Topamax [package insert]. Available at: https://www.accessdata.fda.gov/drugsatfda_docs/label/2017/020505s057_020844s048lbl.pdf.   [Accessed 12 February 2024].
57. Floden L, Taren DL, Muramoto ML, et al. Bmi changes in adolescents treated with bupropion sr for smoking cessation. Obesity (Silver Spring) 2016;24(1):26–9.
58. Nalpropion. Contrave [package insert]. Updated 9/2014. Available at: https://www.accessdata.fda.gov/drugsatfda_docs/label/2014/200063s000lbl.pdf.   [Accessed 12 February 2024].
59. Frias JP, Bonora E, Nevarez Ruiz L, et al. Efficacy and Safety of Dulaglutide 3.0 mg and 4.5 mg Versus Dulaglutide 1.5 mg in Metformin-Treated Patients With Type 2 Diabetes in a Randomized Controlled Trial (AWARD-11). Diabetes Care Mar 2021;44(3):765–73.

Metabolic and Bariatric Surgery for Adolescents

Ihuoma Eneli, MD, MS[a],*, Faith Anne N. Heeren, BA[b],
Rochelle L. Cason-Wilkerson, MD, MPH[a], Keeley J. Pratt, PhD[c,d,e]

KEYWORDS

- Pediatric obesity treatment • Pediatric bariatric surgery
- Adolescent bariatric surgery • Musculoskeletal comorbidities • Psychosocial health
- Micronutrient deficiencies

KEY POINTS

- Metabolic and bariatric surgery (MBS) is a safe and effective treatment option for adolescents with severe obesity.
- MBS results in clinically significant weight loss, for example, 30% decline in pre-operative body mass index and improvements in comorbidities.
- Pre-operative evaluation and post-operative management is important and should be facilitated by an experienced multidisciplinary team in tertiary care pediatric centers.
- Monitoring for post-operative complications, weight regain, psychosocial health, micronutrient deficiencies, and transition to adult care are important and can be conducted in collaboration with the primary care clinician within their medical home.

INTRODUCTION

Metabolic and bariatric Surgery (MBS) is an effective treatment option for youth with severe obesity defined as a body mass index (BMI) greater than or equal to 120% of the 95th percentile for age and sex or BMI greater than or equal to 35.[1–4] Severe obesity is associated with cardiometabolic, psychologic, and musculoskeletal comorbidities.[5] Adolescents with a BMI greater than or equal to 140% of the 95th percentile are 6 times more likely to develop type 2 diabetes (T2D) than peers with a healthy weight[6]

[a] Department of Pediatrics, Section of Nutrition, University of Colorado Anschutz Medical Campus, Aurora, CO, USA; [b] Department of Health Outcomes and Biomedical Informatics, University of Florida College of Medicine, Gainesville, FL, USA; [c] Department of Human Sciences, College of Education and Human Ecology, The Ohio State University, Columbus, OH, USA; [d] Department of Surgery, College of Medicine, The Ohio State University, Columbus, OH, USA; [e] Department of Pediatrics, College of Medicine, The Ohio State University, Columbus, OH, USA
* Corresponding author. Section of Nutrition, Department of Pediatrics, University of Colorado Anschutz Medical Campus, 13123 East 16th Avenue, B270, Aurora, CO 80045.
E-mail address: Ihuoma.eneli@childrenscolorado.org

Pediatr Clin N Am 71 (2024) 981–998
https://doi.org/10.1016/j.pcl.2024.06.007
0031-3955/24/© 2024 Elsevier Inc. All rights reserved, including those for text and data mining, AI training, and similar technologies.

and have a 3 to 5 fold risk of developing cardiovascular disease by age 50.[7,8] Other serious comorbidities include obstructive sleep apnea (OSA), idiopathic intracranial hypertension, slipped capital femoral epiphysis, metabolic-associated fatty liver disease (MAFLD), and Blount's disease.[5] Psychologically, adolescents with obesity have lower health- and weight-related quality of life,[9,10] disordered eating, such as binge eating or loss of control,[11] and higher rates of depression and anxiety,[12] suicidal behaviors, and substance abuse disorders.[13,14] Given these findings, the American Academy of Pediatrics (AAP) and the American Society of Metabolic and Bariatric Surgery recommend MBS as an effective treatment option for severe obesity in adolescents.[1–4] This article will provide an overview of indications for adolescent MBS, pre- and post-operative management, and considerations for future research.

Approach to Adolescent Metabolic and Bariatric Surgery Treatment

Within the last 4 years, the AAP released a guideline and a policy statement emphasizing that clinicians should offer MBS to adolescents with severe obesity and also called out a need for high-quality tertiary care centers with multidisciplinary teams experienced in managing adolescents with severe obesity.[1–3] In addition, the Metabolic and Bariatric Surgery Accreditation and Quality Improvement Program (MBSA-QIP), which was established in 2014 to ensure high-quality standards of care at centers that provide MBS, includes comprehensive recommendations specifically for adolescents.[15] The MBSAQIP accreditation elements cover guidance on treatment protocols, facilities, personnel resources, determining appropriate clinical volume, data surveillances, outcome protocols, and implementing quality improvement processes.

Indications for Metabolic and Bariatric Surgery

The criteria for MBS are similar for adults and adolescents (**Table 1**). Given the association between BMI and fat mass,[16] health morbidity and mortality,[17] elevated BMI is the primary criterion for MBS. Although MBS has been performed safely on children under 12 years with clinically meaningful decrease in BMI, improvement in comorbid conditions, and no linear growth concerns;[18,19] the 2023 AAP Childhood Obesity

Table 1 Indications and contraindications for metabolic and bariatric surgery	
Criteria for Surgery	**Absolute or Relative Contraindication**
BMI $\geq$35 kg/m^2 or 120% of the 95th percentile with significant obesity complications for example, Type 2 diabetes, Obstructive sleep apnea (Apnea Hypopnea Index $\geq$ 5 events/hr), Hypertension, Idiopathic intracranial hypertension (pseudotumor cerebri), metabolic-dysfunction associated steatotic liver disease (MASLD), Blount's disease, Slipped Capital Femoral Epiphysis, Gastroesophageal reflux disease	Medically treatable cause of obesity for example, hypothyroidism Ongoing substance abuse problem (active within the last year) A medical, psychiatric, psychosocial, or cognitive condition that prevents adherence to postoperative dietary and treatment regimen Current or planned pregnancy within 12–18 mo of procedure
BMI $\geq$40 kg/m^2 or $\geq$ 140% of the 95th percentile with any obesity complications listed earlier and impairments in quality of life, active daily living, joint pain, or physical functioning	

Practice Guidelines recommends a lower age limit of 12 years for MBS due to a paucity of studies in younger children.[3]

PRE-OPERATIVE EVALUATION

To adequately address the etiology of obesity and the complexity of pre- and post-operative care, adolescent MBS clinical teams must be multidisciplinary. Evaluation starts with a detailed history and physical examination that screens for the anthropometric criterion, contraindications for surgery, genetic and lifestyle risk factors, physical and psychologic comorbidities, and assesses for family and social support. Recommended screening blood tests include glycosylated hemoglobin for diabetes, a fasting lipid panel for dyslipidemia, a comprehensive panel for liver and renal function, and micronutrient and vitamin profile (eg, iron studies, folate, thiamine (B1), vitamin B12, vitamin A, vitamin B6, calcium, and vitamin D).[1–4] During pre-operative care, these tests are repeated if abnormal or obtained approximately 4 to 6 weeks prior to a planned surgery date. In preparation for surgery, additional blood tests may include a complete blood count and coagulation profile to exclude anemia and bleeding disorders. If pertinent symptoms are present for other co-morbidities or etiology for obesity, a thyroid function test, electrocardiogram, echocardiogram, or a sleep study may be obtained. Most programs screen for high-risk behaviors as part of their psychologic assessment. A laboratory-based nicotine or drug screen is not routine unless required by the insurance carrier. Other tests not usually obtained include imaging studies (eg, dual x-ray absorptiometry [DXA] before surgery) to provide a baseline to track future loss of bone mass or osteopenia, and an upper gastrointestinal fluoroscopy to exclude anatomic or gastric abnormalities (eg, ulcers, gastritis, and helicobacter pylori). Tanner staging or sexual maturity rating, bone age, and history of prior weight loss attempts are no longer routinely required.[1,4]

Dietary, physical activity, and behavioral counseling are the mainstays of the pre-operative course. The dietary goal is to prepare the adolescent to maintain adequate post-operative nutrition, especially protein intake, and minimize micronutrient deficiencies. With the anticipated decrease in calorie intake following surgery, diet quality is optimized by increasing protein intake, vegetables, and fiber while decreasing sugar-added foods and starchy carbohydrates. The average recommended daily intake is 1.1 g per kg of ideal body weight or 60 to 120 g of protein. Daily multivitamin, calcium, and Vitamin D supplementation is often initiated before surgery and remains a lifelong requirement after the surgery to avoid micronutrient deficiencies. Physical activity is essential for weight maintenance.[20] Guidelines recommend a combination of cardio, aerobic, and resistance training. Resistance training can mitigate muscle loss and enhance efficiency of energy expenditure.[21]

Although pre-operative weight loss is not a criterion for MBS, the emphasis on improving diet, physical activity, sleep, and mental health during this period can lead to weight loss or weight maintenance. Decreasing BMI improves perioperative safety of the surgery. Anti-obesity medications (AOMs) can be used as an adjunct to lifestyle interventions if pre-operative weight loss is a desired treatment goal, such as when the BMI is extremely high or in the presence of severe comorbid conditions for example, OSA or MASLD. Food and Drug Administration (FDA)-approved medications for obesity treatment for adolescents include orlistat, phentermine with topiramate, and GLP-1 receptor agonists such as daily-administered liraglutide and once-weekly administered semaglutide.[22,23]

All MBS patients undergo an in-depth psychosocial evaluation as part of the pre-operative course. Preoperative rates of adolescent depressive symptoms range from 15% to 70%, and about a third of adolescents report symptoms of anxiety.[24] The adolescent's developmental stage and cognitive maturity guide the team in assessing the level of support the patient needs, their ability to understand the surgical procedure and complications, and their capacity to adhere to the required post-operative lifestyle changes. As a prerequisite for surgery approval, health insurers require an assessment by a licensed mental health professional (eg, a psychologist) indicating the patient's mental health is stable, the adolescent understands the requirements of the surgery, can give appropriate consent, and can be reasonably expected to follow the post-operative treatment plan. The assessment varies by program but often includes validated instruments such as (i) the *Wechsler Abbreviated Scale of Intelligence,* which screens *for* intellectual functioning and cognitive deficits,[25] (ii) comprehensive behavioral screens using the *Behavior Assessment System for Children,*[26] a parent and self-report measure of both positive (adaptive) behaviors (eg, interpersonal relations, self-esteem, and self-reliance) and negative (clinical) dimensions (eg, depression, anxiety, social stress, and attention problems); (iii) screens for mood disorders with *Beck Depression Inventory-II*[27] or the *Generalized Anxiety Disorder;*[28] and (iv) eating disorders with validated surveys like *Questionnaire on Eating and Weight Patterns-Child.*[29]

Evaluation of social support includes assessment for social drivers of health, family functioning, and household environment. One instrument used in pediatric primary care[30] and pediatric weight management clinics to assess healthy or impaired family functioning is the 12-item *McMaster Family Assessment Device – General Functioning Scale.*[31,32] The instrument is valid and reliable with diverse populations, and endorsed by the Pediatric Psychology Task Force.[33,34] Zeller and colleagues assessed family functioning among caregivers and adolescents undergoing MBS compared to peers with obesity but not pursuing MBS.[35–37] Impaired family functioning, or dysfunctional interactions, occurred in approximately 1 of every 2 to 3 families in the bariatric program. Although preoperative family functioning was not predictive of post-operative weight loss at 1 and 2 years, improvement in family functioning was correlated with higher rates of excess weight loss. Given the importance of psychosocial and family factors for adolescents in the bariatric program, these aspects should be included routinely as part of the preoperative evaluation.

The decision to move forward with MBS can be subjective as it involves a review of psychosocial or cognitive factors that may impair adherence to post-operative recommendations by an experienced interdisciplinary team of surgeons, obesity medicine clinicians, nurses, dietitians, psychologists, social workers, and physical activity specialists. For example, if a patient with intellectual disability meets all other criteria for MBS (eg, BMI, presence of obesity-related comorbidities), withholding the surgery solely because of their intellectual disability may be unethical. In these cases, the MBS clinical team should ensure there is a legal caregiver who understands the procedure, can give consent, and support the adolescent with the required pre- and post-operative changes and a back-up legal guardian. In some instances, input can be sought from the hospital's ethics committee. In addition, programs should modify teaching materials to be responsive to the developmental and cognitive abilities of the patient or extend the pre-operative period to adapt to a different learning style. If these accommodations are not feasible, are unsuccessful, or if the adolescent is able to verbalize a desire not to have surgery based on a reasonable level of understanding of the surgery and expectations, then MBS may be contraindicated. Similarly, psychiatric and mental health diagnoses are not contraindications if the condition is appropriately managed and is stable.

METABOLIC AND BARIATRIC SURGERY PROCEDURES

MBS procedures are gastric bypass (Roux-en-Y), vertical sleeve gastrectomy (VSG), adjustable gastric banding (AGB), and biliopancreatic duodenal switch (BPD). Currently, the latter 2 procedures are rarely performed. Once an intermediate surgical step for BPD or Roux-en-Y in individuals with severe obesity, in the early 2000s, the VSG became a stand-alone MBS procedure. The VSG is now the most-performed MBS, surpassing the Roux-en-Y procedure about a decade ago.[38] The VSG procedure, which is performed laparoscopically, involves excising and discarding approximately 70% to 80% of the stomach through a lengthy incision starting at the lower gastric curvature (**Fig. 1**). The excised stomach leaves behind a tubular or sleeve-like stomach with less volume and fewer fundal gastric cells that produce ghrelin, the hunger hormone. The procedure is irreversible but can be converted to Roux-en-Y or BPD for some patients with inadequate weight loss.

Also often performed laparoscopically, the Roux-en-Y surgery is a more complicated procedure with several anastomotic areas (**Fig. 2**). The stomach is reduced to a 20 to 30 cc volume, about the "size of an egg." In the Roux-en-Y, no portion of the stomach or intestine is excised or removed from the abdomen. The stomach remnant and the duodenum are anastomosed to the mid-distal jejunal part of the Roux limb (jejunostomy) to ensure continued availability of the gastric and hepatobiliary enzymes and hormones for digestion. A gastro jejunostomy connects the newly fashioned stomach to the jejunum, completing the bypass process of the surgery. The AGB surgery involves inserting an adjustable silicone ring around the upper part of the stomach, which can be tightened or loosened by injecting fluid into a port embedded under the skin of the abdomen. The AGB surgery is still not approved

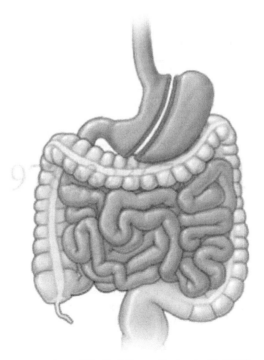

Fig. 1. Schematic representation of Vertical Sleeve Gastrectomy (VSG).

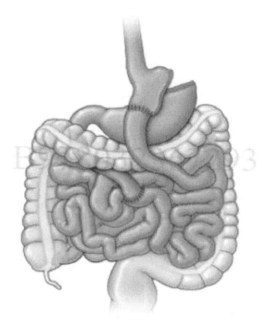

Fig. 2. Schematic representation of Roux-en-Y (Gastric Bypass).

by the FDA for patients aged less than 18 year and has been largely discontinued because of poor weight loss outcomes and high rates of complications.[39]

Overall, the VSG and Roux-en-Y have a low complication profile, are irreversible, and produce comparable and clinically significant weight loss.[40] Weight loss from MBS was initially thought to be due to restrictive or malabsorptive mechanisms; however, recent research indicates a metabolic response to the anatomic changes is more likely the primary driver for the weight loss.[41]

POST-OPERATIVE OUTCOMES AND COMPLICATIONS

In the United States (US), the efficacy and safety of MBS for adolescents is largely informed by the Teen Longitudinal Assessment of Bariatric Surgery study (Teen-LABS), a 5 multi-institutional prospective observational study, which enrolled 242 patients between 2007 and 2012, with a 10 -year follow-up period.[42–46] The median age of the Teen-LABS cohort is 17.1 (1.6) years, and a median BMI of 50.5 kg per m^2 (range 31–88 kg/m2).[47] About 3-quarters of participants are Non-Hispanic White, 22% are Non-Hispanic Black, 76% female, and 60% had at least 2 or more cardiovascular risk factors (high blood pressure, abnormal lipid panel, high sensitivity C-reactive protein levels, prediabetes, or T2D).[47] In the Teen-LABS study, the mean decline in BMI was 13 to 14 kg/m^2 for VSG, compared with a 15 to 16 unit decline in BMI for the Roux-en-Y 12 months after surgery.[48] After 5 years, the mean weight loss was 26% of total body weight[49–51] and 85% and 91% of adolescents had a resolution of their diabetes, and sleep apnea, respectively.[51] In addition, approximately two-thirds had maintained a weight loss of greater than or equal to 20% of total body weight, although about 10% had lost only 5% of total body weight or exceeded their pre-surgery weight.[51] Mean weight loss after 5 years was higher for Roux-en-Y (21%) than for VSG (12%).[52] The reason for the heterogeneity in weight outcomes following MBS is complex and likely due to similar risk factors that led to obesity. AOMs can be beneficial for patients with minimal weight loss or significant weight regain after surgery.[53] Improving retention rates in the bariatric program is helpful, as regular attendance at clinic appointments is associated with greater weight loss.[54]

The results of the Teen-LABS are consistent with the findings from other longitudinal adolescent cohort studies on MBS.[40,45,55–57] In a systematic review of 29 cohort studies (n = 4970) with at least 5 year follow-up post MBS, the mean decline in BMI for all types of MBS was 13.09 kg per m^2 (95%CI 11.75–14.43); and the remission rates were as high as 90% (95%CI 83.2–95.6) for T2D, 76.6% (95%CI 62.0–88.9) for dyslipidemia, 80.7%, (95%CI 71.5–88.8) for hypertension, and 80.7% (95%CI 36.4–100) for OSA.[40] In addition, compared to medical therapy for T2D, adolescents who underwent MBS in the TEEN-LABs study had better glycemic control and improvement in diabetes related comorbidities like albumin-creatinine ratio, dyslipidemia, and hypertension.[58] Finally, adolescents are more likely than the adults to have remission of obesity-related comorbidities such as T2D and hypertension despite similar amounts of weight loss suggesting an additional benefit when MBS is performed at a younger age.[45]

Psychosocial improvements vary by pre-operative psychopathology, weight dissatisfaction, and weight change.[59–63] After MBS, adolescents have significant improvement in health-related quality of life and depressive symptoms over the first year, and these beneficial changes persist for 5 years.[59–63] Compared to their peers with obesity who did not have MBS, anxiety, and depression rates were comparable 2 years after MBS.[64] Also, young adults who participated in the Teen-LABS study as adolescents reported using marijuana (24.6% surgical vs 27.4% surgical) and cigarettes (29.5% surgical vs 41.3% nonsurgical) at lower rates compared to their peers with obesity who did not have MBS.[65]

MBS-related Complications: Gastroesophageal symptoms such as nausea, vomiting, gastroesophageal reflux (GER) are common in the immediate post-operative period as the body heals and adjusts to the new anatomy. The frequency and severity vary and can be difficult to predict for each patient. Adhering to a strict dietary plan and use of antiemetics can help minimize some of these symptoms. By 6 to 8 weeks after surgery, most patients are on a regular diet and are encouraged to eat 5 to 6 small meals. Dietary intake is graduated from clear fluid to full liquids, pureed, and soft and regular foods (**Fig. 3**). The overall goal is to maintain hydration and adequate protein

Stages (Timeframe)[a]	•Examples of Types of Foods
Clear liquids Day 1-3	•Water, Sugar free drinks, Sugar free popiscles, Broth
Full liquids Day 3 to 3-4 weeks	•Protein shakes, Sugar free high protein smoothies, Yogurt- high protein options, sugar -free, Milk- Dairy, Oat, Soy - (all unflavored) Sugar free-hot chocolate, Strained soups or cream soups, added protein supplemnt powders or meal replacement drinks
Pureed/Blended Foods Week 3-4 to 4-5	•Hot cooked cereal (sugar-free), mashed potatoes, naturally sweetened applesauce, cottage cheese, egg substitute or scrambled eggs softly cooked, Stage 1 and 2 Baby food jars (no added sugars), Blended soft meats e.g., chicken, pork, beef, Cream soups, Silken Tofu, packagedTuna
Soft Foods Week 4-5 to 6-8	•Well cooked or blended vegetables/meats, soft pasta/rice
Regular foods Week 6-8 - through Lifetime	•Regular foods as tolerated (emphasis on high protein sources). Raw vegetables. Avoid juices, sugar sweetened drinks and foods, large portions, high fat food options

Fig. 3. Stages of dietary intake following metabolic and bariatric surgery. [a]Times for each Stage are approximate and can differ depending on the patient.

intake. Since the quantity of food is limited by the size of the stomach, the emphasis is on nutritional quality. Patients are also advised to chew their food 20 to 30 times and avoid drinking fluids while eating. Occasional vomiting may occur, often due to intolerance to a specific food, eating too fast, overeating or drinking while eating. It is important that patients are taught to recognize and differentiate these episodes from more serious concerns. Persistent nausea and vomiting need to be investigated to rule out other complications such as a leak, stricture, obstruction from abdominal adhesions, or GER.

Serious surgical post-operative complications are rare but can occur particularly in the first 90 days. In an observational prospective cohort study, major complications such as a gastroesophageal leak, bowel obstruction, and hemorrhage requiring transfusion occurred more often with Roux-en-Y surgery (9.3%) than with the VSG (4.5%).[48] In patients with a history of oral intake intolerance, persistent nausea or emesis, abdominal pain or fever, tachycardia, signs of sepsis, or abdominal tenderness, clinicians should have a high index of suspicion for a gastric leak, an uncommon but serious complication with significant morbidity. The clinical presentation of patients with a leak may vary depending on the position, size, and type of leak. The workup starts with a detailed history and physical examination. Abnormal laboratory tests when present increases the likelihood of a leak. For instance, a complete blood count with leukocytosis, an electrolyte panel with metabolic acidosis, or elevated acute phase reactants like erythrocyte sedimentation rate or C-reactive protein. Free air or increased post-operative air distribution and intraabdominal collections of fluid or abscesses can be seen on a supine abdominal radiograph and a computed tomography, respectively. Depending on the size and position of the leak, treatment ranges from a conservative approach to reoperation. Adjusting nutritional intake during this time is crucial and can include parenteral or oral feeds.

In the Teen-LABS study, about 20% of adolescents required an additional procedure such as cholecystectomy, surgery for bowel obstruction, dilation of strictures, and internal hernia repair within 5 years after surgery.[49] The frequency for re-operation is higher with the Roux-en-Y surgery (16%) than the more commonly performed VSG (5%).[52] There are also higher rates of micronutrient deficiencies with Roux-en-Y. Another long-term complication is GER due to weakening or increased pressure in the lower gastroesophageal sphincter or gastric stricture. Especially after a VSG, screening for reflux symptoms, for example, epigastric discomfort, heartburn, regurgitation of stomach acids, or food into the throat or mouth should be routinely performed at all post-operative visits. GER is often managed conservatively with antacids and proton pump inhibitors. In severe or unremitting cases, conversion from a VSG to Roux-en-Y is recommended.

Micronutrient deficiencies can occur due to inadequate food intake, non-adherence with multivitamin supplementation, persistent vomiting or food intolerance, and fat malabsorption.[66–68] The deficiencies are more common in those undergoing RYGB than VSG.[49,69] In the TEEN-LABs study, nearly half (48%) of adolescents who were 2 years out from surgery had evidence of iron deficiency, 38% had low vitamin D, and 4% had low vitamin B12.[49] Longer-term, there are higher rates, with 46% demonstrating mild anemia and 16% with low B12.[70,71] There is a statistically significant increase in the number of adolescents in the Teen-LABS study with a low ferritin level from surgery to 5 years after surgery, worse with Roux-en-Y surgery (3% vs 71%) compared with VSG (11 vs 45%).[72] In addition, the portion of adolescents with 2 or more micronutrient deficiencies rose 4- to 5-fold over 5 years.[72] As adherence to treatment is a challenging problem in adolescents and young adults, it is important to screen for micronutrient deficiencies at least annually (**Table 2**).

Table 2
Common micronutrient deficiency with metabolic and bariatric surgery

Micronutrient/Vitamin	Screening Labs	Clinical Presentation	Recommended Daily Intake	Food Sources for Supplementation
Iron	Ferritin, Complete Blood count (CBC), Serum iron total iron, iron binding capacity.	Fatigue, Pallor, Tachycardia Dysphagia, impaired learning ability	Ferritin-15–200 ng/mL Iron-50–170 µg/dl	Iron rich foods meats, poultry, fish, eggs, dried fruit, some vegetables and legumes
Vitamin A (due to fat malabsorption)	Vitamin A	Rare but Severe decreases can cause loss of vision and/or night blindness	700 µg/d females, 900 µg/d-males	Liver, dairy products, fish, darkly colored fruits and leafy vegetables
Vitamin D (due to fat malabsorption)	25 hydroxyVitamin D	Decrease in total bone mass, and accrual of bone mineral in developing bone (Osteomalacia) and disorders of Calcium deficiency	>30 ng/mL	Fortified dairy products, fatty fish, eggs, and fortified cereals
Vitamin B1	Thiamine	Early symptoms-anorexia, gait ataxia paresthesia, muscle cramps, irritability Peripheral neuropathy Wernicke's encephalitis	1.1–1.2 mg/d	Meat especially pork, sunflower seeds, grains and vegetables Additional vitamin C helps to absorb thiamine
Vitamin B12 (due to loss of intrinsic factor	Vitamin B12 Methylmalonic acid level	Macrocytic anemia-pale, icteric skin and eyes, fatigue, shortness of breath, tinnitus, palpitations, and numbness and paresthesia. Deficiency will also cause folate deficiency	2.4 µg/d	Meat, dairy, eggs; found in animal products
Folate	Folate	Forgetfulness, irritability, rarely paranoid behaviors Cheilosis and glossitis, and diarrhea	400 µg/d	Vegetables, especially green leafy; fruit, enriched grains, bread, pasta and rice

Data from Refs.[66–68]

SPECIAL CONSIDERATIONS
Role of the Primary Care Clinician

The primary care clinician is a key member of the interdisciplinary MBS team. Within the context of the medical home, the clinician often has a long-standing relationship with the adolescent and their family and can be a trusted liaison between the family and the bariatric program. An informed transition of care hand-off between the bariatric program and the primary care clinician can help identify or prevent long-term complications such as weight regain, micronutrient deficiencies, disordered eating, or gastroesophageal reflux disease. In addition, they are better aware of community resources that can tackle social drivers of health hindering the adolescent's ability to follow through on lifestyle behavior change. **Table 3** summarizes areas for collaborative care between the primary care clinician and the bariatric team.

Age

The World Health Organization age criterion for MBS is 10 to 19 years, which is lower than the AAP guideline that recommends a cut-off of 13 years. Reticence about performing MBS in younger children is driven by concerns about risk for future maladaptive growth or micronutrient deficiencies, limited developmental and intellectual capacity to understand the procedure, provide assent, or adhere to the post-operative requirements. However, there are case studies where MBS has been safely performed in children as young as 5 years.[18] Often, these types of cases have been in children with Prader Willi, hypothalamic obesity, and those at risk for significant weight-related morbidity (eg, optic nerve atrophy from idiopathic intracranial hypertension, esophageal varices due to MAFLD, or severe sleep apnea with pulmonary hypertension). Young age should not be an absolute contraindication. Rather, the decision to perform MBS should be carefully considered and decided upon as a consensus by an experienced multidisciplinary team after weighing the benefits and risks of the procedure for each individual case.[73] In addition, programs must provide adequate psychologic and social support for the child and family and ensure the family does not feel coerced by the process or the team in making their decision.

Disparities and Social Determinants of Health

The availability and acceptability of MBS in the US in the last 2 decades have improved, with over 1700 adolescent procedures performed annually by 2017.[74] Only a small percentage of adolescents who qualify for MBS get the procedure, with apparent gender, racial, and socioeconomic disparities.[74–78] Most adolescents undergoing MBS are female and non-Hispanic White despite the fact that male, Hispanic, and Black patients are likely to have severe obesity or present with higher pre-operative BMIs.[76–78] Adolescents who identify as Black or Hispanic are less likely to undergo MBS compared to their White peers.[76,77] One barrier is insurance authorization for the procedure. In a single site study, only 47% of adolescents who qualified for MBS were approved by their insurer after an initial request for authorization. The most common reason for insurance denial is age younger than 18 years.[79] Also, there is a complicated relationship between socioeconomic factors and race that contributes to inequities in the access and utilization of MBS among adolescents. Perez and colleagues reported that non-Hispanic White adolescents with public insurance were more likely to undergo MBS compared to those with private insurance. However, non-Hispanic Black and Hispanic adolescents with private insurance rather than public insurance were more likely to undergo MBS.[76] Furthermore, the location of tertiary pediatric obesity clinics can exacerbate disparities as many centers that offer multidisciplinary care (eg, MBS) are

Table 3
Collaborative roles for the primary care physician

Stages in Bariatric Program	Clinical Considerations Role for PCP

Pre-operative	• Learn about Adolescent MBS
	• Ensure bidirectional communication with bariatric surgery program
	• Initiate referrals to bariatric program
	• Provide support for adolescent and family
	  1. Counseling on lifestyle behaviors for example, diet. physical activity, sleep, high risk behaviors
	  2. Making an informed decision
	  3. Addressing social drivers of health
	  4. Managing health conditions that may affect their bariatric care for example, disordered eating, anxiety, depression, asthma
	  5. Providing counseling on avoiding pregnancy for example, use of birth control pills, barrier contraceptives for example, condom use for males and females

Immediate post-operative period (first 90 d)	• Be aware of patient's bariatric course and surgery date • Encourage adherence with bariatric program recommendations for example, appropriate hydration, diet regimen • Communicate promptly with bariatric surgery team about any medical concerns for example, vomiting, pain • Encourage multivitamin intake
Post-operative	Monitor of physical and mental health • Encourage adherence with bariatric program recommendations for example, protein intake, avoiding sugar sweetened beverages, avoid drinking fluids while eating, daily vitamin intake, activity regimen • Provide contraceptive care • Screen for mental health concerns for example, disordered eating, depression, high risk behaviors, distorted body image • Screen and provide support for social drivers of health • Assess for medical concerns for example, micronutrient deficiencies, gastroesophageal reflux symptoms, new onset vomiting • Communicate medical concerns with bariatric program

located in urban areas near academic facilities, making it difficult for patients in rural areas to access pediatric obesity treatment.[80]

Despite the well-established safety and effectiveness of MBS as a treatment for severe obesity, providers still are reluctant to refer their adolescent patients for MBS.[81,82] Referral hesitancy has been attributed to a lack of awareness about MBS as a treatment option for adolescents with severe obesity.[81] Interestingly, adolescents report that the recommendation and support of their primary care providers is an important influence in their decision to seek MBS.[83] Educational outreach activities will help primary care providers understand the indications, benefits, and outcomes of MBS, and increase referrals for MBS, particularly for adolescents from minority and low socioeconomic subgroups.

Transition to Adulthood

Adolescents who have MBS are often on the cusp of emerging adulthood, where they are increasingly becoming independent, entering romantic partnerships, "settling down," and potentially forming families. Yet, how transitions are navigated or their outcomes have not been well-explored. Adolescent females in the Teen-LABS study were at a slightly higher risk of contracting a sexually transmitted infection (18.7% vs 14.3%) and of having a child in adolescence compared to adolescents with severe obesity who did not have MBS.[84] Pratt and colleagues reported that being married as young adults or having parents who had ever married were protective factors for sustaining weight loss, suggesting perhaps the positive influence of social support.[85] Conversely, impaired or strained romantic and family relationships led to poorer weight loss outcomes.[85] An area for further study is how undergoing MBS as an adolescent affects partner selection, romantic relationship formation, family planning, and early parenting practices. The results can inform interventions to build healthy adult relationships.

The Lived Experience and the Patient Voice

Qualitatively, adolescent patients share that their experience with MBS differs compared to adults.[86] Before surgery, adolescents often demonstrate a dichotomous thought pattern. While many patients describe a desire to feel 'normal,'[87] they also seem to grasp that MBS is a tool, not a cure, for treating obesity.[88] This discrepancy may be due to gaps in pre-operative education or difficulty comprehending or remembering the information because the process often feels stressful or overwhelming. Tailoring the content and delivery of pre- and post-operative educational materials to provide information in a manner that is acceptable, easy to understand and culturally-sensitive for adolescents may improve their experience and their ability to sustain weight loss and health benefits of MBS.[89] It is also important that programs communicate emerging information on the risks and benefits associated with adolescent to help patients and families make informed decisions about their treatment choices. Finally, current guidelines stress pre-operative assessments of psychologic readiness and post-operative counseling on nutritional deficiencies and avoiding pregnancy,[90] Yet, similar guidance or emphasis on these topics after surgery is limited.

Potential Areas for Future Research

Extant literature on adolescent MBS has largely used longitudinal cohort studies recruited from clinical settings. For example, the majority of our knowledge on adolescent MBS has been developed through the Teen-LABS study[42,45,91] or ancillary studies such as TeenView, which investigates emerging psychosocial health benefits and risks associated with MBS with a group of non-surgical comparators (eg, adolescents with severe obesity who did not undergo surgical treatment).[59,92,93] Although these studies have several methodologic strengths, using other study designs can provide a different perspective. This approach may be more feasible with the newer effective AOMs that can produce similar levels of weight loss. Currently, there is a randomized controlled trial in Sweden on non-surgical treatment versus surgical treatment among adolescents ages 13 to 16.[94,95] Future studies need to incorporate long-term follow-up, include younger children, be sufficiently powered to examine psychologic variables as primary outcomes, focus on weight regain, and investigate the effect of environment (family, society, workplace, and policy) and exposure to bias and stigma on MBS outcomes.

SUMMARY

MBS is a safe and effective intervention when overseen by an experienced multidisciplinary team. Incorporating the primary care clinician into their care is important and can help with adherence to the post-operative regimen, improve retention, and decrease physical and psychologic complications. Other areas for future research include understanding the reasons for disparities with referrals, the impact of family dynamics, incorporating input from lived experience into study design and educational approaches, the use of AOM as an adjunct pre- and post-operative treatment, and expanding the study designs beyond prospective observational cohort studies.

CLINICS CARE POINTS

- Consider MBS as a treatment option for children 13 years and older with severe obesity.
- The primary care clinician is an important part of the MBS care team, and can serve as a bridge between the families and the bariatric team.
- Emphasizing diet quality is important before and after MBS. Ensuring adequate protein intake is a key after MBS.
- Encourage the adolescent to have a physical activity regimen that includes aerobic activity and resistance training. Physical activity helps with weight maintenance and prevents excessive muscle loss.
- After MBS, adolescents need lifelong multivitamin supplementation.
- Screening for mental health conditions and providing psychological support and counseling is helpful for the adolescent before and after MBS.

DISCLOSURES

None.

REFERENCES

1. Armstrong SC, Bolling CF, Michalsky MP, et al. Pediatric metabolic and bariatric surgery: evidence, barriers, and best practices. Pediatrics 2019;144(6).
2. Bolling CF, Armstrong SC, Reichard KW, et al. metabolic and bariatric surgery for pediatric patients with severe obesity. Pediatrics 2019;144(6).
3. Hampl SE, Hassink SG, Skinner AC, et al. Clinical practice guideline for the evaluation and treatment of children and adolescents with obesity. Pediatrics 2023; 151(2).
4. Pratt JSA, Browne A, Browne NT, et al. ASMBS pediatric metabolic and bariatric surgery guidelines, 2018. Surg Obes Relat Dis 2018;14(7):882–901.
5. Kelly AS, Barlow SE, Rao G, et al. Severe obesity in children and adolescents: identification, associated health risks, and treatment approaches: a scientific statement from the American Heart Association. Circulation 2013;128(15): 1689–712.

6. Hubbard RA, Xu J, Siegel R, et al. Studying pediatric health outcomes with electronic health records using Bayesian clustering and trajectory analysis. J Biomed Inf 2021;113:103654.

7. Pratt JSA, Browne A, Browne NT, et al. ASMBS pediatric metabolic and bariatric surgery guidelines, 2018. Surg Obes Relat Dis 2018;14(7):882–901.

8. Michalsky M, Reichard K, Inge T, et al. ASMBS pediatric committee best practice guidelines. Surg Obes Relat Dis 2012;8(1):1–7.

9. Zeller MH, Inge TH, Modi AC, et al. Severe obesity and comorbid condition impact on the weight-related quality of life of the adolescent patient. J Pediatr 2015;166(3). 651-9.e4.

10. Austin H, Smith K, Ward WL. Psychological assessment of the adolescent bariatric surgery candidate. Surg Obes Relat Dis 2013;9(3):474–80.

11. He J, Cai Z, Fan X. Prevalence of binge and loss of control eating among children and adolescents with overweight and obesity: An exploratory meta-analysis. Int J Eat Disord 2017;50(2):91–103.

12. Fox CK, Gross AC, Rudser KD, et al. Depression, anxiety, and severity of obesity in adolescents. Clin Pediatr 2016;55(12):1120–5.

13. Lipari R, Hedden S. Serious mental health challenges among older adolescents and young adults. Rockville, MD: Substance Abuse and Mental Health Services Administration; 2016.

14. Nock MK, Green JG, Hwang I, et al. Prevalence, correlates, and treatment of lifetime suicidal behavior among adolescents. JAMA Psychiatr 2013;70(3):300.

15. American College of Surgeons, American Society for Metabolic and Bariatric Surgery. Optimal resources for metabolic and bariatric surgery: 2019 standards. Available at: https://www.facs.org/quality-programs/accreditation-and-verification/metabolic-and-bariatric-surgery-accreditation-and-quality-improvement-program/standards/. [Accessed 23 February 2024].

16. Freedman DS, Wang J, Maynard LM, et al. Relation of BMI to fat and fat-free mass among children and adolescents. Int J Obes 2005;29(1). 1-8.

17. Di Angelantonio E, Bhupathiraju SN, Wormser D, et al. Body-mass index and all-cause mortality: individual-participant-data meta-analysis of 239 prospective studies in four continents. Lancet 2016;388(10046):776–86.

18. Alqahtani AR, Antonisamy B, Alamri H, et al. Laparoscopic sleeve gastrectomy in 108 obese children and adolescents aged 5 to 21 years. Ann Surg 2012;256(2):266–73.

19. Browne AF, Inge T. How young for bariatric surgery in children? Semin Pediatr Surg 2009;18(3):176–85.

20. Swift DL, Johannsen NM, Lavie CJ, et al. The role of exercise and physical activity in weight loss and maintenance. Prog Cardiovasc Dis 2014;56(4):441–7.

21. Morales-Marroquin E, Kohl HW, Knell G, et al. Resistance training in post-metabolic and bariatric surgery patients: a systematic review. Obes Surg 2020;30(10):4071–80.

22. Weghuber D, Barrett T, Barrientos-Pérez M, et al. Once-weekly semaglutide in adolescents with obesity. N Engl J Med 2022;387(24):2245–57.

23. Kelly AS. Current and future pharmacotherapies for obesity in children and adolescents. Nat Rev Endocrinol 2023;19(9):534–41.

24. Herget S, Rudolph A, Hilbert A, et al. Psychosocial status and mental health in adolescents before and after bariatric surgery: a systematic literature review. Obes Facts 2014;7(4):233–45.

25. Wechsler D. Wechsler Abbreviated Scale of Intelligence (WASI) [Database record]. APA PsycTests 1999. https://doi.org/10.1037/t15170-000.

26. Kamphaus RW, Reynolds CR. BASC-2 behavioral and emotional screening System. Minneapolis, MN: Pearson Assessments; 2007.

27. Costello EJ, Angold A. Scales to assess child and adolescent depression: checklists, screens, and nets. J Am Acad Child Adolesc Psychiatry 1988;27(6):726–37.

28. Mossman SA, Luft MJ, Schroeder HK, et al. The generalized anxiety disorder 7-item scale in adolescents with generalized anxiety disorder: signal detection and validation. Ann Clin Psychiatr 2017;29(4). 227-34a.

29. Johnson WG, Kirk AA, Reed AE. Adolescent version of the questionnaire of eating and weight patterns: reliability and gender differences. Int J Eat Disord 2001; 29(1):94–6.

30. Van Fossen CA, Pratt KJ, Murray R, et al. Family functioning in pediatric primary care patients. Clin Pediatr 2018;57(13):1549–57.

31. Epstein NB, Baldwin LM, Bishop DS. The Mcmaster family assessment device. J Marital Fam Ther 1983;9(2):171–80.

32. Ryan CE, Epstein NB, Keitner GI, et al. Evaluating and treating families: the McMaster approach. New York: Taylor & Francis Group, LLC; 2005.

33. Mansfield AK, Keitner GI, Dealy J. The family assessment device: an update. Fam Process 2015;54(1):82–93.

34. Alderfer MA, Fiese BH, Gold JI, et al. Evidence-based assessment in pediatric psychology: family measures. J Pediatr Psychol 2008;33:1046–61.

35. Zeller MH, Reiter-Purtill J, Ratcliff MB, et al. Two-year trends in psychosocial functioning after adolescent Roux-en-Y gastric bypass. Surg Obes Relat Dis 2011; 7(6):727–32.

36. Zeller MH, Guilfoyle SM, Reiter-Purtill J, et al. Adolescent bariatric surgery: caregiver and family functioning across the first postoperative year. Surg Obes Relat Dis 2011;7(2):145–50.

37. Zeller MH, Hunsaker S, Mikhail C, et al. Family factors that characterize adolescents with severe obesity and their role in weight loss surgery outcomes. Obesity 2016;24(12):2562–9.

38. Reames BN, Finks JF, Bacal D, et al. Changes in bariatric surgery procedure use in Michigan, 2006-2013. JAMA 2014;312(9):959–61.

39. Lanthaler M, Aigner F, Kinzl J, et al. Long-term results and complications following adjustable gastric banding. Obes Surg 2010;20(8):1078–85.

40. Wu Z, Gao Z, Qiao Y, et al. Long-term results of bariatric surgery in adolescents with at least 5 years of follow-up: a systematic review and meta-analysis. Obes Surg 2023;33(6):1730–45.

41. Albaugh VL, He Y, Munzberg H, et al. Regulation of body weight: Lessons learned from bariatric surgery. Mol Metabol 2023;68.

42. Inge TH, Courcoulas AP, Jenkins TM, et al. Weight loss and health status 3 years after bariatric surgery in adolescents. N Engl J Med 2016;374(2):113–23.

43. Michalsky P, Inge T, Teich S, et al. Adolescent bariatric surgery program characteristics: The Teen Longitudinal Assessment of Bariatric Surgery (Teen-LABS) study experience. Semin Pediatr Surg 2014;23(1):5–10.

44. Ryder JR, Gross AC, Fox CK, et al. Factors associated with long-term weight-loss maintenance following bariatric surgery in adolescents with severe obesity. Int J Obes 2018;42(1):102–7.

45. Inge TH, Courcoulas AP, Jenkins TM, et al. Five-year outcomes of gastric bypass in adolescents as compared with adults. N Engl J Med 2019;380(22):2136–45.

46. Dewberry LC, Jalivand A, Gupta R, et al. Weight loss and health status 5 years after adjustable gastric banding in adolescents. Obes Surg 2020;30(6):2388–94.

47. Inge TH, Zeller MH, Jenkins TM, et al. Perioperative outcomes of adolescents undergoing bariatric surgery: the Teen-Longitudinal Assessment of Bariatric Surgery (Teen-LABS) study. JAMA Pediatr 2014;168(1):47–53.

48. Inge TH, Courcoulas AP, Jenkins TM, et al. Weight loss and health status 3 years after bariatric surgery in adolescents. N Engl J Med 2016;374(2):113–23.

49. Inge TH, Courcoulas AP, Jenkins TM, et al. Five-year outcomes of gastric bypass in adolescents as compared with adults. N Engl J Med 2019;380(22):2136–45.

50. Beamish AJ, Johansson SE, Olbers T. Bariatric surgery in adolescents: what do we know so far? Scand J Surg 2015;104(1):24–32.

51. Ruiz-Cota P, Bacardí-Gascón M, Jiménez-Cruz A. Long-term outcomes of metabolic and bariatric surgery in adolescents with severe obesity with a follow-up of at least 5 years: A systematic review. Surg Obes Relat Dis 2019;15(1):133–44.

52. McClelland PH, Kabata K, Gorecki W, et al. Long-term weight loss after bariatric procedures for morbidly obese adolescents and youth: a single-institution analysis with up to 19-year follow-up. Surg Endosc 2023;37(3):2224–38.

53. Stanford FC, Alfaris N, Gomez G, et al. The utility of weight loss medications after bariatric surgery for weight regain or inadequate weight loss: A multi-center study. Surg Obes Relat Dis 2017;13(3):491–500.

54. Lujan J, Tuero C, Landecho MF, et al. Impact of routine and long-term follow-up on weight loss after bariatric surgery. Obes Surg 2020;30(11):4293–9.

55. Durkin N, Desai AP. What is the evidence for paediatric/adolescent bariatric surgery? Curr Obes Rep 2017;6(3):278–85.

56. Inge TH, Jenkins TM, Xanthakos SA, et al. Long-term outcomes of bariatric surgery in adolescents with severe obesity (FABS-5+): a prospective follow-up analysis. Lancet Diabetes Endocrinol 2017;5(3):165–73.

57. Olbers T, Beamish AJ, Gronowitz E, et al. Laparoscopic Roux-en-Y gastric bypass in adolescents with severe obesity (AMOS): a prospective, 5-year, Swedish nationwide study. Lancet Diabetes Endocrinol 2017;5(3):174–83.

58. Inge TH, Laffel LM, Jenkins TM, et al. Comparison of surgical and medical therapy for type 2 diabetes in severely obese adolescents. JAMA Pediatr 2018; 172(5):452–60.

59. Reiter-Purtill J, Ley S, Kidwell KM, et al. Change, predictors and correlates of weight- and health-related quality of life in adolescents 2-years following bariatric surgery. Int J Obes 2020;44(7):1467–78.

60. Zeller MH, Brown JL, Reiter-Purtill J, et al. Sexual behaviors, risks, and sexual health outcomes for adolescent females following bariatric surgery. Surg Obes Relat Dis 2019;15(6). 969-978.

61. Zeller MH, Pendery EC, Reiter-Purtill J, et al. From adolescence to young adulthood: trajectories of psychosocial health following Roux-en-Y gastric bypass. Surg Obes Relat Dis 2017;13(7):1196–203.

62. Zeller MH, Reiter-Purtill J, Jenkins TM, et al. Suicidal thoughts and behaviors in adolescents who underwent bariatric surgery. Surg Obes Relat Dis 2020;16(4): 568–80.

63. Zeller MH, Strong H, Reiter-Purtill J, et al. Marijuana, e-cigarette, and tobacco product use in young adults who underwent pediatric bariatric surgery. Surg Obes Relat Dis 2023;19(5):512–21.

64. Tuli S, Lopez Lopez AP, Nimmala S, et al. Two-year study on the impact of sleeve gastrectomy on depressive and anxiety symptoms in adolescents and young adults with moderate to severe obesity. Obes Surg 2024;34(2):568–75.

65. Zeller MH, Strong H, Reiter-Purtill J, et al. Marijuana, e-cigarette, and tobacco product use in young adults who underwent pediatric bariatric surgery. Surg Obes Relat Dis 2023;19(5):512–21.

66. Aills L, Blankenship J, Buffington C, et al. ASMBS allied health nutritional guidelines for the surgical weight loss patient. Surg Obes Relat Dis 2008;4(5):S73–108.

67. Moizé V, Andreu A, Flores L, et al. Long-term Dietary Intake and Nutritional Deficiencies following Sleeve Gastrectomy or Roux-En-Y Gastric Bypass in a Mediterranean Population. J Acad Nutr Diet 2013;113(3):400–10.

68. Snyder-Marlow G, Taylor D, Lenhard MJ. Nutrition care for patients undergoing laparoscopic sleeve gastrectomy for weight loss. J Acad Nutr Diet 2010;110(4): 600–7.

69. Lamoshi A, Chernoguz A, Harmon CM, et al. Complications of bariatric surgery in adolescents. Semin Pediatr Surg 2020;29(1):150888.

70. Inge TH, Jenkins TM, Xanthakos SA, et al. Long-term outcomes of bariatric surgery in adolescents with severe obesity (FABS-5+): a prospective follow-up analysis. Lancet Diabetes Endocrinol 2017;5(3):165–73.

71. Olbers T, Beamish AJ, Gronowitz E, et al. Laparoscopic Roux-en-Y gastric bypass in adolescents with severe obesity (AMOS): a prospective, 5-year, Swedish nationwide study. Lancet Diabetes Endocrinol 2017;5(3):174–83.

72. Xanthakos SA, Khoury JC, Inge TH, et al. Nutritional risks in adolescents after bariatric surgery. Clin Gastroenterol Hepatol 2020;18(5). 1070-81.e5.

73. Gonzalez DO, Michalsky MP. Update on pediatric metabolic and bariatric surgery. Pediatr Obes 2021;16(8):e12794.

74. Bouchard ME, Tian Y, Linton S, et al. utilization trends and disparities in adolescent bariatric surgery in the United States 2009-2017. Child Obes 2022;18(3): 188–96.

75. Inge TH, Boyce TW, Lee M, et al. Access to care for adolescents seeking weight loss surgery. Obesity 2014;22(12):2593–7.

76. Perez NP, Westfal ML, Stapelton SM, et al. Beyond insurance: race-based disparities in the use of metabolic and bariatric surgery for the management of severe pediatric obesity. Surg Obes Relat Dis 2019;16(3):414–9.

77. Nunez Lopez O, Jupiter DC, Bohanon FJ, et al. Health Disparities in Adolescent Bariatric Surgery: Nationwide Outcomes and Utilization. J Adolesc Health 2017; 61(5):649–56.

78. Inge TH, Zeller MH, Jenkins TM, et al. Perioperative outcomes of adolescents undergoing bariatric surgery. JAMA Pediatr 2014;168(1):47.

79. Inge TH, Boyce TW, Lee M, et al. Access to care for adolescents seeking weight loss surgery. Obesity 2014;22(12):2593–7.

80. Newsome FA, Dilip A, Armstrong SC, et al. Scaling-up Stage 4 Pediatric Obesity Clinics: Identifying Barriers and Future Directions Using Implementation Science. Obesity 2021;20(6):941–3.

81. Vanguri P, Lanning D, Wickham EP, et al. Pediatric health care provider perceptions of weight loss surgery in adolescents. Clin Pediatr (Phila) 2014;53(1):60–5.

82. Woolford SJ, Clark SJ, Gebremariam A, et al. To cut or not to cut: physicians' perspectives on referring adolescents for bariatric surgery. Obes Surg 2010;20(7): 937–42.

83. Ofori A, Keeton J, Booker Q, et al. Socioecological factors associated with ethnic disparities in metabolic and bariatric surgery utilization: a qualitative study. Surg Obes Relat Dis 2020;16(6):786–95.

84. Zeller MH, Brown JL, Reiter-Purtill J, et al. Sexual behaviors, risks, and sexual health outcomes for adolescent females following bariatric surgery. Surg Obes Relat Dis 2019;15(6):969–78.

85. Pratt KJ, Boles RE, Michalsky MP, et al. Associations between marital status and weight loss trajectories entering into early adulthood: a Teen-LABS study. Surg Obes Relat Dis 2024;20(4):376–82.

86. Childerhose JE, Eneli I, Steele KE. Adolescent bariatric surgery: a qualitative exploratory study of US patient perspectives. Clin Obes 2018;8(5):345–54.

87. Doyle J, Colville S, Brown P, et al. How adolescents decide on bariatric surgery: an interpretative phenomenological analysis. Clin Obes 2018;8(2):114–21.

88. Li MK, Regina A, Strom M, et al. It's a tool, not a cure": the preoperative teen perspective on bariatric surgery. Surg Obes Relat Dis 2021;17(6):1190–7.

89. Heeren FAN, Ayzengart A, Menon S, et al. Adolescent bariatric surgery: the need for tailored educational materials. Child Obes 2024;20(4):221–6.

90. Aikenhead A, Lobstein T, Knai C. Review of current guidelines on adolescent bariatric surgery. Clin Obes 2011;1(1):3–11.

91. Inge TH, Zeller M, Harmon C, et al. Teen-Longitudinal Assessment of Bariatric Surgery: methodological features of the first prospective multicenter study of adolescent bariatric surgery. J Pediatr Surg 2007;42(11):1969–71.

92. Reiter-Purtill J, Ley S, Kidwell KM, et al. Change, predictors and correlates of weight- and health-related quality of life in adolescents 2-years following bariatric surgery. Int J Obes (Lond) 2020;44(7):1467–78.

93. Reiter-Purtill J, Decker KM, Jenkins TM, et al. Self-worth and developmental outcomes in young adults after pediatric bariatric surgery. Health Psychol 2023; 42(2):92–102.

94. Janson A, Järvholm K, Gronowitz E, et al. A randomized controlled trial comparing intensive non-surgical treatment with bariatric surgery in adolescents aged 13-16 years (AMOS2): Rationale, study design, and patient recruitment. Contemp Clin Trials Commun 2020;19:100592.

95. Järvholm K, Janson A, Peltonen M, et al. Metabolic and bariatric surgery versus intensive non-surgical treatment for adolescents with severe obesity (AMOS2): a multicentre, randomised, controlled trial in Sweden. Lancet Child Adolesc Health 2023;7(4):249–60.

Statement of Ownership, Management, and Circulation
(All Periodicals Publications Except Requester Publications)

UNITED STATES POSTAL SERVICE®

1. Publication Title	2. Publication Number	3. Filing Date
PEDIATRIC CLINICS OF NORTH AMERICA	424 – 66	9/18/2024

4. Issue Frequency	5. Number of Issues Published Annually	6. Annual Subscription Price
FEB, APR, JUN, AUG, OCT, DEC	6	$290.00

7. Complete Mailing Address of Known Office of Publication (Not printer) (Street, city, county, state, and ZIP+4®)

ELSEVIER INC.
230 Park Avenue, Suite 800
New York, NY 10169

Contact Person: Malathi Samayan
Telephone (Include area code): 91-44-4299-4507

8. Complete Mailing Address of Headquarters or General Business Office of Publisher (Not printer)

ELSEVIER INC.
230 Park Avenue, Suite 800
New York, NY 10169

9. Full Names and Complete Mailing Addresses of Publisher, Editor, and Managing Editor (Do not leave blank)

Publisher (Name and complete mailing address)
Dolores Meloni, ELSEVIER INC.
1600 JOHN F KENNEDY BLVD. SUITE 1600
PHILADELPHIA, PA, 19103-2899

Editor (Name and complete mailing address)
KERRY HOLLAND, ELSEVIER INC.
1600 JOHN F KENNEDY BLVD. SUITE 1600
PHILADELPHIA, PA 19103-2899

Managing Editor (Name and complete mailing address)
PATRICK MANLEY, ELSEVIER INC.
1600 JOHN F KENNEDY BLVD. SUITE 1600
PHILADELPHIA, PA 19103-2899

10. Owner (Do not leave blank. If the publication is owned by a corporation, give the name and address of the corporation immediately followed by the names and addresses of all stockholders owning or holding 1 percent or more of the total amount of stock. If not owned by a corporation, give the names and addresses of the individual owners. If owned by a partnership or other unincorporated firm, give its name and address as well as those of each individual owner. If the publication is published by a nonprofit organization, give its name and address.)

Full Name	Complete Mailing Address
WHOLLY OWNED SUBSIDIARY OF REED/ELSEVIER, US HOLDINGS	1600 JOHN F KENNEDY BLVD. SUITE 1600 PHILADELPHIA, PA ,19103-2899

11. Known Bondholders, Mortgagees, and Other Security Holders Owning or Holding 1 Percent or More of Total Amount of Bonds, Mortgages, or Other Securities. If none, check box ☐ None

Full Name	Complete Mailing Address
N/A	

12. Tax Status (For completion by nonprofit organizations authorized to mail at nonprofit rates) (Check one)
The purpose, function, and nonprofit status of this organization and the exempt status for federal income tax purposes:
☒ Has Not Changed During Preceding 12 Months
☐ Has Changed During Preceding 12 Months (Publisher must submit explanation of change with this statement)

PS Form **3526**, July 2014 [Page 1 of 4 (see instructions page 4)] PSN: 7530-01-000-9931   PRIVACY NOTICE: See our privacy policy on www.usps.com

---

13. Publication Title	14. Issue Date for Circulation Data Below
PEDIATRIC CLINICS OF NORTH AMERICA	JUNE 2024

15. Extent and Nature of Circulation		Average No. Copies Each Issue During Preceding 12 Months	No. Copies of Single Issue Published Nearest to Filing Date
a. Total Number of Copies (Net press run)		282	271
b. Paid Circulation (By Mail and Outside the Mail)	(1) Mailed Outside-County Paid Subscriptions Stated on PS Form 3541 (Include paid distribution above nominal rate, advertiser's proof copies, and exchange copies)	159	156
	(2) Mailed In-County Paid Subscriptions Stated on PS Form 3541 (Include paid distribution above nominal rate, advertiser's proof copies, and exchange copies)	0	0
	(3) Paid Distribution Outside the Mails Including Sales Through Dealers and Carriers, Street Vendors, Counter Sales, and Other Paid Distribution Outside USPS®	105	91
	(4) Paid Distribution by Other Classes of Mail Through the USPS (e.g., First-Class Mail®)	14	19
c. Total Paid Distribution (Sum of 15b (1), (2), (3), and (4))		278	266
d. Free or Nominal Rate Distribution (By Mail and Outside the Mail)	(1) Free or Nominal Rate Outside-County Copies included on PS Form 3541	3	4
	(2) Free or Nominal Rate In-County Copies Included on PS Form 3541	0	0
	(3) Free or Nominal Rate Copies Mailed at Other Classes Through the USPS (e.g., First-Class Mail)	0	0
	(4) Free or Nominal Rate Distribution Outside the Mail (Carriers or other means)	1	1
e. Total Free or Nominal Rate Distribution (Sum of 15d (1), (2), (3) and (4))		5	5
f. Total Distribution (Sum of 15c and 15e)		282	271
g. Copies not Distributed (See Instructions to Publishers #4 (page #3))		0	0
h. Total (Sum of 15f and g)		282	271
i. Percent Paid (15c divided by 15f times 100)		98.37%	98.15%

* If you are claiming electronic copies, go to line 16 on page 3. If you are not claiming electronic copies, skip to line 17 on page 3.

PS Form **3526**, July 2014 (Page 2 of 4)

16. Electronic Copy Circulation	Average No. Copies Each Issue During Preceding 12 Months	No. Copies of Single Issue Published Nearest to Filing Date
a. Paid Electronic Copies ►		
b. Total Paid Print Copies (Line 15c) + Paid Electronic Copies (Line 16a) ►		
c. Total Print Distribution (Line 15f) + Paid Electronic Copies (Line 16a) ►		
d. Percent Paid (Both Print & Electronic Copies) (16b divided by 16c × 100) ►		

☒ I certify that 50% of all my distributed copies (electronic and print) are paid above a nominal price.

17. Publication of Statement of Ownership
☒ If the publication is a general publication, publication of this statement is required. Will be printed in the OCTOBER 2024 issue of this publication.   ☐ Publication not required.

18. Signature and Title of Editor, Publisher, Business Manager, or Owner

Malathi Samayan - Distribution Controller   *Malathi Samayan*   Date 9/18/2024

I certify that all information furnished on this form is true and complete. I understand that anyone who furnishes false or misleading information on this form or who omits material or information requested on the form may be subject to criminal sanctions (including fines and imprisonment) and/or civil sanctions (including civil penalties).

PS Form **3526**, July 2014 (Page 3 of 4)   PRIVACY NOTICE: See our privacy policy on www.usps.com

Printed and bound by CPI Group (UK) Ltd, Croydon, CR0 4YY

08/05/2025

01864751-0005